FEVERED MEASURES

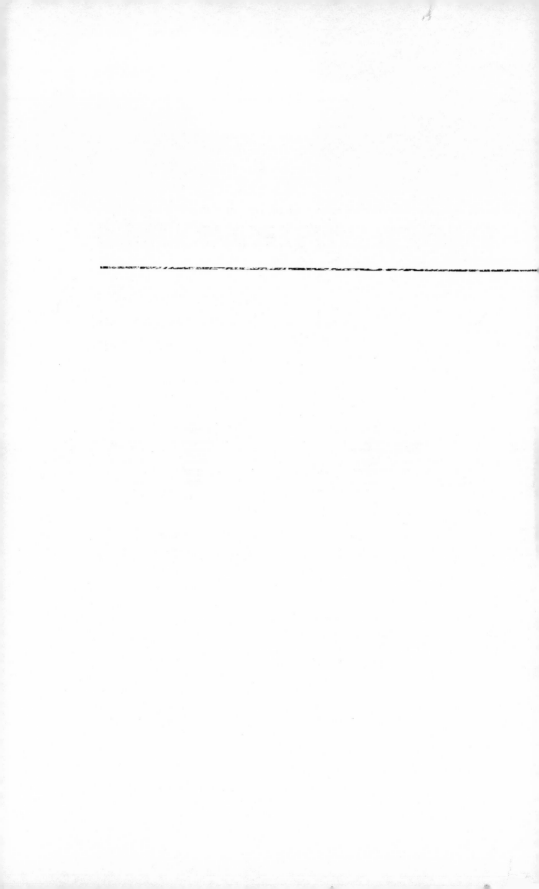

FEVERED MEASURES

PUBLIC HEALTH AND RACE
AT THE TEXAS-MEXICO BORDER,
1848–1942

John Mckiernan-González

Duke University Press | Durham and London | 2012

Library of Congress Cataloging-in-Publication Data
appear on the last printed page of this book.

Duke University Press gratefully acknowledges the support of
the Office of the President at The University of Texas at Austin,
which provided funds toward the publication of this book.

In celebration of
Feliciano Enrique Mckiernan Cordova,
se hace camino al andar

CONTENTS

NOTES ON LABELING PLACES,
PEOPLES, AND DISEASES

A Note on Places, Peoples, and Labels

Shared borders don't necessarily mean shared labels. In Mexico, most people call the river connecting Mexico and the United States El Rio Bravo. In the United States, most U.S. Americans use Spanish words in English to describe the same river: they call it the Rio Grande. The use of "Rio Grande" instead of "El Rio Bravo" in the United States might also remind readers that the present political border between Mexico and the United States was one of the outcomes of the war of 1846. Moreover, the presence of Spanish words in English should remind readers that Mexico and Mexicans still shape the use of English and Spanish in Texas. The different names and the enduring presence of Spanish words for the same river highlights an ongoing contention over the local and national meaning of a shared landscape.

On the other hand, most people agree on the names for cities on the north bank of the Rio Grande and the south bank of El Rio Bravo. The current Texas-Mexico border begins in the city that once was El Paso del Norte and is now both Ciudad Juárez, Chihuahua, and El Paso, Texas. The river wends its way south and east, through Big Bend National Park, past Presidio, Texas, and Ojinaga, Chihuahua, and by the town of Del Rio, Texas. The cities of Piedras Negras, Coahuila, and Eagle Pass, Texas, follow. These two cities house the main rail hub linking the industrial centers of Torreon, Durango, and Saltillo to San Antonio, Texas, and the rest of the United States.

If one were to follow the river's flow, Laredo, Texas, and Nuevo Laredo, Nuevo León, would be the next destination. These two cities have long been the busiest crossing between Mexico and the United States, the site of the first railroad linking Mexico and the United States, and the connection between U.S. consumers and Monterrey, Nuevo León—Mexico's second-largest but most industrial city. The river then makes its way through the lower Rio Grande Valley, drifting past Harlingen, Ciudad Reynosa, and Rio Grande City and ending in the Gulf of Mexico. Brownsville lies on the north side, and Matamoros, Tamaulipas, on the south. These seventeen cities are often set pieces for a place called the border. Whenever possible, this book will refer to these cities by these names.

These cities are key parts of the Texas-Mexico borderlands. I follow Gloria Anzaldúa's use of the term "borderlands"—"a borderland is in a constant state of transition"—because this term allows for an emphasis on the ongoing unequal power dynamics.[1] I prefer "borderlands" to "the border" because it places the political border between Mexico and the United States within the creation of a variety of borders. This is better than having "the border" stand in for the variety of national, racial, cultural, political, and medical borders still being drawn across the upper and lower Rio Grande Valley.

If the name for the river is open to dispute, the term "American" is similarly fraught. Originally used to describe the people living on the lands claimed by Spain, "American" can refer to someone from North, South, or Central America, all in the American continents; someone who grew up in the United States of America; or someone who resides in the United States; someone who is a citizen of the United States; or the term can be used to exclude people Americans believe should not be living in the United States. In the 1930s in Texas, people started using the terms Mexican American and Latin American to claim their belonging and their rights in the political community of Americans in the United States.[2]

"Mexican" has also been a point of conflict. The term entered into Spanish when Cortes and his Tlaxcaltecan and Nahua allies met with Emperor Moteuczoma Xocoyitl and learned of the label that members of the Aztec empire used to describe themselves.[3] In 1580, the Spanish crown granted Coronado authority to establish a New Mexico among the Pueblo in the lands north of the Rio Grande. During the wars of independence that started in 1810, Mexico became the banner under which many different forces fought Spanish rule. In 1824, Mexican forces ousted Spanish military authority from the territory of New Spain and claimed the lands between Oregon and Panama for Mexico. In Texas, Mexicans negotiated the boundaries of their political authority with France and the United States to the east, Comanche nations to the northwest, and the various Apache nations in their midst. In

1845, the U.S. Senate annexed this land as the state of Texas, which many in Mexico considered to be an act of war. The subsequent war between Mexico and the United States helped create the Mexican/American binary.

The Treaty of Guadalupe Hidalgo accelerated the connections between Mexico and the United States and further complicated the designation of Mexican and American for people on both sides of the border. Between 1845 and 1945, residents and citizens, men and women in both republics, drew new national boundaries, confronted the relationship of Indian nations to their body politic, found uneven ways to address the presence of slavery and the process of emancipation, and fought over the boundaries and privileges of citizenship through various civil wars. In Mexico's case, people there also experienced U.S., Spanish, and French military occupations. The enduring contrast between Mexican and American obscures the entanglement of Mexico and the United States. Over the last 150 years, Mexican and American became simultaneous national, racial, and ethnic designations.

Each chapter will touch on the variety of ways people define Mexican and American in the midst of epidemics. The process of establishing public health at this border demonstrates the ways that "the notion of race does not just consist of ideas and sentiments; it comes into being when these ideas and sentiments are publicly articulated and institutionalized."[4] Public health campaigns and interventions were not simply a way to prevent illness. The act of deciding who to protect became key to establishing what it meant to be Mexican or American.

When American public health officers claimed the authority to detain, bathe, and vaccinate any Mexican crossing into the United States, their interpretation of who was Mexican mattered more than the actual health status of every person—American or Mexican—walking across or taking a streetcar into downtown El Paso from Ciudad Juárez. When a long-term resident in El Paso remembered that the U.S. Public Health Service "disinfected us as if we were some kind of animals that were bringing germs," she marked the difference between her self-definition as a member of a shared community of humans and the definition of Mexican enforced by these American public health officers.[5] She also demonstrated her familiarity with the language of modern medicine. When public health authorities prevented any movement of people between South Texas and the rest of Texas, their authority trumped other forms of political authority or forms of citizenship. Public health, as much as formal politics, shaped the encounters between people and the states

that took shape in the Texas-Mexico borderlands. As public health formation is an ongoing political process, the assumption that labels hold the same
meaning over time is problematic.

The use of designations to describe people with different access to power
is always complicated. A flurry of terms developed in Mexico to calibrate
the relationships among people indigenous to Mexico; the people enslaved
in Africa, Asia, Mexico, and the Americas and imported to Mexico; and the
established Spanish elite, soldiers, and other Spanish migrants. The reality of
sexual liaisons across these lines and the establishment of a variety of households led to the adaption of names to designate the privileges of a given individual. *Criollo* referred to people born of Spanish parents, or to people born
to *criollos*. *Indio* referred to someone who was indigenous, or someone who
looked indigenous to the observer. *Mestizo* referred to the children of Spanish and Indian parents. *Mulato* referred to children of African and Spanish
parentage. *Chino*, *lobo*, and *zambo* referred to children of black and Indian
parents. In northern Mexico, *coyote* referred to people who had family on
different sides of the Spanish/Indian divide. *Esclavo* and *pieza* were words
people used to describe slaves and enslaved war captives. *Genizaro* described
slaves and war captives brought into Spanish households at a young age. The
names give the impression of timeless categories.

Nothing could be further from the truth in Mexico. Historian Dennis
Váldes completed an analysis of court records in Mexico City and found that
people frequently disagreed with their legal caste designation on the record
and that the same people often had different designations accompany them in
the court records.[6] The majority of people in New Spain chafed under these
designations, and after they wrested control of Mexico from Spain, they abol-
ished slavery and officially frowned on the presence of these racial designation in the legal record. The words disappeared from much of the legal record,
though the inequalities were much more difficult to end. In Texas and New
Mexico, *indio*, *mestizo*, *mulato*, *moreno* (black), and *negro* (black) continued
in use, partly because the Comanche, Apache, Pueblo, Yaqui, and Navajo
Nations actively shaped the economics and culture of these once Mexican
regions.[7] I will use the relevant national terms for various Indian Nations
because they reflect the diplomatic dimension of the history of displacement,
war, and persistence. In Texas, *esclavo* stayed in the record because the Texas
Revolution reestablished slavery in towns and ranches that were once Mexican. For these Spanish-language terms, I use *indio* to refer to indigenous

people based in Mexico or in Mexican communities in the United States whom other people considered indigenous or who used the term to refer to themselves. I use it to remind readers of the layering of racial inequality in the United States and Mexico. Currently, people use "Afro-Mexican" to refer to people from communities who trace their existence to African slavery and emancipation in colonial and postcolonial Mexico. I prefer to use "white," "brown," or "black" to designate situations where *blanco, mestizo,* or *moreno* were used to distinguish racially between Mexicans.

The presence of racial slavery in the Republic of Texas made "white" mean "citizen," "black" mean "noncitizen" or "slave," and "Mexican" mean "someone of Mexico who belonged in Mexico." Mexicans in the Texas Republic started using the term "Tejano" in English to designate their long-term presence in Texas. In Spanish, people used Mexico-Tejano to refer to long-standing Mexican communities as well as Mexicans born in Texas who still participated in Mexican communities on both sides of the border. "Texas-Mexican" appeared as a term during the Mexican Revolution to help Americans distinguish between recent arrivals displaced by the Mexican Revolution and the people who lived in Texas before the Revolution. In West Texas, people started using "Hispano" and "Hispanic" during the New Mexico statehood debates to distinguish themselves from immigrants displaced by the Mexican Revolution. Community activists in the 1930s pushed the adoption of the terms "Latin American" and "Mexican American" to refer to the political communities of Mexican descent with roots in the United States. People used "Mexicano" to refer to people with a deep level of participation in Mexican communities in Texas or Mexico. This book will use Tejano, Hispano, and Mexicano throughout, will use Mexico-Tejano and Mexicano for the time before the Mexican Revolution, and will start using the terms Texas-Mexican and Mexican American for the Progressive Era and the New Deal.

Americans in Texas also used "Anglo-Saxon" or "Anglo" to refer to white people in counterpoint to the American racial designations "black" and "Mexican." "Anglo" has also come to mean "Anglophone," which means people who grew up using English most of the time—in other words, most people born in the United States. I use the second version for people of European descent who do not have strong ties to Mexican societies in the United States and who can probably claim legal whiteness in the United States. Anglo earned this meaning because of the political subordination in Texas of Spanish-language dominant communities with ongoing personal and economic ties to Mexico. I will use the terms black, African American, or black American to refer to people who are part of the communities that still face political and social hostility after the abolition of slavery and who have taken up residence in the United States. I will use the term "black" when cultural or social issues seem the most relevant and "African American" when the political relationship to American citizenship is at issue. I will use "black American" to refer to cultural or social situations in Mexico, because there are also black Mexican nationals. The terms "Negro" and "colored" appear in both capitalized and lowercased forms in many historical sources, of course, and quotations from those sources are reproduced without alteration to respect the formal conventions in the United States before 1970.

I will also use national designations to refer to people or communities with ties to additional nations or cultures. In Texas, "German" means "ethnic German" or "German," "Irish" means "ethnic Irish" or "Irish," "French" means "ethnic French," and "Czech" means "ethnic Czech," not "Austro-Hungarian." I will use "Algerian," "Syrian," and "Lebanese" to refer to the people with Arabic surnames in English whose families left these countries when they were under French control. When necessary and also possible, I will use "Jewish" to refer to Ashkenazi Jewish communities with ties to Russia and Eastern Europe and "Ladino" to refer to Sephardic communities with ties to the Middle East, Spain, and Mexico. I will try to modify "Chinese" with national designations when possible, using "Chinese Mexican," "Chinese American," or "Chinese national" to refer to people at the border negotiating the racial category "Chinese." I will use the ethnic and national designations when they were politically relevant to the situation or when they help complicate racial designations like white, black, Chinese, Jewish, Indian, or Mexican.

A Note on Diseases

People suffer from illnesses. Doctors evaluate symptoms and diagnose diseases. The act of naming a cluster of symptoms a particular disease helps organize individual, medical, and community responses. These names for diseases emerge at particular times and reflect both current medical theories and the general culture of the time.[8] In the case of cholera, the loss of fluids through diarrhea is so quick and severe that the diagnosis should follow the immediate treatment for fluid loss. People used "cholera" to describe a deep melancholy, a loss of bodily control, and an uncontrollable heaving. The nineteenth-century appearance of *vibrio cholera*, the bacterial infection, in Europe and the Americas was so dramatic that in English the term applies only to bacterial infection, not to the rage or the deep melancholy previously associated with cholera.[9]

"Smallpox" refers to the small pus blisters (pox) that appear on the outside of the full body during the trajectory of the illness. The pox can damage parts of the nervous system, and the spread of the pox adds to the pain and internal tissue damage associated with the disease. If the pox grow close enough, they merge and turn an already painful and disfiguring disease into *variola major* or hemorrhagic smallpox. This almost certainly leads to death from the internal blisters and bleeding. Smallpox infections did vary, which led people to think temperature, humidity, barometric pressure, or patient disposition or racial background might be relevant to the diagnosis and the treatment. We now know that there were two major strains of smallpox, *variola major* and *variola minor*. The pain, cramps, fevers, internal bleeding, and pox for *variola minor* were nearly identical to *variola major* with one exception: most people survived *variola minor*. Families and doctors sought to find ways to distinguish between them, but death or survival provided the best diagnosis.[10] In the nineteenth century, most people recognized the arrival of smallpox.

The arrival of typhus, on the other hand, is difficult to diagnose by symptoms. The symptoms start with intense headaches and hallucinations. The spirochetes that cause the infection begin to pierce cell walls, which leads to internal bleeding of tissues and damage to veins, muscle tissue, and intestinal walls. At the height of the infection, the intracellular bleeding will cause a red coat to form on the back and shoulders of the patient. Patients who survive may still suffer relapses and hallucinations. However, the initial pains, cramps, high fevers, hallucinations, and subsequent relapses can be very similar to malaria or typhoid fever. Doctors used the term "typhomalarial fever" to describe the ways the symptoms overlapped yet varied. When typhus grew less common in the United States, the typhomalarial diagnosis lost its clinical utility, and after the Civil War it died out.[11] The discovery of specific patterns of intracellular bleeding on intestinal walls during an autopsy helped doctors determine that typhoid and typhus were two different diseases, though this distinction was not helpful to live patients. This did mean that they were infections, and once clinicians started identifying bacteria and accepting that germs could cause diseases, clinicians started searching for typhoid and typhus bacilli. Clinicians identified typhoid bacilli in the 1890s. The Weil-Felix test used bacteria that responded to the presence of typhus and thus allowed doctors to diagnose typhus directly. Nearly thirty years after Robert Koch identified the cholera bacilli, doctors were finally able to use laboratory tests to support their diagnosis of typhus.

A severe case of typhomalarial fever in the mid-nineteenth century could also shade into yellow fever. Here, patients suffer from cramps, muscular pain, and high fevers. However, the diagnosis of yellow fever became clear once patients started vomiting digested blood, hence the name *vomito negro*, "black bile," in many of the nineteenth-century records. Most frightening for observers and family members, the older and healthier patients tended to have far more severe and deadly bouts of yellow fever. Survival, however, guaranteed immunity against yellow fever.[12] Unfortunately, there is still no reliable treatment for yellow fever. The best remedy still dates back to the beginning of the twentieth century: mosquito eradication and patient isolation. There are temporary vaccines with potentially dreadful side effects.[13] Fortunately, mosquito vectors for yellow fever no longer tend to concentrate in urban areas, though there are still occasional outbreaks.[14]

FEVERED MEASURES

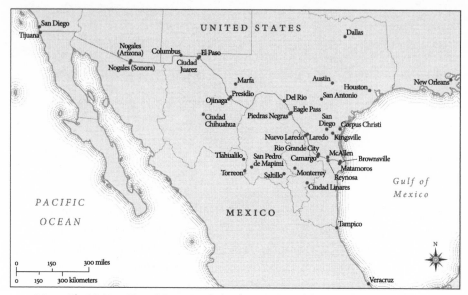

Map 1. The Mexico–United States Borderlands. Courtesy of the University of Wisconsin Cartography Laboratory, 2011.

INTRODUCTION

Laredo's political culture troubled Gregorio Guiteras. The United States Marine Hospital Service had detailed him to coordinate the yellow fever quarantine in Laredo, Texas, in 1903. The distinguished Cuban American doctor probably expected the credentials he earned by ending yellow fever in Cuba to translate into professional respect in Laredo. But the people there publicly ignored his medical authority throughout the yellow fever epidemic. According to Guiteras, locals "seldom called in a physician, fearful that they might be quarantined or sent to a hospital."[1] Even more frustrating to Dr. Guiteras was that Laredo's political and military authorities reported that "the very class of cases I wished to remove to a hospital would absolutely refuse to go, and that there was no authority to force them to do so."[2] In Havana, Guiteras sent in armed American soldiers alongside Cuban and American medical personnel to move people with yellow fever symptoms directly to American field hospitals.[3] Laredo authorities confounded Guiteras's desire to exercise unconstrained sovereign authority over other people in the name of public health.

People at the border learned to negotiate the desire to exercise unconstrained medical authority to enforce national boundaries. In 1917, Miguel Barrera complained to the local Mexican consul that the United States Public Health Service (USPHS) doctor at the immigration station in Camargo, Texas, treated him like a medically suspect foreign national. "In spite of having my residence in Sam Fordyce [Texas], the doctor refused to hear my arguments and vaccinated me." As he explained, "When a boy I was vaccinated at the age usually done in Mexico, said vaccination having taken; but to be vaccinated at the age when the danger of infection may be said to have passed is in my opinion altogether unnecessary." Barrera reported, "The doctor appears insensible to the just reasons that may be exposed to him by persons like myself that are used to deal with the truth."[4] Most important to Barrera, Dr. John Hunter's refusal to recognize Barrera's experience and expertise challenged Barrera's sense of self, as did the subsequent vaccination against Barrera's direct will. National public health authority worked at two levels in this encounter. First, Hunter decided who deserved to be an American, who did not fully belong in the United States, and ultimately whose borders mattered. In Barrera's case, the boundaries of his person and the experience of his body were immaterial to the importance of the medical boundary between the United States and Mexico, even in tiny Camargo, Texas. For Barrera and Hunter, the medical border they shared and re-created meant Hunter's vaccination needles turned Barrera's body into a site to redefine citizenship.[5]

As these two anecdotes suggest, public health campaigns provide a rich staging for encounters between medical professionals, political authorities, and working-class residents; for processes that expose the interplay of local and national identities; and for the forging of ethnic identities at places where two nations staged and built their own changing identities. Moreover, Guiteras and Hunter were part of a larger drama at the Rio Grande border over the political and social implications of modern public health measures. In 1804, King Charles V of Spain charged Dr. Francisco Javier de Balmis with the task of disseminating vaccine lymph from Spain to every corner of the larger Spanish empire.[6] Within four years of the announcement, towns and presidios across the state of Coahuila y Tejas (one of the far reaches of the Spanish empire) had started registering and vaccinating the children of military families, Mexican families, and enrolled Apache families.[7] Imperial incorporation and ethnic subordination through public health measures pre-dated the creation of the Mexican Republic and the American-Mexican border. Public health matters at the Texas-Mexico border were as much a question of national belonging as of medical authority.[8] Public health measures came with the process of creating political communities in the Texas borderlands.

By drawing a medical line between Mexican or American bodies, public health officers helped "reinforce territorial identities, symbolize and protect an image of state authority, and relegitimize the boundaries of the imagined community."[9] This medical border—the line public health service officers drew to protect American citizens—played an important role in "the medicalization of the general public."[10] Medical historians, drawing from Michel

Foucault, emphasize the way medicalization subjected the autonomy of individual men and women to medical scrutiny and gave physicians an often-challenged public authority over the intimate boundaries of private life.[11] This authority also gave a medical dimension to inclusion within the nation: the power to determine whether people at the border were potentially, in historian Natalia Molina's words, "fit to be citizens."[12] Medical norms, like the ideal place to treat people with yellow fever, became an implicit part of the staging of citizenship. Public health provided another theater for people to demonstrate their ability to participate in national society—to show that they were indeed worthy of citizenship.[13] In both Mexico and the United States, people still struggle to define the relationship of public health measures to the creation of a meaningful national identity.

Public health policies emerge from the ways people understand their relationship to the world just beyond their immediate selves.[14] Early nineteenth-century people did not draw the boundaries we draw between illness and identity. Historians roughly agree that for most nineteenth-century residents of the Americas, "health or disease resulted from cumulative interaction between constitutional endowment and environmental circumstance. . . . The body was always in a state of becoming—and thus always in jeopardy. . . . This was a system which had necessarily to remain in balance if the individual were to remain healthy."[15] Moreover, the dynamic balance meant that bodies were dangerously porous. People had to monitor and regulate the movement of air, food, sweat, blood, and other excretions across their personal boundaries.[16] Town residents in nineteenth-century Mexican Texas, the Republic of Texas, Mexico, and the United States sought ways to monitor and possibly contain the dangerous airs and humors in their immediate environments. Smallpox vaccination, one of the few translocal disease-specific prevention measures available in the early nineteenth-century Americas, depended on local families' willingness to undergo the painful arm-to-arm transfer of vaccine lymph and on strong political and commercial relationships to places that offered steady supplies of vaccine lymph, such as central Mexico or New Orleans. This was a dynamic balance, for the relationships that made smallpox vaccine lymph available across political boundaries also helped smallpox move from one locale to another.[17]

Political boundaries in the nineteenth-century Texas borderlands followed the dangers of this dynamic and porous model of borders. Living within and working across Mexican, Comanche, and American spheres of influence,

Tejanos and Anglo-Texans plotted new borders and drew on outside allies to gain power and control over their political and commercial destinies. These competing desires led to the War of Independence (1810–22), the Texas Revolution (1834–36), the Cordova Rebellion (1837), the Cherokee War (1838), the Council House Fight (1840), the Mier Expedition (1842), the U.S.-Mexico War (1846–48), the Cart War (1857), the French Intervention (1862–67), and the American Civil War (1860–65). By the end of the American Civil War, Spain, France, Mexico, the Comanche, the Apache, the Republic of Fredonia, the Cherokee Nation, the Republic of Texas, the United States, and the Confederacy had all laid competing claims for parts of what are now the states of Texas, Tamaulipas, Nuevo León, Coahuila, and Chihuahua.[18] The Rio Grande border, once tentatively fixed by the Treaty of Guadalupe Hidalgo, now marked the place where Mexico and the United States agreed to start exercising their political sovereignty in 1848.

For medical professionals, 1848 and 1849 probably marked the low point of their cultural authority. Cholera effectively demonstrated their inability to predict or treat a disease with a lightning-quick trajectory.[19] Moreover, rampant illness and medical anxiety accompanied the American occupation of Mexico and the Rio Grande border in 1846; medical authorities found it difficult to treat these illnesses and thus to translate these far-ranging anxieties into federal medical policies. Americans and Mexicans both looked to France for ways out of this medical conundrum. In the medical schools and hospitals of Paris, doctors emphasized observing before treating. In the United States, people expected race-, place-, and person-specific treatments. Watching an illness develop threatened to sink even further the low financial status then associated with American medical identities.[20] Doctors had to produce "phenomena which all—the physician, the patient, and the patient's family—could witness and in which all could participate," and watching doctors simply observe the course of an illness frustrated patients and family.[21] When research minded medical practices undercut the participatory dimension of doctor-patient encounters, doctors found it hard to explain their special role in society. Moreover, people were deeply suspicious of professional authority. Local participation in the vast political transformations that shook Mexico and the United States had given people and communities experience managing their own affairs in a time of crisis. The democratic culture that encouraged the abolition of slavery, local elections, and local militia in both countries also helped generate forms of local cooperation during epidemics. Doctors had to learn to conform to local mores to survive.

The presence of the political border at the Rio Grande complicated these forms of medical community and regional identity. In Texas and New Mexico before and after 1850, people changed national identities at the border; more subtly, national identities themselves also changed at the American-Mexican border.[22] The threat and presence of various epidemics raised the already high stakes involved in creating and maintaining national identities. The material strain of public health campaigns and the human cost of epidemics forced many men and women living along or moving through the Mexico-U.S. border to go beyond their local resources and engage federal public health policies and policy makers.[23] When public health measures started adding specific diseases and, later, specific germs to their policy goals, public health officers started searching for ways to protect members of their political communities from the threat of other diseases, peoples, and germs. The forms of racial exclusion that often accompanied the establishment of national health policies at the border complicated local border engagement with federal authorities, especially in their demands for federal health resources.[24] When people remembered feeling that the USPHS "disinfected us as if we were some kind of animals that were bringing germs," demanding more public health resources would not address this demeaning dimension of border health encounters.[25] The border context also complicated the extent of racial exclusion in public health. Public Health Service officers continually commented on the dangerous independence of border residents during the course of illness, expressing variations on the statement that they "do not limit their movements on account of it, but continue to mingle freely as ever with other people."[26] Placing more doctors at the border simply made more doctors aware of this general attitude among border families and neighborhoods. The increased medical presence could not guarantee additional cooperation by locals with medical norms.

In the 1880s, federal medical officials gained the authority to implement a variety of cultural and medical projects in the Texas-Mexico borderlands. These projects helped shape national and international debates in public health. These projects also sparked a long-term, fractious, and occasionally violent dialogue among federal health officers, locals, and migrants over the connection between disease, citizenship, and state action. Federal authorities then became the people connecting medical politics at the border to the politics of public health. The case studies in *Fevered Measures* track the changing medical and political frameworks U.S. federal health authorities used to treat the threat of epidemic disease to Americans.

Thus the book makes it clear how medical borders differ from political borders. After 1850, public health authorities moved. The international border in the Rio Grande/Rio Bravo stayed in place. The medical borders public health officers created responded to rumors of outbreaks, followed the movements of people, and often seemed to work far outside local political frameworks. The long federal medical presence in the Rio Grande borderlands made public health matters more visible and present in local politics. The movements around questions of disease and state action exposed how concepts of illness were folded into categories of citizenship, how emerging political identities changed the demands made on public health authorities at the border, and how processes at the border confounded the easy designation of Mexican and American. By the start of the twentieth century, public health measures became key points of struggle over the privileges of citizenship.

Public Health and the Promise of History

Unlike Dr. Guiteras, I was pleasantly surprised by the power that people at the border exercised over the thoughts and actions of American public health officers. This study began with my experiences as a glorified HIV/AIDS epidemiologist with the Cook County Department of Public Health, working a beat in suburban Chicago. In addition to drawing blood and interviewing people with AIDS, I listened to others wrestle with the potential changes in the self-identity that they might create in response to a positive or negative HIV antibody test. I had committed to a bilingual-bicultural practice in public health as a way to implement social justice in the United States or, alternatively, expand Latino cultural and political access to publicly funded medical services. But I grew frustrated with the way Latinos seemed outside the immediate concerns of the public health department. What particularly irked me was the way most of my colleagues separated medical matters from "Mexican" matters, implying that somehow public health had never reached Mexico or Latin America. Their ignorance of history—or their idea that Mexicans are "new" to the United States—justified their attitude toward many residents of Cook County, which meant real difficulties with Latino clients. I pointlessly sought articles that connected the long Mexican presence in the United States to the institutional history of American public health. I wanted to show that Mexicans, Mexican Americans, and Mexican immigrants were also part of the drama of American public health.

In the 1980s and 1990s, the drama of American public health could not have had a larger stage. The AIDS epidemic in North America galvanized new forms of political mobilization in gay and lesbian communities across the United States.[27] AIDS and HIV advocacy brought public health professionals and diverse coalitions of everyday people together.[28] These political struggles created medical and political encounters feared and desired by all involved.[29] AIDS activists worked on two different fronts, exposing the general indifference of the public medical response to the pain of HIV and AIDS and confronting the homophobic and racist dimensions of the American cultural response to AIDS and homosexuality.[30] In our working-class and ethnically diverse sexually transmitted diseases (STD) department, history provided a number of ways to discuss our relationship to the worlds beyond the doors of our STD clinics. We discussed the USPHS's untreated syphilis study in Macon County, Alabama (the Tuskegee study), the experience of gay men and lesbians in Germany under the Third Reich, Japanese American internment, the Second World War military purge of gays and lesbians, and the general experience of Jim Crow as cautionary tales about the power of state agencies to create minority identities.[31] On reflection, Latinos were generally invisible in these American narratives about civil rights and public health. Moreover, I find it unsettling that I remember no Latino public health civil rights narratives or case studies discussed by public health professionals based in greater Chicago in the mid-1990s, even though Latinos represented close to 20 percent of Chicago's population.[32] I decided that historical work could help paper the gap between the long presence of Latinos in the United States and the relative absence of popular narratives about race, Latinos, history, and American public health. So I marched off to the archives to document the encounters between Latino communities and public health institutions.

However, the archival traces of these public health encounters were surprisingly difficult to track down. A partial record of these debates and discussions exists in medical research libraries, partly because American public health authorities have been publishing weekly updates on communicable diseases in specific places since 1888.[33] However, I was surprised to find that many of the records for the Eagle Pass, Laredo, and Brownsville epidemics were under correspondence for Southern Quarantine Stations. This archival designation was geographically correct, as the Rio Grande border is south of the (American) South.[34] Clearly, the U.S. Marine Hospital Service drew regional boundaries that reflected a different logic. The National Archives did keep records for the different Rio Grande border stations in the central files for the USPHS, but the more historically compelling correspondence often lay buried in the surgeon general's massive files regarding specific diseases like smallpox, yellow fever, and typhus.[35] Some of the conflicts in the various epidemics and quarantines involved Mexican consular representation in the United States, which placed the legal record in the State Department diplomatic archives in College Park, Maryland. State Department specialists in the National Archives in College Park, because of their initial skepticism, were always surprised to find that "complaints against quarantine" did exist and had their own decimal file.[36] This project owes these archivists an enormous debt, for they helped make these once-classified records available to me and to the scholarly public.

The reason the State Department regarded memoranda involving smallpox, typhus, and yellow fever in the Texas-Mexico borderlands as matters of national security remains a mystery to me, especially given that public health officers gave regular updates on these diseases in the surgeon general's *Public Health Reports*. The records themselves revealed that American citizens as well as Mexican nationals used Mexican consular advocacy to challenge and negotiate the actions of American health authorities in the United States. That this U.S.-based medical and diplomatic record is undocumented—or hidden in plain sight—speaks to the ways multiple archives push Mexicans in the United States out of the main currents of American historical experience, helping them become, in Mae Ngai's term, "alien citizens."[37] The foreign dimension of this public archival record is a reminder of the long-obscured relationship between Latino communities and U.S. federal authorities. These diplomatic records provide a privileged way to understand how locals, migrants, and national public health authorities understood the medical dimensions of national identity, citizenship, belonging, personhood, and public space at the border.

Simply finding these records was not enough. The research process also complicated my initial framework explaining medical encounters at the border. I began my preliminary research looking for interactions between American health officers and border residents. I started with the telegraphs, memos, and reports generated by the USPHS in El Paso, Laredo, and Brownsville. I sought evidence of unequal treatment and Mexicano awareness of these inequalities. I ran across memos and news stories about the 1917 El Paso Typhus Bath Riots, a conflict that, up to that point, was not included in any history of El Paso or Ciudad Juárez.[38] The women involved in these riots defied the USPHS demand that they enter the clinic by the bridge, disrobe, place their clothes in a cyanide mixture, and then place themselves in a kerosene and vinegar bath.[39] For the next three days, women living in Juarez and working as domestics and laundresses in El Paso shut down traffic across the Santa Fe Bridge. This riot confirmed the importance of Mexican resistance in the history of American public health. The daily presence and potential anger of working-class Mexican women who crossed the border on a daily basis limited the sphere of action for American public health officers at the El Paso border.

However, my search for Mexican or American responses to public health practices at the border also restricted my understanding of the ebb and flow of a complex and multiethnic social world in formation in the medical encounters. When I started researching the Laredo Smallpox Riot of 1899, I believed that it stemmed from *Mexican* resistance to violent *Anglo*-American medical policies enforced by the Texas Rangers.[40] I was intrigued when I found that the (white) (Anglo) Texas Rangers depended on the (African American) Tenth Cavalry to defend the Rangers from Laredo's working-class residents. When I started seeing Spanish surnames among the police officers and volunteer inspectors who were forcing their way into working-class households in Laredo, I realized that my American/Mexican binary—my initial narrative tracing Anglo-American modernity and ethnic Mexican resistance—did little to explain the variety of responses in the multiethnic world of twentieth-century Laredo. These unexpected situations in El Paso and Laredo underscored the ways public health at the border can both contribute to our understanding of how racial formations move across borders and complicate nation-bound narratives about state building.[41] They inspired me to dig deeper and find a larger story through these public health encounters, which I hope to tell here.

Marked Bodies and Moving Medical Borders, 1848–1942

Medical borders moved to respond to the perceived threat of illness, not the establishment of political borders. In 1848, the drafters of the Treaty of Guadalupe Hidalgo included a medical exception to the new political border they drew between Mexico and the United States. Article III stated that

American troops could stay in their highland locations in central and northern Mexico for an additional six months to avoid malaria and yellow fever
during the May to November sickly season (*la estación malsana*) in the Gulf of
Mexico.[42] The treaty signers acceded to the U.S. Army's demand to extend the
occupation in order to keep American troops and volunteers alive in Mexico.
After the establishment of the political line between Mexico and the United
States, federal actions followed news of illness in the greater Texas-Mexico
borderlands, not simply on the Rio Grande border. In the 1882 Mexico-Texas
epidemic, the U.S. Marine Hospital Service (USMHS) drew a 146-mile-long line
from Laredo to Corpus Christi and quarantined everyone south of the Texas-
Mexico railroad. This effectively erected a medical border between Mexico
and the United States, 150 miles north of the Brownsville border. During the
same yellow fever epidemic, the USMHS hired mostly Anglo local cowboys to
man the line and prevent any river crossings from Laredo to Brownsville.[43]
This mounted medical guard preceded the Border Patrol by forty years.

Federal public health officers also crossed into Mexico to treat and address the potential threat of smallpox, yellow fever, and typhus to U.S. nationals. In 1895, the U.S. Army and the USMHS helped escort American citizens
three hundred miles north, from Torreon, Coahuila, to a detention camp in
Eagle Pass, Texas.[44] After 1899, the USMHS stationed public health officers in
key ports and cities in northern Mexico to review the progress of any yellow fever epidemic and invoke quarantine if necessary.[45] In the process of
crossing borders to protect American citizens, the health services defined
who was going to be an American citizen and who was going to be a threat
to American citizens. The USMHS (1797–1902), the National Board of Health
(1879–1883), the United States Public Health and Marine Hospital Service
(USPHMHS) (1902–1912), and the USPHS (1917–present) authorized border health
work in places far from the Rio Grande border. The public health services
drew medical borders and crossed political borders to protect American citizens. The ongoing movement of American medical officers across state and
international borders made medical borders different from political borders.

Most medical border work after 1903 happened around the key hubs of the
Rio Grande. The main foci of federal health attention were the bridge stations by the Rio Grande, the detention camps for medical quarantines, and
the people in the streets and houses of Brownsville, Rio Grande City, Laredo, Eagle Pass, and El Paso. Public health service officers treated the various
communities in formation at the border in medically distinct ways. Far too

often, they considered the many Mexican communities along the border to be one population.[46] They placed (white) Americans outside their medical surveillance.[47] They evaluated the illnesses in their midst at the border by their relative threat to places beyond the border, not by the danger to people at the border.[48] Much of the political authority of the medical border derived from its mobility and its power to control traffic—other people's mobility—across the border region.

Though the American medical border had mobility and power, the distinct complexities of Texas-Mexico border societies troubled that mobility and challenged the power of the disease labels and racial categories that medical officers brought to the Texas borderlands. The presence of an established working-class Mexican and Mexican American population with land bases in Texas and northern Mexico gave locals a sense of power and authority over their own affairs. The construction of a railroad network between northern Mexico and the United States accelerated the growth of a racially diverse and highly mobile regional labor force on both sides of the Rio Bravo. Finally, a modernizing Mexican and Mexican American middle class ripped apart remaining racial generalizations regarding expected Mexican attitudes toward public health measures.[49] These three different classes developed divergent expectations of official authority. As residents of the most affluent and educated region in Mexico, many border migrants and residents prided themselves on their education, their health, and their commitment to progress. To put it simply, people at the border—Mexicans, Americans, Mexican Americans, African Americans, and other minorities—expected American medical officers to honor shared concepts of disease, health care, and autonomy. This expectation troubled the exercise of medical power at the border.

Working-class Mexican, Mexican American, and African American demands for mutual medical recognition from public health authorities on the border complicate the sense that doctors were the agents of medicalization on a submissive population.[50] In an 1892 article on vaccination, journalist-in-exile Justo Cardenas equated vaccination with civilization and demanded universal vaccination and, by implication, universal civilization at the border. This modernist impulse implied that public health and equal citizenship were part of national progress. Cardenas's writings shared the many visions of medical modernity and national community that men and women were developing within their ethnic and national communities.[51] However, late nineteenth-century public health measures also meant quarantines, inspections, detentions, and forced treatment regimens.[52] The demands for mutual recognition and equal treatment conflicted with the exclusion and humiliation that came with inspection, detention, compulsory vaccination, and quarantine. These contradictory tensions made public health matters potentially dramatic and volatile; at the border, ongoing questions of national belonging accelerated the potential drama of public health.

The process of defending a nation's health meant distinguishing "Mexican" from "American" within deeply interconnected border communities. If, as George Sánchez has argued for Mexican Americans in Los Angeles, ethnicity is "not a fixed set of customs surviving from a life in Mexico, but is a collective identity that emerged from the experience of living in the United States," the collective identities that emerged in public health crises at the Texas-Mexico border expose the uneasy relationship between ethnic and national identities.[53] When communities came into being to demand changes in public health policies, the public health encounter "played an active role in formulating, articulating and acting on the pressing issues facing [what would then be defined as] their communities."[54] Moreover, the sense of shared crisis in an epidemic also forced individuals who participated in multiple communities to choose and define their immediate community.[55] The responses by national health authorities actively helped define what was American or Mexican about this encounter. National public health interventions required local participation; national public health interventions also amplified local patterns of exclusion. The simultaneous engagement and exclusion that accompanied public health interventions at the border made it difficult for border residents and sojourners to fully participate in American or Mexican identities. That people arrived at different conclusions about the value of these political identities—even given shared circumstances—was as true then as it is now. When public health concerns melted into questions of race at the border, public health measures tracked along racial lines and redefined the experience of shared circumstances.

Public health crises implicated white Americans in this alchemy of race at the border. The federal sanitary cordon around South Texas and northern Mexico during the yellow fever epidemic of 1882 forced white Americans in South Texas to reconsider their relationship to their Mexican neighbors and their white colleagues in Central Texas. Laredo mayor Santos Benavides—a Texas Mexican, a southern Democrat, and a Confederate veteran—arrested and detained Texas State Health Officer Robert M. Swearingen, another southern Democrat and Confederate veteran, for breaking the Texas state quarantine of Brownsville that Swearingen himself had ordered.[56] This ended up being just one of multiple detentions Swearingen experienced; they troubled his unmarked mobility and authority as a white state professional and forced him to seek political measures to reclaim his hold on his challenged national identity.[57] Swearingen thundered in his telegrams against the political authority of Rio Grande City, Peña, and Laredo that if the mayors "refuse to obey your orders, they are not being more nor less than organized mobs and the state should not pay one dime of the expenses incurred by them."[58] Swearingen equated the exercise of the law (he mandated) by democratically elected Tejano authorities with democracy run amok. The spatial restriction of public health policies forced some white people confronting medical borders to reaffirm a white American class identity among Mexican others. Quarantines could expose, trouble, or reaffirm the privileges of whiteness along the border.

Public health measures could also expose and trouble the national performance of African American identity at the border. The interventions became flashpoints where observers recognized, incorporated, rejected, and modified particular ethnic scripts and national identities. For example, in 1895, a group of black southern workers from Alabama started a labor rebellion on a cotton plantation in northern Mexico. They demanded that the United States intervene to end "the conditions akin to bondage" on the Tlahualilo plantation and insisted on being treated as American citizens who suffered from a foreign company's breach of contract.[59] However, the presence of smallpox among some of the workers' family members complicated their labor dispute with the Tlahualilo Agricultural Company. The U.S. Army and the U.S. executive branch used these cases of smallpox to define the workers as "Negro refugees with smallpox" as they moved the workers three hundred miles north to the U.S. border. The USMHS then treated some of the workers as "an opportunity not to be lost to test the serum therapy" and placed them in a smallpox detention camp called Camp Jenner.[60] The workers' experience with federal authority highlighted the ambivalence of transnational American belonging. The workers' negotiations shifted with each change in the public label—workers, exiles, colonists, citizens, workers, refugees, detainees—that defined their relationship to American national identity.[61] The threat

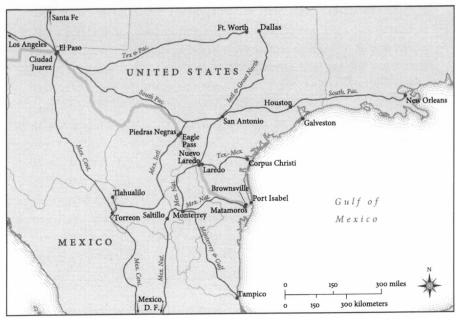

Map 2. Railroad Lines Connecting the Texas-Mexico Borderlands. Courtesy of the University of Wisconsin Cartography Laboratory, 2011.

and stigma of illness and state action forced the black colonists to forge collective identity that emerged from their experience with illness and exclusion at the political edge of two nations.

Public health measures themselves provide deeply resonant metaphors for state intervention. Vaccinations require medical authorities to touch and breach the boundaries that define the beginning and end of each individual. Quarantines create boundaries around homes, households, cities, countries, and even full regions. The presence of quarantine may be a visible reminder of the ongoing labor that members of their community perform to protect, and thus define, the outer edges of their communities. Sanitary inspections can restrict access to publics and public spaces, and the spectacle of sanitary inspection at the border stations can foster the impression that certain groups of people are always medically suspect. These inspections can also guarantee subsequent access to the general community. Developments during the Mexican Revolution and the Progressive era helped make these federal health measures part of the urban landscapes of the Rio Grande.

The federal dimension of these intimate encounters between doctors and people meant that local tensions moved into the national arena and that national tensions shaped local politics. Racial tensions in the USPHS germ control campaign in El Paso made the urban spaces occupied by women visible, public, and foreign to American observers in El Paso. Their avid and potentially hostile embrace of germ control affected residents and commuters in Ciudad Juárez, many of whom resisted the generalization of these germ control measures to streetcar riders, to residences in Chihuahuita and South El Paso, and to bridge-crossing commuters. Using germ control as their lens, public health officers saw and separated *Mexicans*—people who had been considered part of the general landscape of West Texas—from the suddenly *American* landscape in which they lived and worked.[62] Rather than treating "Mexican" afflictions as an important part of life on the border, this newer "dangerous bodies" approach treated domestic laborers in El Paso as the medical threat that needed regulation, symbolically cleaning the people cleaning El Paso.

American political pressures could transform the physical meaning of the body. Between 1910 and 1915, state health authorities in California, Arizona, Texas, and Tennessee could—and did—respond to local smallpox outbreaks by demanding more rigorous and invasive inspections in El Paso and Laredo.[63] After five years of these pressures, USPHS officers started actively dismissing the presence of vaccination scars on Mexican bodies as evidence of vaccination. Mexican consular representatives organized against this rite of state medical exclusion to help the Carranza regime demonstrate their commitment to Mexican residents of all nationalities living and working in these border hubs. If, in the artist Barbara Kruger's words, your body is a battleground, Mexican consular authorities turned these scars into places to make the revolution real in the United States.[64] Public health practices turned the body itself into a site of postrevolutionary national sovereignty.

The border quarantines established during the Mexican Revolution shaped the political culture of the Texas border through the Second World War. As the frequency and severity of smallpox, yellow fever, and typhus—and the associated disease prevention campaigns—receded from popular memory, USPHS officers began to lose hold of their exclusive authority over the definition of disease. Counties across South and West Texas expanded the initial smallpox vaccination requirements to create full-fledged medical justifications for separate schools. The children of a generation of Mexican nationals who crossed the border and started lives across South and West Texas now faced segregation because of an ongoing medical response to the dislocations of the Mexican Revolution. Local school authorities justified the separate and unequal facilities on the basis of the medical danger that "lousy" and "dirty" *Mexican* (American) children posed to American children. The techniques ostensibly established against lice proved very effective at erecting boundaries around white privilege. South Texas county officials appropriated the medical border and the border quarantines for their own racial purposes.

Progressive Texas New Dealers sought to find ways to expand the medical border line into a medical border zone. Texas state legislators sought to create an international border medical district. Here federal authorities would be responsible for the health outcomes among the Mexican majority living in the border counties along the Rio Grande. Just as the USMHS did in the Mexican-Texas epidemic of 1882, the state of Texas sought to create a space *in* Texas but not *of* Texas. For Texas state authorities leading to the Second World War, border health meant *Latin America*, not Texas, and the answer lay in federal or diplomatic responsibility. State health officials turned the sense that medical conditions were different along the border into a disavowal of state responsibility for the outcomes along the border. Again, the mobile and porous medical border was designed to separate and isolate a population with strong ties to the Texas economy. Legislators sought to draw medical boundaries between citizens and their political representatives.

Community-based medical authorities sought political means to challenge these medical boundaries. El Paso was the site of two such actions: in 1925 Dr. Laurence Nixon initiated the two-decade-long NAACP campaign against the white primary in Texas; and in 1936 Juan Carlos Machuca and other medical professionals who were members of the League of United Latin American Citizens (LULAC) successfully beat back the attempt by the El Paso City-County Health Unit to reclassify and place Mexican and Mexican American residents in the colored category for vital statistics purposes. By 1942, Dr. Hector Garcia saw the importance of organized citizenship claims in transforming the health conditions of Mexican American communities. Civil rights mobilizing provided an emerging strategy to counter the political effects of the medical border.

This project started with the desire to connect Latinos to the making of American public health. I was interested in writing a historical analysis of public health measures that would demonstrate that Mexicans at the border were in an ongoing conversation with state medical personnel over common diseases. I found multiple examples of these conversations as I made my way through the archive. I also began to see the traces of a different project. Federal medical personnel had started a dialogue with people in the Rio Grande borderlands over the meaning of citizenship. The dialogue did not happen in courtrooms, schools, or churchyards. Rather, public health officers started these conversations when they knocked on people's doors and offered to bring quinine to suffering patients. Their actions on bridges and streetcars reminded people at the border of the basic privileges of citizenship. As health officers moved from one place in the borderlands to another, people responded to the ways the USMHS and the USPHS implemented their public health project. The original project about popular understandings of typhus, yellow fever, and smallpox would turn into a long conversation about the proper medical boundaries of citizenship at the Texas-Mexico border.

The fundamental point of anchorage of power relationships,
even if embodied and crystallized in an institution, is to
be found outside the institution.—Michel Foucault, "The
Subject and Power"

ONE

From the U.S.-Mexican War to the Mexican-Texas Epidemic

Fevers, Race, and the Making of a Medical Border

In 1847, public health matters concerned Americans in Mexico. The advent of fevers and disease among soldiers turned the initial military victories over Mexico into medical disasters. American soldiers and volunteers had started dying from typhomalarial fevers, dysentery, and yellow fever even before the American invasion of Port Isabel and Matamoros, Nuevo León, in May 1846. There was agreement regarding why Mexico was so harmful to Americans when the United States was supposed to be the healthier, more physically vigorous and energetic nation.[1] For Samuel Curtis, the American military governor of Matamoros, Nuevo León, the American occupation of the lower Rio Grande Valley meant "sustaining a position where the loathsome diseases of the south carried off hundreds around us."[2] The Veracruz campaign in the summer of 1847 exposed another set of troops and volunteers to the sickly season (*la epoca malsana*) in lowland Mexico. By the winter of 1847, the U.S. Army calculated that there had been more hospital visits than troops in Mexico and that approximately one of eight American troops died of illness during the occupation. Facing the same conditions after the winter of 1847, American military authorities warily prepared for another season of fevers and agues.

The American military reality of illness shaped diplomatic proceedings in Mexico. Nicholas Trist, the U.S. agent for negotiations between Mexico and the United States, had developed a close working relationship with General

Winfield Scott in Mexico City. Everyone was aware of the high level of illness and deaths among the troops stationed in Matamoros, Veracruz, and Monterrey. General Scott and the Mexican negotiator Manuel Peña y Peña wanted to end the American presence in Mexico as quickly as possible, but the reality of fevers during the summer gave the U.S. military pause. Trist and Peña agreed that, according to Article III, "the final evacuation of the territory of the Mexican Republic, by the forces of the United States, shall be completed from the said exchange of ratifications, or sooner if possible."[3] The clause spelled out the ways the Mexican military would help American troops avoid *la temporada malsana* in lowland Mexico:

> If, however, the ratification of this treaty by both parties should not take place in time to allow the embarcation of the troops of the United States to be completed before the commencement of the sickly season, at the Mexican ports on the Gulf of Mexico, in such case a friendly arrangement shall be entered into between the General-in-Chief of the said troops and the Mexican government, whereby healthy and otherwise suitable places, at a distance from the ports not exceeding thirty leagues, shall be designated for the residence of such troops as may not yet have embarked, until the return of the healthy season. And the space of time here referred to as comprehending the sickly season, shall be understood to extend from the first of May to the first day of November.[4]

This language dramatically illustrated the way the public health concerns of the American military became diplomatic concerns between Mexico and the United States. The high medical casualty rates among American troops in Mexico created a medical exception to the new political border.[5] Public health exercised its own state of exception across America's new international border.[6] Matamoros military governor Samuel Curtis, two months into his occupation of Matamoros, after nearly a third of his regiment had spent time in the makeshift camp hospital and he had weathered his own bouts of fever and agues, had already concluded that "the malignant diseases of this climate appear unconquerable."[7] The treaty language moved medical concerns into the language of diplomacy and provided for an extended temporary occupation in the name of American public health. Article III of the Treaty of Guadalupe Hidalgo provides a graphic example of the way American fears of disease forged a set of medical and political practices that transcended immediate political borders. This power and associated mobility defines the American medical border since 1848. The visible presence of state medical authority in the Texas borderlands throughout the nineteenth century challenges the assumption that American medical authority at the Mexican border began with the Mexican Revolution.[8]

American military leaders were not the first people to search for ways to make northern Mexico and South Texas medically safe for national purposes. Men and women in the Texas-Mexico borderlands had been grappling with the political and social implications of modern public health measures for nearly half a century before Winfield Scott composed Article III in the Treaty of Guadalupe Hidalgo. Spanish, Mexican, and American authorities all sought to create policies to contain smallpox, typhus, cholera, pneumonia, and yellow fever at the nation's outer edges. This chapter begins at the end of the Spanish empire in Mexico and traces the interactions between local people and national health initiatives up to the establishment of a U.S. Marine Hospital Service presence at the Texas-Mexico border through the aptly named Mexican-Texas epidemic. Conditions in the Mexican towns of northern Mexico and South Texas encouraged people to rely on each other, to draw on commercial and political resources beyond immediate national borders, and to create a sense of local autonomy in the midst of an epidemic. Locals, immigrants, and soldiers shaped the local contours of public health within the Texas borderlands.

Civil wars and foreign military interventions also shaped conditions for public health practice in the Texas borderlands. The Texas Revolution and the U.S.-Mexico war of 1846–1848 installed new political authorities over already existing commercial relationships. The aftermath of the U.S.-Mexico war of 1846–1848 led to open conflicts over slavery in the new territories acquired by the United States, which in turn led to the American Civil War.[9] In Mexico, conservative opposition to liberal economic and political reforms led to an open civil war and to French intervention after the passage of the Leyes de Reforma.[10] The French occupation of Mexico and the Confederate allegiance in Texas disrupted any consistent relationship with a federal public health service during both civil wars.[11] A concern over public health accompanied national reconstruction efforts after each nation's civil wars.

Civilian federal medical authority followed the military medical presence to the Texas-Mexico border. After the devastating Mississippi Valley yellow fever epidemic in 1878, the U.S. Congress created the first national civilian health authority, the National Board of Health (NBH), to outline the necessary policies to prevent future yellow fever epidemics. Four years later, the U.S. Marine Hospital Service (USMHS) wrested this authority from the NBH. When news of yellow fever in Brownsville hit Washington in 1882, the USMHS adopted two very different approaches to the challenge posed by the disease. At the heart of the yellow fever epidemic in Brownsville, the USMHS employed Spanish-speaking ethnic Mexican nurses, established free dispensaries and an open grocery, and treated the majority of patients in their own homes, beyond the boundaries of the USMHS field hospital.[12] The USMHS also deployed their first military quarantine around what they ultimately called Mexican Texas. The 190-mile-long quarantine line, set along the Texas-Mexico railroad connecting Laredo and Corpus Christi, medically separated and segregated the region from the rest of Texas. The USMHS trumpeted its experience incorporating communities outside the quarantine and containing goods and people within the quarantine to demonstrate to Congress that it had found the administrative means to contain yellow fever. The USMHS turned Brownsville and South Texas into the first American communities to wrestle publicly with the simultaneous medical outreach, political loss of autonomy, and federal exclusion that came with an American federal quarantine.

Making It Stick: Vaccination and Belonging in Late-Colonial Spanish Texas

The encounters among Tejanos, Mexicans, Anglo-Texans, European Americans, and African Americans in national public health ventures in the Rio Grande borderlands began at the end of the Spanish era in Texas and Mexico. A royal mandate brought vaccination, the quintessentially modern public health intervention, to the Texas borderlands.[13] There had been an ongoing demand and hunger for an effective smallpox prevention measure since a disastrous regionwide epidemic struck New Spain in the 1780s.[14] Edward Jenner published his experience with cowpox and the creation of vaccine lymph in 1798.[15] Writers and publishers quickly copied and translated Jenner's work for wider distribution, and by 1803, Dr. Francisco Javier de Balmis had translated Jacques-Louis Moreau's writings on Jenner's vaccination techniques into Spanish.[16] In early 1804, King Charles IV charged Dr. de Balmis with transferring vaccine lymph and implementing vaccination techniques to the Americas, China, the Philippines, and other overseas dominions.[17] On May 2, 1804, the military governor of Coahuila y Tejas ordered every military doctor in Texas to follow the vaccination procedure spelled out by the Balmis expedition and Charles IV. The military outpost nature of Spanish Texas shaped the Texas phase of the world's first immunization campaign.[18]

> To this end His Majesty wishes that in imitation of what has been done in the peninsula, you should destine one room in the hospital of the city and another one in each of these provinces of his district where the vaccine can be preserved fresh and administered precisely from arm to arm to all that may come, furnishing it free to the poor. The doctor appointed for this purpose must make periodical and constant operations at intervals and on a limited number of persons. It shall be furnished to the children born in a year in that place and on other places of the capitals of his orders. In this manner the inhabitants of the capitals as well as those of the respective provinces will have secured resources in order to avoid destroying or altering the vaccine.[19]

This was a burdensome order for Mexican and Native families in Texas. The forts housed the only hospitals in San Fernando de Bexar, Laredo, and Matamoros, and the doctor's primary responsibilities were to the troops in his care. Families had to bring their children into the hospital on a staggered basis to ensure the potency of the vaccine lymph for each arm-to-arm vaccination. They had to stay in the general vicinity for at least ten days to ensure that there was a good take: an immune response to cowpox lymph. Vaccination in Texas required a public commitment to stay by the army doctor.

Viceroy Don Felix Maria Calleja, concerned with keeping his subjects alive against the threat of smallpox epidemics that might emerge during the wars for independence in Mexico, circulated a medical handbill to all military governors describing "the proper way to administer the vaccine, the only means to prevent the contagion of smallpox."[20] The handbill describes the painful effects of a successful vaccination:

> From the first to the third day, there will be no real discomfort. On the fourth and fifth day the incisions made by the lancet will begin to burn. A sunken pox [pus blister], accompanied by a heightened burning sensation will begin to form between the fifth and seventh day. By the seventh day the pox will grow. The borders of the pox will contain a clearer more transparent matter. The center of the blister will begin to sink and a fleshy colored areola will form. On the eighth day, the pus blister will itch. This is the time to remove the clear fluid lymph for the next vaccination. This can

be removed by lancet or incision. On the tenth day a yellowish scab will begin to form in the middle of each incision. This material is now useless for vaccination. The scab will fall off by the twenty-fifth or thirtieth day. If the original incisions were too deep or the boy scratched too frequently, there will be a permanent scar.[21]

The doctor and the procedure required substantial cooperation from child and family. The length of cooperation extended far past the initial incision, all the way to the point of maximum irritation, when the doctor had to start removing the vaccine lymph from the pus blister or pox. The intimate yet public nature of this complicated vaccination procedure turned into a public performance of military belonging. The town residents witnessed the involvement of a now-registered member of the community in this high-level medical matter. The vaccinated child and family, on the other hand, performed their belonging—down to the painful extraction of vaccine lymph from the cowpox blister—for the rest of the fort's community. This public health measure forced individuals, families, and local communities to weigh the costs and benefits of belonging in the Spanish imperial community. The isolated conditions on the northern Spanish frontier turned vaccination into, in historian Natalia Molina's words, a way to delineate social membership.[22]

Vaccinations could go awry for a variety of reasons and complicate this form of national belonging. There could have been a previous exposure to smallpox. The level of cowpox in the vaccine lymph might be too low to generate an immune reaction, and the patient might be responding to another disease in the lymph. The circular explained that if the pus blister was irregular, the course of the inflammation seemed quicker, or the lymph in the pus blister was cloudy there had been no immune reaction to cowpox.[23] In this case another vaccination was required. If the doctor was vaccinating one child at a time, the unsuccessful vaccination meant the end of that particular chain of vaccinations. Thus the doctor needed ongoing access to vaccine lymph from other sources.[24]

The threat of smallpox gave vaccination a presence on the Texas edge of the Spanish imperial borderlands. Towns and presidios across Coahuila y Tejas started registering and vaccinating the children of military families, local families, and enrolled Apache families.[25] Jaime Gurza requested additional personnel familiar with vaccination "to observe the personnel and the transport of recently vaccinated children, to ensure the quality and the spread of vaccination."[26] Vaccination practices started to reflect military hierarchies among soldiers, settlers (*gente de razón*), and recently settled Indian families (*indios civilizados*). General Antonio Cordero y Bustamante recorded that four hundred additional points (units of vaccine lymph) arrived in San Fernando de Bexar, some of which would be shipped to Nacogdoches to be a *regalo de yndios*, part of the tribute given to keep peaceful and profitable relations with the Caddos, Wichitas, and Comanches around that northern trading post.[27] Manuel Salcedo reported that he started the process of vaccinating mission Indians around San Fernando de Bexar (contemporary San Antonio) with the cooperation of mission priests.[28] Originally, vaccination was an imperial imposition, but doctors, soldiers, and families in Texas quickly turned vaccine lymph and vaccination into tools that strengthened the military outposts' position relative to American settlers and emerging Indian nations like the Apache and the Comanche.

In 1810, early Mexican victories over Spanish and Creole forces in the War for Independence shook Spanish trust of local political authorities. In Texas, Spanish military authorities responded by arresting residents with close ties to central Mexico, including Dr. Jaime Gurza. San Antonio residents circulated an anonymous petition asking for clemency, "because of the zeal with which he attended them during the most dangerous epidemics," and requesting that the viceroy grant Dr. Gurza "his liberty so that the people may enjoy his faculties."[29] Gurza's work with patients and vaccines embedded him in the everyday life of San Antonio. An anonymous petition in a small military outpost brought out the ways people in San Antonio embraced Dr. Gurza and took him as their own in the face of a violently imploding Spanish empire. Dr. Gurza and San Antonio residents transformed vaccination from an imperial imposition to a matter of local belonging in six short years. The Spanish counterinsurgency efforts turned public health into a site of dissent.

The Challenge of Independence: Making Public Health Local in Mexican Texas

The reappearance of civilians in public health matters in Texas became one of the legacies of Mexican independence. Texas, for Spain, had been the place to project Spanish military strength against French and American incursions. The joint Mexican and American commercial development of cattle and cotton enterprises after 1821 turned Texas into one of the few commercially vibrant territories in war-ravaged Mexico.[30] Mexican authorities feared

Americans would turn their commercial presence into something else. Colonel Jose María Sanchez believed that Tejanos, "accustomed to the continued trade with the North Americans, have adopted their customs and habits, and one may say truly that they are not Mexicans, except by birth."[31] For Mexican onlookers, the local initiative taken in San Fernando de Bexar during an epidemic of intermittent fevers, possibly malaria or yellow fever, demonstrated the extent of Tejano dependence on the United States. The onset of the fevers was so extreme, and the cases so severe, that Juan Padilla, the military commander of San Fernando de Bexar, hired an American physician despite the near state of war with the United States. Padilla had him treat first the officers and their families, and then the troops. He then asked the American physician to offer his services to the residents of San Fernando de Bexar for fifty pesos a month.[32] The doctor's presence was part of Tejano autonomy and initiative in community medical affairs.

Residents and city councils started to exercise their growing power in an independent Mexico by developing their own public health measures. When smallpox struck San Antonio in 1831, the police chief of Bexar, Ramón Musquiz, formed an emergency board of health. He explained, "Recognizing that smallpox was one of the greatest scourges to humanity, the municipality had initiated a vaccination campaign so that the people who needed the measure could be vaccinated."[33] The extent of smallpox among San Antonio's residents required public measures that went beyond vaccination and emergency medical employment. The members of the board divided the city into five parts. Armed with handbills and doctor's instructions, the board members, "because of the absence of medical professionals," identified and treated people with smallpox in their division.[34] Dr. Alejandro Vidal, the only doctor on the board, agreed to consult on individual cases. The board provided food to indigent patients and subsidized the other families. Musquiz asked each head of household to inform the board members when "they smell any aroma of smallpox in their midst."[35] The emphasis on smell underscored the ways humors and excretions still framed the way most people understood illnesses. Musquiz also asked everyone to search for a higher quality of vaccine lymph, as the previous lymph did not ensure successful vaccinations.[36] For these men, public participation and a certain level of literacy gave them a measure of medical authority in the epidemic.

There was an additional democratic measure in this epidemic. Musquiz and the city council encouraged residents to start inoculating their children, a procedure otherwise known as variolation. In this procedure, family members took little scabs, mucus, or dried fluid from a patient who had not yet fully recovered from smallpox and transferred the material into shallow knife cuts on the person being variolated. Because smallpox might weaken at the end of recovery, the subsequent infection in the variolated person would also be minor. This was a risky procedure. The small-scale infection of smallpox could also become far stronger and potentially fatal. Inoculation quietly took place outside immediate medical authority; after vaccination appeared, inoculation started losing medical legitimacy. Mayor Musquiz asked all families considering variolation to ensure that the smallpox patient was suffering from an officially benign or attenuated case of smallpox.[37] This decision gave official sanction to an alternative, community-based, and less official mode of smallpox prevention. The board of health officially sanctioned medical tolerance.

The appearance of the temporary board of health mirrored the expansion of the local political elite after independence.[38] Musquiz and the board of health implemented policies that challenged the ideal of one single medical authority. The city council in San Antonio called on and trained local citizens to provide smallpox treatment, recruited and hired American doctors, and emphasized various means of smallpox prevention to protect the residents of Mexican San Antonio.[39] They even used American "vaccine lymph produced in the city of Nacogdoches." White emphasized its qualities: "The general effect has been strong. There have been no epidemics of smallpox in Austin, and the inhabitants are generally in good health."[40] This multitude of public health responses reflected participatory and border-crossing political cultures of Mexican Texas.

The 1836 revolution in Texas upended commercial relationships connecting townships across the state of Coahuila y Texas with Central Mexico. Tejanos and Texians (Anglo-Americans who became Mexican citizens) declared their independence from Mexico and dared the central Mexican government to reassert political authority over Texas. Ongoing Mexican and American military assertions of control over San Antonio and South Texas after the battles of the Alamo and San Jacinto cut Tejano and Texan relationships with Mexican federal authority. By 1842, many Tejanos felt they were "the first to sacrifice their all in our glorious revolution . . . and the last to receive the benefits."[41] Anglo-Texans turned local medical and commercial ties across the southern border into a threat to the Republic and thus a danger to the individual health of Tejanos in Texas.[42]

Medical Consensus and National Disarray
after the U.S.-Mexico War, 1846–1877

The American annexation of Texas in 1845 moved the contact zone between Mexico and the United States from the Louisiana border to the Nueces River. President Polk believed Texas expanded all the way to the Rio Grande Valley. He ordered General Zachary Taylor to march three thousand troops south from Corpus Christi to build Fort Texas on the banks of the Rio Grande. This was an act of war. General Mariano Arista moved his troops across the Rio Bravo to lay siege to Taylor's troops. The forces met in Palo Alto, Texas, and Polk used news of casualties in the Battle of Palo Alto to claim that Mexico had "shed American blood on American soil."[43] He demanded that Congress declare war on Mexico. General American opinion, despite eloquent and significant opposition, pushed Congress to endorse the war and invade Mexico.[44] Thus Americans used the blurry boundary zone between the states of Texas, Coahuila, and Tamaulipas as the spark for American expansion.

The Rio Grande was one of the main channels for this military expansion. General Taylor used Matamoros as the main supply port for his campaigns in the northern cities of Saltillo, Coahuila, and Monterrey, Nuevo León. However, Mexican irregulars and guerrilla forces lay siege to American supply lines on both sides of the Rio Bravo. The American defeat of Mexican federal forces in 1846 and 1847 led to the occupation of the main cities in central and northern Mexico, and this urban settlement challenged the capacity of the United States to keep soldiers healthy. Military success did not translate into medical victory, and military success in Mexico did not assure political peace in the United States. Expansion into once-Mexican territories forced the U.S. government to redefine its relationship to Indian peoples, slavery, and the incorporation of Mexicans as citizens.[45]

For the American troops guarding the supply lines to Monterrey, Nuevo León, the threat of fevers along the Rio Grande far outweighed the threat of skirmishes along the supply lines into Mexico. Samuel Curtis, the American military governor of Matamoros, wrote in August 1846 that "there can hardly be found a well man in camp."[46] Three months later, sickness was "still continuous [and] severe. . . . The climate is evidently unfavorable to our men, even in this month of November."[47] Curtis decried the reluctance of military authorities to build permanent hospital facilities in Matamoros and mourned the absence of clear flowing water in the lower Rio Grande Valley. The diary also reflects his regular doses of quinine and his ongoing battle with malaria.[48] His final diary entry as he debarked in New Orleans remarked, "The ague remains a dull memento of the campaign in Mexico."[49] For the people charged with the general welfare of the camp, the inability to deal with fevers and agues (malaria) among American troops occupied their mental energies. Smallpox vaccination, on the other hand, provided a public display of American military generosity to the people whose land they occupied.

Colonel Curtis and General Taylor decided to make vaccinations available to anyone. This included any Mexican willing to enter the camp outside Matamoros. The *American Flag* stated, "Dr. P. H. Craig offers his services to the inhabitants of Matamoros, and would inform them that he is prepared with vaccine matter to operate for the prevention of smallpox. He is to be found at his tent, near the headquarters of General Taylor."[50] The threat of additional epidemics reminded the Ohio-based Republican that "the dangers that surround us must create the greatest anxiety among our friends at home and the idea of smallpox in the army must no doubt add very much to that anxiety."[51] The offer to vaccinate everybody demanded that Mexicans in the middle of a violent occupation walk unannounced to the tent next to General Taylor's and ask for the vaccine matter. Americans also had to treat the people who underwent vaccination as patients, not potential saboteurs. Dr. Craig's gesture turned a medical tent into dramatic colonial political theater, partly because controlling smallpox was part of the image of American authority in Mexico.

For Mexican authorities, American control—the invasion, the ongoing low-intensity warfare, and the American occupation—disrupted relationships across states and regions. American troops moved into Mexico with numerous cases of smallpox.[52] Local authorities in northern Mexico could not make contact with any authority in central Mexico because of the American occupation of Saltillo and Monterrey. Thus, for those two years, the U.S. Army became the central purveyor of vaccine lymph in northern Mexico. The U.S.-Mexican war forced communities along the Rio Grande to rely on their relationships with American military authorities. Moreover, the epidemic of smallpox that started with the arrival of Mississippi troops continued after American troops left Mexico.

After 1849 Mexican governors were able to communicate directly with Mexican federal authorities, but recurring civil wars between liberal and conservative forces confounded this line of communication. Serapio Vargas, governor of the state of Coahuila, repeatedly requested glass containers of dried lymph from President Mariano Arista.[53] Vargas pled for "the *pus vacuno* because the lymph is completely unavailable in the neighboring states."[54] By the mid-1850s, only Jalisco and the state of Mexico had ongoing vaccine farms. The central location of these vaccine farms meant that the quality of access to *paquetitos de pus vacuno* depended on the quality of the individual relationship between federal and state authorities.[55] The personal ties connecting governors to the highest levels of political authority guaranteed the presence of vaccine points in northern Mexican towns. The ability to intervene and prevent smallpox epidemics in the aftermath of the U.S. occupation depended on the quality of personal ties between national-level politicians.

The 1849 gold rush in California increased the number of people using Mexico's ports as well as the possibility of yellow fever and cholera in Mexico. In Brownsville, Dr. Jarvis noted that cholera cases started in the *resaca* (tide flats), but the majority of cases were concentrated among the "transient and floating population always found in a new and rapidly increasing town, and especially on the frontier, consisting of California emigrants, travelling merchants and traders, gamblers, Mexicans, etc, who fled on its first approach." Surprisingly, "the Mexicans inhabiting the ranches where these occurred escaped entirely at the time."[56] Jarvis ascribed this to the interaction of the "poison" and the "sudden changes of climate that were so common" in the South Texas winter.[57] Cholera also struck Cabo San Lucas and Mulege (Baja California) after the landing of the California-bound English ship *Gazelle*.[58] People fled the presence of cholera in both towns and became internal medical refugees. Governor Pedro Manuel Amaya's reports detailed the demands he placed on missions to treat the refugees. He mentioned local attempts to reform the butcher shops to guarantee cleaner meats, and he put in a request for tax abatement for the funds used to treat and host internal medical refugees.[59] Gobernación, the Mexican equivalent of the executive branch, did not have the resources to coordinate any response to either illness.[60] In the United States, priests and doctors led local village and town responses to cholera and poverty.[61] Gobernación, but not the American federal government, provided tax abatements almost equivalent to their municipal expenses during the epidemic.[62] The disease theories emphasized the regionally specific

organic origins of diseases. The absence of specific federal public health policies reinforced the medical understanding that epidemic diseases were merely
regional matters.

Civil wars turned disease outbreaks in military theaters into national matters. The military conflict between the United States and the Confederacy
changed the nature of commerce and federal authority along the Rio Grande
borderlands. The conservative overthrow of the duly elected Mexican president Benito Juarez and the French establishment of Maximilian I as the emperor of Mexico in May 1864 turned the United States into a place of exile for
liberal forces. France turned Mexico into an unofficial ally of the Confederacy. The U.S. Navy tried to prevent Confederate cotton shipments through
Mexico to France and England. The Texas secession turned the Rio Grande
Valley into a low-level battlefield between cotton growers, mule train operators, navy boats, the Texas Rangers, and Union regulars. There was no federal health presence in the Rio Grande until the United States reestablished
control over the Rio Grande in 1865, one month after General Lee's surrender
to General Grant at Appomattox.[63] With this surrender, the U.S. Army became the American federal presence in the valley, and the river towns of Rio
Grande City, Brownsville, and Bagdad, Tamaulipas, returned to their roles
as the commercial centers of the Rio Grande Valley and northern Mexico.

Disease on the Rio Grande border achieved a temporary prominence in
Mexico after the end of the American Civil War. News of cholera in Brownsville and Matamoros in 1867 made its way to Mexico City. Memories of the
death and disruptions of cholera epidemics in Paris and Mexico in 1849
prompted Emperor Maximilian to call together a national medical convention on cholera. Dr. Jose María Reyes, one of the founding members of
the Asociacion Medica Mexicana and coordinator of research publications
for the *Boletin de la Asociacion Medica Mexicana*, remembered that "both
French and Mexican doctors agreed that no quarantine should be imposed.
Despite that decision, cholera did not spread into Mexico."[64] This decision
ratified the sense that epidemics of cholera were local matters and—more
important—that containing people in specific places did little to address the
underlying environmental causes of cholera. French and Mexican doctors
rejected Emperor Maximilian's offer to create a federal-level disease-specific
policy along the Mexican side of the Rio Grande.

The U.S. Army camps in Brownsville and Brazos Santiago, Texas, became
the site of another visible public health failure. Army policies created the first

border health crisis of the Reconstruction era. The army stationed African American troops at the mouth of the Rio Grande to prevent Confederate cotton smuggling and general cross-border cattle rustling. Army medical officials knew how to prevent scurvy in 1865, but General Godfrey Weitzel did not budget for enough supplies of vegetables from New Orleans. As a result, these troops suffered some of the highest death rates of the Civil War. These deaths, however, were from scurvy and diarrhea, and they followed the end of armed conflict: they were clearly preventable. As African American soldier Garland White wrote to his editor in Indianapolis, "No set of men in any country ever suffered more severely than we in Texas. Death has made fearful gaps in every regiment. Going to the grave with the dead is as common as going to bed."[65] Since the U.S. Army was no longer at war with Texas, the army prohibited any foraging from the surrounding farms. The troops stationed at Brazos Santiago faced a Gulf Coast island with very little fruit, vegetables, or meat, and, unlike many of their poor neighbors in Brownsville and the surrounding ranches, the troops did not have the time to go deep into the chaparral to hunt and forage. The high death rate among the troops stationed at the Rio Grande in the immediate aftermath of the Civil War resulted from a combination of insufficient food, the South Texas heat, difficult living conditions, and inadequate drainage.

The American defeat of the Confederacy allowed the U.S. Army to support Benito Juarez and the armed insurgency against Maximilian. The informal joint Mexican/American military effort strengthened the commercial ties between Monterrey, Saltillo, Laredo, Bagdad, Brownsville, Tampico, and New Orleans. Brownsville and Cameron County went from 6,028 people in 1860 to 10,999 people in 1870 to 14,959 people in 1880. Webb County and the city of Laredo grew from 1,397 people in 1860 to 5,273 people in 1880.[66] The steamships that moored in Rio Grande City, Brownsville, and Brazos Santiago led a wool- and cattle-driven boom economy in the South Valley. The troops stationed at Fort Mcintosh and Fort Brown shifted from supporting Mexican efforts against Maximilian to becoming the troops that prevented cross-border cattle raids and insurgent movements across the Rio Grande.[67] Military deployment during the Civil War and the French Intervention changed the meaning of local initiative, as both federal troops and a growing Mexican immigrant and European immigrant community established themselves as soldiers, merchants, laborers, muleteers, and day laborers in the South Texas borderlands. The border seemed to provide a new home.

By the late 1870s, American policy makers considered black troops to be at home on the Rio Grande border. The conflicts between local farmers, towns-people, smugglers, and the U.S. Army acquired a racial tinge during Reconstruction. At the border, local hostility to black troops followed from their role monitoring traffic across the Rio Grande. However, local communities did not treat black federal troops as a fundamental challenge to the racial status quo in the same way that black federal troops in the Deep South constituted an open challenge to the white racial structure after slavery. When President Garfield decided to move more divisions to the West, General Sherman uttered a note of concern. The general hesitated to move black troops away from the border because "the death rate in that climate is greater among the white troops than among the Black, and there was an implied understanding when we employed the black troops that they were better qualified for southern stations than troops of our Anglo-Saxon race."[68] Sherman's comment demonstrated the commonplace acceptance of a racial geography: that some ethnicities are better suited for some climates. That this alleged medical geography became a policy reason to keep black troops along the Rio Grande demonstrated the extent to which officials forgot the deaths from scurvy and diarrhea at the end of the Civil War. When Sherman used the phrase "our Anglo-Saxon race," he was probably referring to the European immigrants and northern European ethnics who made up the majority of troops in the U.S. Army. For Sherman, the border was medically different, suited to people "of that climate." Still, American investors, despite the perceived medical threat, continued to invest in South Texas.

The economic growth of northern Mexico and the Rio Grande Valley led to additional capital investments in railroad construction in Nuevo León, South Texas, and Tamaulipas. By the late 1870s, South Texas and northern Tamaulipas lay at the center of a wide triangle of railroads being built between Monterrey and Tampico, San Antonio and Laredo, Corpus Christi and Laredo, and Nuevo Laredo and Monterrey, Nuevo León. However, actual railroad construction brought workers from across Texas, Mexico, and the Caribbean to northern Mexico and South Texas. Railroads provided a quicker connection to the wider nation for people living in South Texas and northern Mexico. The price of the ticket and the prerogative of the conductor determined the extent to which Mexicans and others at the border could physically participate in the life of the nation. Conversely, states and communities across the United States and Mexico now felt they had a greater stake in public health matters at the Texas-Mexico border.

Yellow Fever, Political Unrest, and the National Board of Health

The year 1876 was one of the most violent and contested election years since the end of the Civil War.[69] The Hayes-Tilden compromise that followed the standoffs across the South required that Congress withdraw troops from southern states. The following year, workers and working families joined "the Great Strike" to challenge the railroads and steel mills' hold over their everyday lives. Governors across the midwestern and northern states called for army troops to put down the labor insurrection, local police cooperation, and wildcat strikes that accompanied the railroad strike. The Battle of Greasy Grass (Little Big Horn) led to questions about the extent to which the American military had imposed order in the American West. American narratives about South Texas faced a middle-class suspicion of local and working-class initiatives.

In the summer of 1878, yellow fever cases started appearing north of New Orleans, spreading into Memphis and making their appearance as far north and west as Iowa, Illinois, Indiana, and Ohio. Towns and cities across the Midwest and Plains states imposed shotgun quarantines on steam, rail, and canal traffic and brought all traffic connected to the Mississippi River to a halt. The yellow fever epidemic of 1878 shocked the entire country.[70] Authorities across the middle Mississippi River Valley reported approximately 100,000 cases of yellow fever and 20,000 deaths from the disease. The U.S. Congress estimated that public authorities spent approximately $200 million trying to deal with the disruptions, deaths, and disorder that accompanied this epidemic in the middle of the industrial Midwest. For the Senate, the 1878 Mississippi River Valley epidemic was "so destructive to human life, and the interests and prosperity of the whole country as to make it a subject of gravest public concern."[71] President Hayes used his State of the Union address in 1879 to call for national responses to public health crises. "The fearful spread of this pestilence has awakened a very general public sentiment in favor of national sanitary administration."[72] As Congress stated in the legislation that brought the National Board of Health (NBH) into existence, "Public health is second in importance to no question which addresses itself to the consideration of the legislator."[73] As Representative McGowan stated, "If $100,000 expended upon a national board of health would diminish by *one day* the duration of an epidemic such as that of 1878, the *nation* would be repaid many times over."[74] A broad consensus demanded that doctors and medical professionals prevent the horrors and economic chaos of another epidemic in the middle of the American heartland.

This national concern with the future of yellow fever in the United States framed the next movement of the Texas-Mexico border into American consciousness. The NBH first sought to learn the general medical lay of the land and commissioned sanitary surveys from doctors active in their regional medical associations. The sanitary survey required medical professionals to examine the general landscape of disease and review the underlying geological, sanitary, and meteorological conditions that contributed to yellow fever and other potential epidemics. The survey was the first step toward a much larger national project, creating the "means of ushering in a new era when sanitary science would triumph over the diseases of the tropics."[75] The NBH assigned Dr. John Hunter Pope, the long-term president of the Texas State Medical Association and the head of the research section in the Texas state medical journal, to complete the survey and identify any issues that might affect the return of yellow fever at the Texas-Mexico border.[76] Pope needed to investigate whether malaria and yellow fever were endemic and explore what that might mean to the possibility of (white) American settlement and commercial development in South Texas.[77]

This open question regarding epidemics and commercial development framed Pope's approach to the question of yellow fever. Dr. Pope needed to see whether the local populations were, like those in the Gulf South, relatively immune to yellow fever or whether their general immunity to yellow fever paralleled the majority of the white American population.[78] He needed to determine whether the local soil, temperature, and atmospheric conditions in South Texas approximated the yellow fever belt in Veracruz, Tampico, Havana, and Louisiana. Pope also needed to determine whether the health conditions in South Texas might affect the rest of the United States. The survey meant to answer the questions of whether South Texas provided the conditions for a yellow fever outbreak and whether this mattered to the United States.

Pope left for South Texas with questions about conditions that foster yellow fever. He returned from South Texas with a different question: how will Mexicans in South Texas affect the nation's health? Pope wanted to make the

American Public Health Association (APHA) aware that "the large majority of the people of that section is Mexican. Much the largest part of them belong to the lower class. They seem to differ in some respects from the other nativities in the state of Texas, and some of these differences have an important bearing on public health."[79] His focus on Mexican difference, "the more prominent of these peculiarities," probably came from his professional encounter with Anglo-Americans and Anglo immigrants in South Texas, not Mexicans. In Brownsville, he consulted with Dr. Combe, Dr. Mellon, army surgeon William Crawford Gorgas, and Irish immigrant and mayor Tom Carson. In Rio Grande City, he met with Judge Livingston, and in Laredo, with Dr. Montgomery and the city physician, Dr. Arthur. Canadian-born Dr. Spohn, the physician for the King Ranch, the Texas-Mexican railway, and the city of Corpus Christi, coordinated his work in Corpus Christi. He corresponded with army surgeons and doctors in Ysleta (El Paso) and Del Rio. This Anglo elite shared a sense of difference from the local Mexican majorities, even though—with the exception of the army surgeons—they worked within a political milieu with a substantial Mexican participation. Pope trusted his Anglo informants to provide enough reliable material to discuss "the condition of the Mexican population of western Texas in its relation to public health."[80] The term "Mexican" framed his description of disease conditions in South Texas; concern with "filth diseases—those which are the result of removable causes"—informed his Anglo-American encounter with Mexicans in the region.[81] Pope was looking for situations that could be amenable to public intervention.

Pope used a lurid and sensationalist travelogue to communicate his sense of difference in South Texas, beginning with the sounds of the region. For Pope, this was like being "on a foreign shore, in the midst of a foreign people. And we would hear little of any language among the laboring classes except Spanish . . . and their everyday business language is Mexican—a corrupt Spanish."[82] This sense of a degrading Mexican difference translated into his depiction of housing, food, access to water, and the population's general response to the presence of illness. Housing was more "overcrowded than the tenement-houses of New York," Baltimore, and even the Chinese quarter of San Francisco, but Mexican difference overshadowed a discussion of the different kinds of housing available in South Texas. Each smaller individual residence became a *jacal*, whether stone, adobe, or wood, roofed or unroofed.[83] The food provided evidence of an ongoing *mexicanidad*. The bread, too, was different: "Indian corn ground by a primitive machine [*metate*] and made into a kind of thin pancake—a tortilla." The diet relied primarily on tortillas and spiced meat, primarily beef, goat, and sheep, "highly seasoned with peppers and onions and garlic." He emphasized this peculiarity, even though in the matter of food, "the Mexicans are more careful than any of the 'other' lower classes" he had the opportunity to observe.[84] The sounds, smells, and sights of Mexican South Texas provided a sense of cultural difference.

Pope also worried about the racial nature of Mexican bodies in South Texas. Did their experience with fevers in South Texas reveal a deeper connection with or alienation from the tropical environments of South Texas? Pope catalogued the perceptions of local Anglo physicians and reported: "Some physicians of long experience and practice among Mexicans in western Texas, state they are not so liable to malarial diseases—that is, intermittent, remittent and typhomalarial fevers—as are whites or negroes in the same locality. Others say they notice no difference in favor or against them, while others report that the Mexicans are much more liable to such diseases." Pope tested this generalization by reviewing the medical records of doctors practicing in the two main towns on the Gulf Coast of South Texas. His findings troubled his racial assumptions about local Mexican populations. As he stated, "We might naturally infer from their nativity that they would enjoy some immunity, but the result of my special investigations in some towns is that the Mexicans furnish a larger proportion of malarial fevers than do whites or negroes. In August 1879, there was scarcely a fever among the white population of Corpus Christi, while physicians reported not a few such cases amongst Mexicans there. During the same season in Brownsville, the largest proportion of such diseases was in the Mexican settlements."[85] Pope—or the original attending physicians—did not note the birthplace, work history, or recent migration history of people suffering from their first exposure to tropical fevers. Without this information, Pope could only say that, contrary to the general belief regarding the biological homogeneity and tropical roots of Mexicans in South Texas, malaria was more frequent among Mexican residents.

The situation may have arisen because a significant number of Mexican families moved to the gulf towns of South Texas from the towns and villages in the foothills and prairies of Central Texas, inland South Texas, Nuevo León, and Tamaulipas as adults.[86] They may have followed opportunities or fled their displacement from their lands in South Texas and northern Mexico. This labor migration exposed them to the fevers associated with the Gulf of Mexico. Their Mexican ethnicity obscured this death-by-migration because Brownsville and Corpus Christi already had a large resident working-class Mexican majority.[87] Public health historians Marcos Cueto and Miguel Bustamante noted a similar social impact of malaria on Peruvian and Mexican internal migrants.[88] Labor historians Aviva Chomsky and Julie Greene traced similar patterns among migrant *mestizo* (racially mixed background, predominantly indigenous and Spanish) and *ladino* (Spanish identified, predominantly indigenous) workers in medical records for the United Fruit Company in Costa Rica and the Canal Zone.[89] Pope's report troubled racial assumptions about native Mexican immunity. The racial basis of his labels obscured the ongoing movement of Mexicans into Mexican South Texas.

The culture of illness among Mexican families created a more disturbing portrait for American readers. The portrayal of Mexican responses to illness emphasized "loose morals," "indifference to exposure," and "neglect of treatment," all of which related to the public dimensions of Mexican life in South Texas. Pope assumed that "loose morals" followed from the overcrowded housing. Historians agree that this class anxiety about the sexual morals of working-class communities pervaded many middle-class depictions of American working-class life as well.[90] This ubiquity may be why loose morals did not rate as a particularly Mexican peculiarity in his report. Pope found indifference to illness and neglect of treatment in Texas-Mexican communities to be much more threatening and disturbing to the United States. Mexicans "neglected" vaccination because of the expense and trouble. They "neglected" isolation because they prefer "to mingle as freely as ever," with "neighbors and relatives visit[ing] and assist[ing] in nursing them." They opposed quarantines and pesthouses, "because they prefer to care for their own sick and they do not think it has any influence in checking the spread of disease." This Mexican embrace of shared public spaces carried through to the troubling news that, unlike Americans, "Mexicans are fond of entertainments, shows and all sorts of public gatherings."[91] Pope's report demonstrated discomfort with Mexican mores in American public spaces.

Pope was also uncomfortable with American mores in South Texas. He decried the landowners and ranch owners who owned the sites where working-class Mexicans built their homes. He reported that "these *jacales* are not generally owned by the poor Mexicans who live in them, but by others who could supplant them with healthier abodes without becoming paupers." He charged that the landowners were creating "a foul ulcer on the body corporate of these cities" and were responsible for "the crime of menacing the lives of citizens by harboring serious contagious diseases."[92] His critique detailed how landlords and city officials refused to provide the residents of Mexican neighborhoods with access to water. He described the mule-driven wagons that brought water directly to each residence, and the water storage jugs and barrels that residents of the *jacales* made to collect rain. He noted the absence of privies and sewage services in the neighborhoods. He mentioned that the residents of houses with regular access to water bathed regularly, while those without any access did not bathe as often. He noted, "If cities and counties would supply good virus and free vaccination, an energetic city and county physician would leave very few unvaccinated in his territory. If compulsory vaccination were deemed best, no class of citizens would more freely submit to it than these Mexicans."[93] Most importantly, he stressed that even though the residents of the *jacales* found ways to live in "overcrowded conditions," town ordinances allowed landlords and landowners to profit from this unhealthy state of affairs. The solution to the health crisis in South Texas lay in a drastic reform of available housing, the gradual abolition of the *jacal* as an urban residence, and the provision of basic preventive medical services. American mores created the Mexican health problem in South Texas, and American mores should change to intervene in the health conditions there.[94] The change, however, should come from within the same communities.

Railroads were the catalyst for communities in South Texas to change their American attitudes toward Mexican health conditions. Pope declared to all who would read, "Many lines of railways are vying each other as to which shall be the first to reach Mexico. Nearly everyone passes through the section of which I write."[95] This meant that South Texas, "which now seems so remote, will soon be at the very door of the commercial centers of the entire union."[96] Pope hoped that railroad-enabled contact with public opinion would change the attitudes of the "best men" in South Texas. Exposure to "public opinion" in other places might help them see the benefits of investments in the health and housing of the urban Mexican majority in South Texas. The local economy relied on Mexican workers, as they "were the chief laborers of that country, handling the thousands of bales of wool or other freights destined for our *metropolis*"—they were the "porters, the boat-men, the hack-men, the hotel-waiters."[97] The local political elite had to invest in general access to basic health reforms to guarantee the safety of American consumers. Otherwise, without this larger change in South Texas mores, "the

Mexican cannot then indulge his peculiar ideas of epidemics without involving some of the rest of us."[98] Public health reforms were necessary to isolate and contain the threat of Mexican culture to the United States.

Pope confronted the ambiguities that American capital investments created in South Texas in the process of surveying Texas west of Corpus Christi. Shocked by the ease with which local doctors and professionals conversed in Spanish, he ignored the fact that a plurality of Spanish speakers in South Texas were born in the United States, and—unlike Dr. Pope in his Confederate youth—had never waged war on the United States. When he expressed surprise at the ubiquity of Mexican workers in Brownsville, he ignored the fact that Mexican and American employers hired local Mexican labor. These forms of active ignorance and overt hostility shaped his analysis as much as his experience and commitment to public health interventions did. Pope's report was the first civilian-based federal survey of health conditions in Mexican American communities in the United States. It reflected the concerns and commitments of a generation of American medical professionals who believed deeply in the potential of public health interventions, sanitary transformation, and the environmental origins of epidemic disease. This reform orientation framed Pope's lurid and frightening depiction of health conditions across South Texas and the Mexican border, and it led him to suggest making basic health services and housing conditions accessible to all residents of South Texas.

Practice without Theory: The USMHS, the Mexican-Texas Epidemic, and the Medical Border

In 1882, the Department of the Treasury charged the USMHS with the orderly prevention of yellow fever. The deepest ambiguity of this campaign lay in the national process of defining American bodies and American landscapes in South Texas. The Mexican-Texas epidemic of 1882 shifted the federal terms of the medical conversation about the Texas borderlands away from the cooperation invoked by the NBH. Pope's report on the health conditions of Mexicans in West Texas recommended public health policies that would incorporate the Mexican residents as full citizens of the United States and mitigate the public health threat they posed to American consumers. The process and politics of containing yellow fever in the Mexican-Texas epidemic moved to make everyone, especially the Texas-Mexican residents of South Texas, noncitizens. Various communities in South Texas happily cooperated with

American public health authorities, but the USMHS turned their local politi-cal autonomy and transnational connections into evidence of a foreign pub-lic health threat. The USMHS set up a 190-mile-long quarantine line between Laredo and Corpus Christi, quarantining a region larger than Maryland, Delaware, Rhode Island, eastern Pennsylvania, and New Jersey combined. Even the moniker "Mexican-Texas" reminded Americans that South Texas was a foreign place, home to a foreign people. The Mexican-Texas epidemic provided a convenient Mexican foil against which to build a shared American identity between southern and northern enemies.

The federal quarantine on South Texas caused different political ripples in Laredo, Corpus Christi, and Brownsville. In Laredo, a number of local pro-fessionals volunteered their services and fund-raising contacts and publicly aligned themselves with the USMHS. In Corpus Christi, the city council rested on the unsanctioned quarantine (known as a shotgun quarantine) established by Dr. Spohn before the federal intervention took place. In Laredo and Cor-pus Christi, the local quarantine aligned with the federal sanitary cordon. In contrast to Laredo and Corpus Christi's exclusionary popular investment in the quarantine, political activities in Brownsville made the federal effort vastly more inclusionary. This democratic mobilization led to open conflicts with the federal government, when the Brownsville city council and town residents also attempted to protect its transportation network by lowering the federal quarantine. The popularity of the Mexican-Texas quarantine in Texas became clear when the democratic nominee for the Senate, Tom Ochiltree, included the demand for a permanent quarantine guard as part of his plat-form.[99] By the time the quarantine ended in mid-November of 1882, Laredo, Corpus Christi, and the USMHS comfortably aligned themselves with the uses of quarantine; South Texas lay outside America's medical boundaries.

Bureaucratic conflict at the federal level enhanced the national impor-tance of yellow fever in South Texas. Ever since Congress had created the NBH in the wake of the great yellow fever epidemic of 1878, the USMHS had been struggling to gain the authority that Congress had granted to the civil-ian-run board. The institutional infighting between the USMHS and the NBH turned yellow fever in South Texas and northern Mexico into a matter of intense national scrutiny. The surgeon general of the USMHS, John Hamilton, had just convinced the president and the secretary of the treasury to trans-fer authority over the epidemic fund from the NBH to his service.[100] News-papers framed this transfer with an aura of victory: "National Board of Health

Suppressed—Marine Hospital Service to Fight Infectious Disease."[101] In order to maintain USMHS control of these funds, the attempt to control the spread of yellow fever had to achieve certain objectives: contain the spread of yellow fever; maintain the air of professional legitimacy; and create a variety of constituencies for USMHS quarantine support. The USMHS effort had to avoid the types of costly conflicts that had ensued between local officials, businesses, and federal authorities in previous yellow fever prevention efforts.[102] Furthermore, the USMHS had to avoid any perception that their efforts might lead to a white southern backlash against American federal authority.[103]

Informal town-based quarantines followed the news of yellow fever in Brownsville. On August 6, Texas State Health Officer R. M. Swearingen diagnosed four cases of yellow fever in a six-member Mexican household in Brownsville and recommended a modified quarantine against the town.[104] Three days later, on August 9, the city council of Corpus Christi established a quarantine against Brownsville.[105] By August 10, Galveston and Indianola, Texas, declared quarantines.[106] On August 13, the mayor of Corpus Christi demanded a statewide quarantine against Brownsville.[107] The next day, Governor O. M. Roberts declared a full state quarantine against Brownsville and any other points along the Rio Grande that might harbor yellow fever.[108] Competition from other Gulf Coast port towns and inland fears of the chaos that accompanied yellow fever drove the quarantine against Brownsville.[109]

The local quarantine established by the Mexican-majority towns along the border troubled the State Health Office's administration of their quarantine along the border. Swearingen decided to return to Austin by going up the Rio Grande to Laredo once he realized the ports of Corpus Christi, Indianola, and Galveston would refuse entry to any ship from Brownsville.[110] The trip up the river to Laredo ended up being politically frustrating to Swearingen. In Rio Grande City, Judge Tugwell ordered Swearingen's detention because the good doctor broke the state quarantine.[111] Governor Roberts ordered his release, and then the sheriff escorted Swearingen to the Starr County line, where the sheriff of Roma (the county seat of Starr County) promptly detained him.[112] Two days later, the city of Roma released him and escorted him to the Webb County line. There, Laredo mayor Porfirio Benavides placed Swearingen in jail for breaking the yellow fever quarantine on Brownsville.[113] On August 23, Benavides released Swearingen "under protest," by direct order from Governor Roberts.[114] For the previous week, Swearingen had been in direct defiance of his own instructions.

That same day, in Rio Grande City, "an armed mob" refused to allow people and goods on the boat that carried Swearingen to enter Rio Grande City. County judge Tugwell, who had given the ship permission to disembark after the completion of the ship's quarantine, "feared for his life" and asked the governor "to please send the rangers to enforce the law."[115] The sheriff of Rio Grande City called up a posse to defend the judge and the boat. The armed mob and the detentions were independent exercises of local political authority and, in the case of Rio Grande City, popular will. They exposed the general weakness of the Texas State Health Office: Swearingen could not convince these towns to break quarantine for the office itself. The independent actions by the residents of these Mexican-majority towns along the Rio Grande posed a potential challenge to the exercise of quarantine power by the USMHS.

The welter of yellow fever quarantines became the biggest challenge for the state of Texas and the USMHS. In San Diego, County judge James Luby and the commissioner's council—under pressure from Corpus Christi and Laredo—ordered a quarantine against Starr County and set up four mounted guards to police any movement across the county line.[116] San Patricio County commissioners set up a mounted quarantine at three different ferry stations on the Nueces River because "Mexican refugees [were] coming by these routes to avoid the guards of the city of Corpus Christi."[117] Nueces County set up nine different quarantine stations and hired fourteen health inspectors to monitor any traffic between suspected Mexican people and Nueces County.[118] All four of these mid-Texas counties demanded financial support for their quarantine guards and health inspectors from the state of Texas. On August 19, the secretary of the treasury responded assertively to this financial controversy, telegramming Governor Roberts that "this department will muster quarantine guards into service and pay them. We will also take charge of the hospital at Brownsville and proper inspection stations if you desire."[119] Secretary of the Treasury French's decision to take financial control of the various quarantines placed the USMHS at the center of the relief and quarantine efforts in Texas.

Surgeon General Hamilton took immediate advantage of the Treasury Department's offer of financial control of the yellow fever effort in South Texas. He had recently wrested control over the $100,000 of the congressionally mandated epidemic fund from the National Board of Health. Now he needed to prove to Congress and the president that the USMHS was far more effective than the NBH in coordinating local yellow fever efforts and, ultimately, confining the medical and economic devastation of yellow fever to the place where the first cases appeared. South Texas became a key battlefront in the turf war between the NBH and the USMHS over national responsibility over interstate disease. He sent surgeon Robert Drake Murray to administer and manage these delicate relationships. Murray was a good choice and an interesting one. He was a good choice because he had extensive experience working in three different yellow fever epidemics with Cuban and West Indian tobacco and fishing communities in Key West. He had also been visible treating people with yellow fever in Memphis and Vicksburg in the great Mississippi Valley yellow fever epidemic of 1878. He was an interesting choice because he was a volunteer with the Army of Ohio at the age of sixteen, was wounded and left for dead in the battle of Saltville, Virginia, and spent the rest of the war in a Confederate prison in Richmond.[120] Murray's establishment of the Florida Medical Society in 1875 placed him among the many Republicans who sought to modernize and transform southern culture through Reconstruction. He had to learn to work with Governor Oran Milo Roberts, a leader of the Secessionist movement in Texas, a Democratic senator in the Texas delegation that Congress refused to seat because of the disenfranchisement of black citizens, and a governor who actively sought to reduce state responsibility for everyday affairs in Texas.[121] Surgeon Murray's commitment to increasing the professional visibility and state authority of doctors lay at cross-purposes with Governor Roberts's alliance with large landowners and white rural smallholders.

Support for federal yellow fever efforts had to come from the grass roots so that demands for (northern) federal intervention seemed to emerge from everyday Texans. First, Murray had to turn towns with independent quarantines into firm supporters of a possible central federal quarantine.[122] He also had to get people in Brownsville, the epicenter of cases, to cooperate with federal authority. There he set up a hospital station to provide treatment to people with yellow fever and possibly intervene in the conditions that were encouraging yellow fever across South Texas. This created an air of solidarity. Murray and the USMHS also financed the efforts of mounted guards, who regarded any "Mexican refugees" as a potential source of infection. Funding and administering the various quarantines and providing direct relief in Brownsville worked against each other. The hospital and quarantine became actual spaces where people could connect the Mexican presence in South Texas to yellow fever. The residents of Brownsville—Mexican and otherwise—

had concrete reasons to reject this racialized working understanding of yellow fever. Quarantining Brownsville put the USMHS at the center of a medical conflict between South Texas and the rest of the state.

The quarantine reinforced a particular understanding of the cause of yellow fever, even if the causes were still widely debated. The key question facing Murray, since the USMHS was now financially responsible for the salaries of all county quarantine guards, was where the USMHS would draw the line between infected and noninfected districts. Tejano involvement in labor matters in Mexico complicated this decision. E. H. Goodrich, the acting customs agent in Brownsville, claimed that "railroad tramps from Tampico" who arrived at the port of Bagdad, Mexico, a month earlier had brought yellow fever to Matamoros.[123] Furthermore, Goodrich reported that a local Mexican steamer had dropped forty more railway workers in Bagdad, and, despite a number of deaths in temporary detention, Mexican authorities had released the laborers after three days.[124] Sixteen of these railway workers made their way home to their (ethnic Mexican) families and small ranches in Texas. The remaining few were French and American workers "tramping" their way back to Corpus Christi.[125] Murray's actions to contain yellow fever strengthened the imaginary links between the fever, South Texas Mexicans, international migrant railroad workers, and refugees in Mexico.

Medical officers also fretted over the land-based and family connections of the railway workers. Dr. Spohn wanted to make Murray aware that "many of the ranches south of the Texas-Mexican railroad are full of people from Brownsville and Matamoros."[126] Moreover, Spohn argued, because Mexican ranch families had settled across South Texas, "a cordon around Brownsville [was] now impracticable and useless."[127] As the city health officer in Corpus Christi, the head physician for the recently completed Texas-Mexican railroad, and the doctor for the 825,000-acre King Ranch, Spohn's political responsibilities made him fairly anxious that the "death of these tramps will create a panic in the ranches."[128] Spohn considered the family connection between railway workers in Mexico and their ranches in South Texas to be the most difficult challenge. Murray himself reported rumors that the labor recruitment and workplace practices of the Monterrey & Mexican Gulf Railroad were responsible for yellow fever in Tampico.[129] He noted, "Large numbers of laborers for railroads were carried from Havana and Jamaica to work in swamps north of Tampico."[130] The conditions in the Tampico swamps brought yellow fever to the fore among these Mexican and Caribbean workers. According to the rumors, "the men were not housed, were ill fed, and suffered much hardship, so that by scores they left the camps, and from exposure or starvation, many lost their lives in efforts to reach the United States."[131] The labor decisions of the U.S.- and British-owned, and Texas-managed, Monterrey & Mexican Gulf Railroad in northern Mexico brought Tejano workers south to Mexico and West Indian workers west to Tampico.[132] These corporate decisions in Mexico turned Matamoros, Tamaulipas, and Brownsville, Texas, into refuges for Mexican, Tejano, American, French, Cuban, and Jamaican workers fleeing the fevers and swamps around Ciudad Victoria.[133]

Officials in Texas treated the movement of these ethnically diverse workers as a Mexican threat. R. H. Wood, the mayor of Rockport—a town on Aransas Bay north of Corpus Christi and 190 miles away from the border—demanded quarantine because of the Mexican presence in his town. "We have a considerable Mexican population in and near Rockfort and owing to the fact of other points on the coast as well as inland towns being quarantined strictly many of the Mexicans are making their way to this point."[134] Wood's demand for quarantine "for the protection of the citizens" assumed a mutual solidarity among all Mexicans living in Texas and, because of these imagined ties, excluded Mexicans from U.S. citizenship. The Mexican residents of Rockfort were therefore medical threats.[135] Dr. Wilcox in Laredo had already declared quarantine against Brownsville. Dr. Spohn, on his side, emphasized that yellow fever was probably present in the small *Mexican* ranches in South Texas. These people pushed Dr. Murray to treat yellow fever as a dangerous *internal* Mexican threat inside American borders.

Murray had difficult choices. He confronted a possible yellow fever outbreak in a South Texas built from the labor of an ethnic Mexican majority involved in steamboat links, railway construction, and the wool trade. Moreover, providing medical attention with a focus on Mexican laborers implied starting a smaller and more multihued Reconstruction in South Texas. Federally isolating Brownsville from its South Texas hinterlands, Mexican trade networks, and Gulf Coast sea routes also seemed to be a difficult long-term proposition. As of August 20, Murray did not have a way to coordinate all the different town quarantines abutting the Texas-Mexican railroad.

Murray turned the different quarantines at the Texas-Mexican railroad into the "Corpus Christi–Laredo Cordon." Spohn modestly stated that, "as Corpus Christi health officer and chief medical officer of the Texas-Mexican railroad," he himself was best positioned to supervise the quarantine."[136] The railroad company provided telegram operators and coaling stations at regular intervals between Corpus Christi and Laredo, and the railroad line allowed for ready access to supplies for any guard along the railroad. With Spohn as the Corpus Christi–Laredo Cordon coordinator, the USMHS effort became tied to the interests of the Texas-Mexican railroad, the King Ranch, and the city of Corpus Christi. The railroad and the King Ranch were central to the emerging geography of power that built on the expected rail connection between Laredo, Monterrey, and Corpus Christi.

The USMHS map makes the Texas-Mexican railroad seem like an obvious delineator for the Mexican-Texas quarantine. Dr. Wilcox and Dr. Spohn had already called for mounted medical police to prevent the movement of potentially dangerous Mexicans in South Texas, and in Laredo Wilcox mustered a large number of volunteers to staff the quarantine.[137] Spohn fired the railroad workers who volunteered because they knew "nothing about the country and if sent out into the bush would never get back without assistance."[138] Spohn argued instead for the use of hands from the King Ranch, because "my men are nearly all 'Cow Boys' who know every path, water hole and crossing between the gulf and the Rio Grande by night and day and can be relied on."[139] Like many other cowboys, Spohn's quarantine guards learned their skills riding herds and working in mule trains alongside Mexican ranch hands and vaqueros.[140] Some probably learned their policing skills by herding cattle and terrorizing neighboring smallholders, coercing title transfers from neighboring Mexican ranches to the King Ranch.[141] Staffing the quarantine guard with King Ranch cowboys turned the USMHS sanitary cordon into another instrument of intimate domination over local Mexican rancheros.

The quarantine was also an ironic opportunity for the ranch hands. The completion of the Texas-Mexican railroad made detailed knowledge of South Texas terrain irrelevant to the transportation of cattle and other goods. This made the hard-won skills of mule train drivers and cowboys obsolete.[142] The threat of cattle-tick quarantine on Texas longhorns and the invention of barbed wire were also rendering cattle-herding skills irrelevant.[143] The quarantine guard provided three months of employment for Anglo ranch hands and mule train drivers. Murray spent a large percentage of the $26,000 budgeted for the epidemic fund on these guards.[144] By placing armed medical police authority in Texan cowboy hands through the establishment of the mounted quarantine guard, Murray and Spohn reinforced white labor privileges through federal

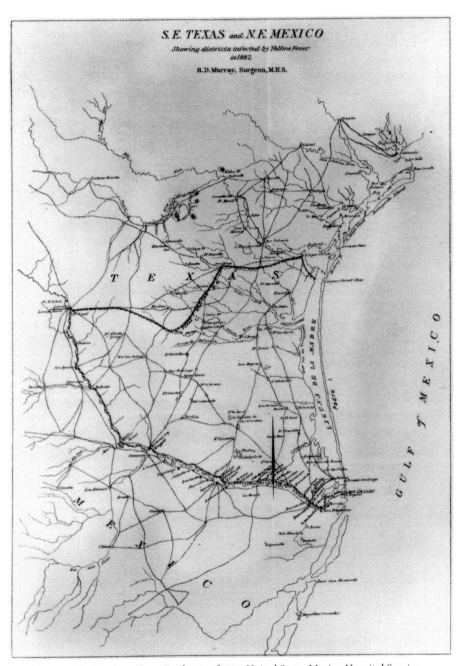

Figure 1. The Mexican-Texas Epidemic of 1882, United States Marine Hospital Service.

wages and the imprimatur of federal authority.[145] Moreover, they gave the same cowboys who rode along the railroad the medical and political authority to decide who did or did not belong in this South Texas landscape. Every medical detention of a South Texas resident or ethnic Mexican seeking to cross the Texas-Mexican railroad added an air of medical illegality to a Mexican presence north of Brownsville.[146] The soon-to-be-ex ranch hands literally embodied the quarantine when they enforced the medical border around the Mexican-Texas epidemic.

The quarantine guard was more than just "the first time military force was employed by the Marine Hospital Service."[147] The cowboy dimensions of the guard affected the ways USMHS officers asserted their medical manliness. Dr. Murray recalled more than a decade later, "For months I was dependent on my wits and willingness to pull a trigger in order to save the cause I upheld. Once a mob of three hundred men called to hang me."[148] Murray's words highlight the way the military dimensions of the quarantine fostered a violent and threatening air around his presence in South Texas. The conclusion of his "Once a mob" story—"but a few sentences in Spanish and a careless air turned the curses into *vivas!*"—reframed a group of aggrieved residents inside the United States into a foreign, Mexican, easily swayed group of people outside an Anglophone consensus. The policing dimensions of the quarantine added a violent federal edge to the public health encounters between doctors and patients on the South Texas border. This was the first time mounted guards enforced a federal border that fully matched a line on the map of Mexico and the United States.[149] This was the leading edge of a militarized civilian border in the United States.

Mounted guards and medical borders were not in Dr. Pope's citizen-based investigation of yellow fever conditions across South Texas. Instead, the ongoing presence of the armed USMHS quarantine guard provided visual evidence that—regardless of the causes of yellow fever—Mexicans were a dangerously diseased, potentially criminal, and transnationally connected population that required either expulsion or violent supervision. Both Dr. Spohn, the coordinator of the cordon between Corpus Christi and Laredo, and Dr. Fisher, the Rio Grande City health officer, maintained a "Mexican" label to describe Mexican health behavior. Dr. Fisher found that "Mexicans are great fatalists and were ill disposed to assist in the quarantine."[150] Dr. Spohn collapsed a distinction between body, environment, and behavior, arguing that the USMHS should maintain the mounted quarantine guard because "the Mexican people (in the lower class) are a filthy set and pay no attention to cleanliness or sanitary matters."[151] In their final report to the USMHS, Dr. Spohn and Dr. Fisher used this alleged "fatalist," unhygienic, and antimodern attitude to argue for a continued quarantine on Brownsville after the federal quarantine ended. The armed guards added weight to the medical threat Texas-Mexicans posed to Texas.

Life under the Brownsville Quarantine

In Brownsville, Murray used federal resources and authority to provide material and political support for a different argument: that the dislocations caused by the USMHS quarantine were an important medical matter of federal responsibility.[152] The quarantine disrupted Matamoros's position as a key import hub for northern Mexico and Brownsville's position as the premier place to ship livestock and woolen goods to New Orleans from the Rio Grande Valley. For people living in Brownsville, yellow fever and starvation by unemployment were the two greatest threats to life under the federal quarantine. This city of five thousand people incurred major expenses maintaining the hospital as well as local sanitation and disinfection measures. The quarantine meant that over two thousand people in Brownsville lost their jobs. By August 19, the ten days of quarantine and sanitary cordon had overwhelmed the funds raised by the relief committee in Brownsville. Carson demanded more funds from the USMHS "as, if we have to care for the destitute, we cannot deal with the sick, and neglect of either will bring about an immediate and most probably uncontrollable increase of the disease for the citizens of Brownsville."[153] In response, Surgeon General Hamilton again informed the governor of Texas and the mayor of Brownsville that the USMHS was not in the business of providing relief to the destitute.[154] But he was wrong.

USMHS surgeon Murray defied the surgeon general on this very point. The relief committee and the hospital service distributed free groceries to the sick from the emergency hospital grounds, the St. Joseph school building.[155] Dr. Murray hired a number of Spanish-speaking attendants, stating simply that "the vast majority of patients being of Mexican origin, it was necessary to have persons to attend them who could be understood, and vice versa."[156] The community objected to the separation of family members, so he "admitted the companion as a temporary attendant" and allowed family members to stay with the patient in the yellow fever field hospital.[157] Dr. Finney and Dr. Murray distributed quinine and calomel to local doctors and began a program of house-to-house consultations to diagnose yellow fever and distribute USMHS remedies.[158] This community-based pattern of financial and medical relief in Brownsville included relief to everybody economically affected by the yellow fever quarantine, not just to the people with yellow fever.[159]

This federally coordinated support of local well-being in Brownsville challenged the surgeon general's restrictions by extending hospital care to people in their own households. Surgeons Murray, Burk, and Finney treated 486 patients with cases of yellow fever on an outpatient basis, and consulted on 429 cases with local physicians. He hired a number of Spanish-speaking doctors and attendants and began a house-to-house outdoor relief program. In Brownsville, yellow fever funds went to prevention as well as relief and medical treatment.[160] In the neighboring towns of Point Isabel and Santa Maria, USMHS surgeons also treated a number of other diseases. The prevalence of other illnesses (see table 1.1) marked a political reality for the USMHS surgeons. "As the people were generally poor," Murray found that "it saved time and prevented misunderstanding and complications to treat anything that came up."[161] His decision to expand and democratize medical aid within the Brownsville quarantine resonated with Dr. Pope's call to make medical services conform to local Mexican ideals. Brownsville's residents and Dr. Murray pushed effectively for a wider definition of community.

The outer reaches of Brownsville's community became visible in the national relief campaign. The funds for this generous form of economic relief came from the Treasury Department's epidemic fund as well as a national donation campaign. People raised money for yellow fever relief in San Antonio, Eagle Pass, Dallas, Austin, Houston, and New York City. The firm of Bloomberg & Raphael raised $920 in two days from twenty-eight donors.[162] There were two $100 donations and ten $50 donations by various export-import firms. Even the Little Havana Lottery donated $100 to the city of Brownsville.[163] The National Cotton Planters Association, perhaps recalling Santos Benavides's previous cotton-smuggling relationship with the Confederacy, donated $200 to the relief effort.[164] The wide field of relief subscriptions highlighted Brownsville's place in a wider national community, linked by empathy and, perhaps, experience.

The visibility of relief subscriptions for Brownsville residents in Texas newspapers challenged some Americans' visions of the proper place for Mexicans in Texas. San Antonio resident Roy Landgridge thought the provi-

Table 1.1. Patient cases and patient days, Brownsville area, August 26–October 2, 1882

	Yellow Fever	Other Diseases	Patient Days	Yellow Fever Deaths
Brownsville Hospital Cases	90	0	533	14
Brownsville Outpatient Cases	486	230		n/a
Point Isabel	2	37	223	0
Santa Maria	208	137	547	6
Total	*786*	*404*	*3,682*	*20*

Source: Robert Murray, "The Texas-Mexican Epidemic," *Annual Report of the Supervising Surgeon General of the United States Marine Hospital Service, for the Fiscal Year of 1882* (Washington, D.C.: Government Printing Office, 1883), 307–9.

sion of relief fostered too much independence among Brownsville's working classes. According to Landgridge, "the free grocery tickets made [Mexicans] exceedingly lazy and impudent—no more work and the free grocery allowed the situation to exist," and impudence among potential employees had to be suppressed.[165] Murray, on the other hand, thought the free groceries and the house-to-house distribution of medical care meant that "very soon all repugnance to the hospital was obliterated and, but for the prompt out of door relief given, the hospital would have been overcrowded."[166] Murray cooperated with the Brownsville relief committee and made sure people who suffered from the hardships of the quarantine, and not only from the illness of yellow fever, received a level of relief that would allow them to stay alive. Brownsville's medical demands and Murray's receptive ear democratized the practice of American medical norms.

The contradiction in Brownsville between being trapped by USMHS quarantine guards and being treated and fed by the USMHS grew increasingly obvious. By mid-September, the number of cases began to fall. Although the USMHS distributed relief in Brownsville, it also staffed the barrier to any contact outside of Brownsville. On September 14, the USMHS moved the sanitary cordon south from the Texas-Mexican railway, tracing a hundred-mile-long line from Rio Grande City to Brownsville. It established another line along the Arroyo Colorado, the main link between Brownsville and Corpus. Finally, the service had a number of patrols guard the main paths around Brownsville.[167] The USMHS drew this latent contradiction into manifest conflict when they moved the cordon from the Texas-Mexican railroad to the paths connecting Brownsville to the surrounding countryside.

With this redeployment, the USMHS released one hundred quarantine guards from its payroll. The sudden disappearance of the federal resources that created a line between South Texas and the rest of the state caused a stir in Laredo and Corpus Christi. J. C. Whitehead and C. C. Pierce formed a citizens' council in Laredo to staff the positions recommended by the USMHS surgeon, but the citizens' council dismally failed to get people to volunteer to become the mounted quarantine guard. In Corpus Christi, the city council reaffirmed their willingness to staff the federal quarantine. The mayor claimed, "Her citizens, before the United States took charge of quarantine affairs, joined themselves into a protective guard—every merchant's clerk and mechanic volunteering for services. Now that it devolves on her citizens to protect themselves, there is no doubt that they will again."[168] The mayor of Corpus reaffirmed their own earlier quarantine using the rhetoric of citizenship and skilled labor to claim authority over it. For Laredo and Corpus, modern disease prevention now meant a mounted quarantine guard.

Inside Brownsville, residents began to agitate for another solution to the quarantine. Brownsville's aldermen convened a number of "indignation meetings" to address the increasingly rigid conditions around the quarantine.[169] On September 19, 1882, the mayor of Brownsville and seven of the eight aldermen requested that Murray and city health officer Combe lift the quarantine on Matamoros.[170] Lifting it there would permit traffic from Brownsville into the inland trade networks that connected Matamoros to Tampico and Monterrey. This would allow residents to engage in the steam trade from Bagdad across the river, and from Bagdad to Tampico and Veracruz. When Murray refused to obey the request, local doctors challenged USMHS's medical authority over Brownsville's boundaries.

The challenge to Murray's authority came from within the ranks of relief physicians in Brownsville, who used their experience with yellow fever patients as the basis to dispute the medical justification for the quarantine.

The undersigned physicians practicing having treated the epidemic which has prevailed here and considering that the disease has nearly run its full course, we beg to state that in our opinion the quarantine installed because of infection against the intercourse of our people with those of the city of Matamoros are [sic] useless and should be at once discontinued. In as much

as we are satisfied that the disease in Matamoros has almost entirely disappeared and no danger from a free intercourse with the people of Matamoros needs to be apprehended for the inhabitants of Brownsville.[171]

At this point, elected officials, public opinion, and medical authorities in
Brownsville openly challenged the rigors of the federal quarantine. The city
council ordered the arrest of anyone who attempted to prevent ferry traffic
between Brownsville and Matamoros. This was in direct defiance of Governor Roberts, the surgeon general, and the coordinator of the federal quarantine. On the morning of August 20, Sheriff Aristeo Brito arrested two quarantine guards employed by the Department of the Treasury at the ferry landing
and placed them in the local jail.[172] Brito also warned the governor that he
expected more violence, since "we are informed quarantine will be reestablished by said doctors and [we] fear our excited populace cannot be prevented
from forcing said quarantine if reestablished under authority of these physicians."[173] The arrest placed the customs collectors and the USMHS in a difficult
position. As E. H. Goodrich told Governor Roberts, the quarantine guards
had "been placed subject to orders of Health officers Murray and Combe.
City authorities have arrested and placed in jail customs officers for obeying
their orders."[174] Murray recognized the decision taken by the city council as
an "attack on the legality of the cordon."[175] Murray may have remembered
the meeting on August 19, where he and Dr. Combe were "criticized for their
stubborn propensities in keeping on quarantine when seven or eight aldermen, the mayor and a great majority of citizens want quarantine restrictions
lifted."[176] The council had expected the USMHS to cooperate, as Murray had
worked closely with Mayor Carson and the council's earlier demands for assistance. His rejection of their demands shocked them and pressed the city
into open political conflict.

Murray responded to the political challenge to his medical authority by
ensuring that a Brownsville-managed quarantine would be politically and
medically problematic to Texas. To Governor Roberts, he emphasized that
the USMHS would withdraw all of its resources if "mob law was permitted to
rule."[177] The term "mob law" attacked the democratic process through which
Brownsville doctors, the city council, and local citizens arrived at their conclusion that the federal quarantine was illegal. Murray also stopped enforcing
the quarantine and claimed that the lifting of the quarantine turned Brownsville into a "city full of Matamoros people."[178] Without a federal quarantine,

no one would "prevent the ingress of paupers and new material and prog-ress of disease into ranches."[179] Murray added "new material" (people unex-posed to yellow fever conditions in Brownsville) to his previous concern with tramps and ranches.[180] Labor control in the South Texas countryside became another benefit of a reimposed federal quarantine.

Governor Roberts endorsed this understanding of the relationship among the intrastate sanitary cordon, Mexican labor mobility, and the federal inter-national and interstate quarantine. Sheriff Brito warned Governor Roberts, "We fear our excited populace cannot be prevented from forcing said quar-antine if reestablished under authority of these physicians."[181] On September 21, H. F. French informed Murray that Governor Roberts gave Murray full authority over the quarantine, then fired Dr. Combe from his commission in Brownsville and named Arthur Wolff as the new health officer in Browns-ville. All of these actions voided the city council declaration on quarantine. The *Express* depicted the conflict over the rule of law and the sovereignty of the city of Brownsville as a "difficulty between the Mayor of Brownsville and Governor Roberts" and cooperation between federal and state authorities as "a victory for the governor."[182] The many people who used the ferry, attended the indignation meeting, and attended to family and friends who did cross over from Matamoros disappeared into a Mexican town engaged in "the forc-ible breaking of quarantine."[183] The "mob law"—organized political dissent against federal quarantine enabled by the resident Mexican majority in South Texas—brought a devoted U.S. Army veteran and liberal modernizer into a working rapprochement with a Confederate Democrat who instigated seces-sion in Texas. South Texas political assertions brought the North and South together against an internal (allegedly) Mexican threat to federal authority.

The actions in Brownsville required a hard hand. Governor Roberts, Dr. Murray, and Surgeon General Hamilton made it clear that the rule of law and the federal quarantine both emanated from and protected the state of Texas. Murray requested that the quarantine guard at Rio Grande City take a loy-alty oath in front of the local county judge because "our men owe it to Texas to perform their duties with extra vigilance."[184] In Murray's view, Governor Roberts's measures guaranteed that instead of mob rule, "law seems to be re-established here."[185] The state of Texas and the government of the United States stepped in to contain the disorderly, diseased, and unruly, essentially Mexican, residents of Brownsville.

Murray used his new authority to place himself and the USMHS in author-

ity over any movement across the Rio Grande. Again he followed the demands placed on him by officials in Brownsville. He implemented a modified quarantine, allowing traffic across the river. Once the state of Texas
gave Murray authority, he opted to allow ferry traffic—after a careful federal
inspection—between Matamoros and Brownsville. He implied that any traffic would be scrupulously inspected, and probably restricted, but that the
system was guaranteed to keep Brownsville orderly. The request went not to
Surgeon General Hamilton but to Governor Roberts.[186] The only difference
between this modified federal quarantine and the Brownsville city council
proposal was the locus of authority. Local medical opinion, coupled with
local democratic initiatives at variance with federal public health practices,
had no place in establishing who could and who could not enter Brownsville;
only federal medical opinion guaranteed the safety of South Texas.

Between September 15 and September 25, 1882, the movement of the sanitary cordon southward caused different political ripples in Laredo, Corpus
Christi, and Brownsville. In Laredo, a number of local Anglo professionals
volunteered their services and fund-raising contacts and publicly aligned
themselves with the USMHS. In Corpus Christi, the city council rested on the
shotgun quarantine established by Dr. Spohn before the federal intervention
took place. In Brownsville, the city council and populace also attempted to
protect its transportation network by lowering the quarantine. In contrast
to Laredo and Corpus Christi's individual quarantine, Brownsville's emphasis on local sovereignty led to a direct conflict with the federal government.
The popularity of a medical border in racially exclusionary politics in Texas
became clear when Tom Ochiltree, the independent nominee for the Senate,
included a demand for a permanent quarantine guard as part of his stump
speech and platform. By the time the Mexican-Texas epidemic ended in mid-
November, Laredo, Corpus Christi, and the USMHS had comfortably aligned
themselves with Texas's uses of quarantine. Brownsville residents ended up
being far less understanding of this definition of national interest.

1882: From Sickly Seasons to Quarantine

Surgeon General Hamilton successfully banked on the spectacle of the
Mexican-Texas epidemic when Congress granted the USMHS continued authority over the epidemic fund.[187] Governor Roberts told the secretary that,
"all things considered, the effort made to protect the state of Texas from a
general epidemic was a perfect success."[188] Hamilton mailed a copy of an

article in *Appleton's Annual Cyclopedia* that described how the USMHS used the epidemic fund "to drive yellow fever out of Texas" to the chair of the National Board of Health.[189] As the Mexican-Texas epidemic demonstrated, the increased federal investment in disease prevention sanctioned a temporary exclusion of South Texas from the new southern railroad economy. This exclusion of South Texas was done, in R. Murray's words, "to disturb commercial relations as little as possible." The quarantine along the river and the Corpus Christi–Laredo cordon drew a line around all of South Texas. The process of building the quarantine enabled an institutional rapprochement between southern and American federal institutions in Texas. Dr. Murray, the prisoner of war and U.S. Army veteran; Dr. Swearingen, the ex-Confederate Texas State Health Officer; and Governor Oran Milo Roberts, the president of the Secession Convention, worked together to prevent the movement of Mexican yellow fever farther into Texas. Fifteen years later, Joanna Nicolls emphasized that the internal medical border drawn "on the American side and three hundred mounted guards (Texan Cowboys) [prevented] any further importation of the disease while medical officers were engaged in stamping it out in Brownsville."[190] The Mexican-Texas epidemic prompted officials to draw a medical line around South Texas to deter the risk of unruly Mexican behavior and thus provided a convenient Mexican foil against which one-time American enemies could build a shared American identity. In the eyes of Texas, the political actions in Brownsville justified the exclusion of Mexican Texas from this new national community.

The Texas-Mexican railroad became the dividing line for the new South Texas. Jovita Gonzalez said as much in her thesis: "For a period of twenty years nothing much was heard of in the lower Rio Grande valley country in the United States. This may be due to two factors. First, the yellow fever epidemic devastated the country. Second, the construction of a railroad from Corpus Christi to Monterrey . . . killed all the trade which had heretofore gone to the states of Chihuahua, Durango and Zacatecas by way of the Brazos de Santiago."[191] Laredo became the next new economic hub of South Texas. In Webb County, both the U.S.-born Anglo population and the foreign-born Mexican population nearly tripled; the county's total population rose from 5,274 to 14,842. The majority of these new Anglo residents were concentrated in the city of Laredo. Around Corpus Christi, Nueces County's population increased from 7,673 to 8,093 people, but the number of Mexican-born residents fell from 2,734 to 1,759.[192] In Cameron County, where Brownsville was located, the general population dipped slightly, to 14,424; the Mexico-born population fell by 2,300, to 5,403; and the number of non-Mexican immigrants fell from 700 to 300 people. The Texas-Mexican railroad and the Mexican Central Railway insulated trade between northern Mexico and the southern United States from the vagaries of the sickly season and its accompanying quarantine. The railroads drew a medical boundary between old and new South Texas just as they were connecting northern Mexico and the United States.

People in Brownsville bore the brunt of the quarantine, especially since both the sanitary cordon and the federal mounted quarantine guard was new to Texas, Mexico, and the United States. Governor O. M. Roberts had "advised scattering people in camps" to hold the medical refugees who were escaping the particular conditions that fostered yellow fever along the coasts.[193] Even R. D. Murray voiced his displeasure with quarantine, stating in the preface of his report, "I have been and am yet opposed to quarantine, because of the unnecessary restrictions and encumbrances."[194] At the 1882 American Public Health Association meeting in Boston, Agrippa N. Bell, one of the nine members of the National Board of Health, described the use of armed guards and federal funds to keep people in a dangerous yellow fever district equal to "the murdering of people" that happened in the Philadelphia yellow fever epidemic one hundred years earlier.[195] Bell held the USMHS sanitary cordon responsible for nearly two thousand cases of yellow fever and the 114 deaths in Brownsville that year.[196] The debates in Brownsville over the harm of the USMHS quarantine became deeply embedded in the politics of race at the border.

Catarino Garza, the border revolutionary of the 1890s, voiced his revolutionary rage and his sense of the relative value of Mexican life at an indignation meeting in late September. Garza first recounted a statement at an indignation meeting given by Russell, a local Anglo-American lawyer: "Gentlemen. I have been assured that there are still cases of yellow fever in Matamoros. We should not raise the quarantine for any reason, even if it is starving or harming the working poor. We must stop any invasion of yellow fever to prevent any American deaths. Since 'one white man is worth ten Mexicans,' I stand against any attempt to raise the quarantine."[197] The Brownsville community ignored Russell's pleas and openly defied the quarantine. Garza used this anecdote to show the ways an Anglo minority identified with a white American identity over and against their Mexican neighbors. Garza was so offended by Russell's statement that he published a letter challenging him to a duel, to prove to him that he was one Mexican who was equal to at least one American. This was Garza's first use of the Spanish-language press to send out a call for arms to surrounding Mexican communities.[198] For him, the quarantine exposed American feelings about the Tejano presence in Texas. His demand for a duel demonstrated that he could be publicly defiant and continue working in South Texas. Garza used the lesson that he learned in the Brownsville quarantine to build a career organizing armed insurrections against Porfirio Díaz from his base in South Texas.[199]

The Mexican-Texas epidemic provided a medical dimension to the expulsion of Brownsville and South Texas from a more assertive, confident, and military American medical community. In Robert Drake Murray's obituary in the Report of the State Board of Health, they remembered that "he commanded the first armed cordon sanitaire in the United States, one hundred miles in length, and he conducted the first detention camps for the security of people outside the infected region. He was so successful, there was not a case of fever outside the cordon."[200] By 1910, the memory that Brownsville residents actively cooperated with the USMHS medical efforts, that the USMHS hired Spanish-speaking Mexican American nurses, and that the USMHS provided medical treatment within people's residences had become irrelevant to the service's national identity. The cordon, and not the people, symbolized the new identity of American federal medical efforts. South Texas and the Mexican-Texas epidemic simply became a stage in the USMHS struggle for national authority.

TWO

The Promise of Progress

Quarantines and the Medical Fusion
of Race and Nation, 1890–1895

In 1882, most medical authorities in Mexico and the United States considered quarantines medically unacceptable. Agrippa Bell, the head of the American Public Health Association, called them "akin to the murdering of people."[1] Dr. Jose María Reyes, the head of the Central Health Council in Mexico, called them blunt and inefficient and maintained that "only good hygiene can prevent or attenuate the presence of epidemics."[2] By 1892, the medical consensus on quarantine had undergone a dramatic shift. The Texas State Board of Health, the American Public Health Association, the U.S. Marine Hospital Service (USMHS), and the Asociación Médica Mexicana made quarantines central to their political projects. This medical unanimity and shared commitment to medical lines in the sand exacerbated existing political tensions among public health officials. Politics turned the joint American Public Health Association / Asociación Médica Mexicana meeting in the Palacio Nacional in Mexico City in 1892 into a staging ground for debates about sovereignty and the place of modern medical borders.[3] This chapter argues that the political debate over public health authority over goods and people at the Texas border became a way to assert state sovereignty and, in the process, make unsettling claims about Mexican peoples in the Texas borderlands. The debates over border quarantine in the 1890s point out how "modernity, on the one hand, promotes ideas of universality and, on the other, obsessively objectifies difference."[4] The public health debate in Mexico City over quarantine at the Texas border made it very clear that medical authorities could not separate "Mexican" as a Mexico-based national citizenship from "Mexican" as a subordinate ethnic community in Texas, even leading to assertions that Mexicans had a strange lack of fear regarding epidemic disease.

National quarantines went hand in hand with a renewed public investment in laboratory techniques associated with the germ theory. Quarantines provided an opportunity to apply and emulate the clinical practices forged in France by Pasteur and in Germany by Koch and his followers.[5] The USMHS created the National Hygienic Laboratory in 1887 to look for and identify new germs and to test and implement new vaccines and serums.[6] The USMHS was eager to apply the latest clinical techniques in bacteriology to identify the germs and create the treatments that would roll back the fearsome epidemics and communicable diseases that still marked the nineteenth century. Bacteriology promised to add effective diagnosis and new medical treatments to the judicious application of quarantines at America's borders.

The economic importance of American ports and border hubs connected American domestic reforms to the U.S. commercial presence abroad.[7] The 1878 Quarantine Law required that American consulates prepare regular reports on the local prevalence of key epidemic diseases. The 1893 Immigration Act demanded medical inspections of incoming goods and people; this inspection turned American ports and railroad hubs into laboratories for effective public health interventions. Quarantines had become relatively new and popular sites of American medical progress. Their approval went hand in hand with Pasteur's antirabies vaccine.[8] New York City cut its fatality rates from diphtheria through the free distribution of domestically produced diphtheria antitoxin serum.[9] The USMHS had sole federal authority over the response to epidemics that might have an international or interstate dimension. Surgeon General Walter Wyman and Surgeon General George Miller Sternberg opened an additional international front and initiated an ongoing commission-level investigation of yellow fever conditions in Veracruz, Mexico, and Havana, Cuba.[10] A growing American faith in government's ability to contain illness added a public health dimension to U.S. expansion, as when Americans called for the invasion of Cuba to end yellow fever in the United States.[11] For others, the rail lines connecting Mexico to the American South and U.S. Southwest made disease in Mexico seem uncomfortably close.[12]

For public health officers, this was an era of hope and political progress.

Public health activist and public intellectual Cyrus Edson hoped that the microbe would work as a social leveler, forcing elite and middle-class society to fund public health measures in poor and working-class areas.[13] Americans would finally recognize that "disease binds the human race with an unbreakable chain."[14] Edson was not unique. Historian Nancy Tomes argues that many Progressive era reformers used germs as a "common ground for debating the relationship of public health to social justice."[15] The growing faith in the application of the germ theory to field conditions expanded the political landscape for the USMHS.

The expanding promise and appeal of public health to the American public overlapped with large movements to shrink access to politics in the United States.[16] Across the southern states, white racist southerners used legal and extralegal means—open electoral violence, lynching, constitutional conventions, and political disenfranchisement—to remove African Americans and Mexicans from public and political spheres.[17] The U.S. Supreme Court transformed the Fourteenth Amendment. They restricted the due process to freedmen and their descendants in the United States, a process capped by the "separate but equal" language in the *Plessy v. Ferguson* decision.[18] The same amendment struck down unions, strikes, collective bargains, and labor legislation.[19] The U.S. Army repeatedly intervened in railroad, steel mill, and mining strikes. The army's violent actions and the subsequent thirty-four deaths in the Pullman strike illustrated the extent to which the federal government valued order over working-class assertion.[20]

This decade also marked a high point for federal involvement in Native American lives. The Department of the Interior actively forced men and women in Indian nations to comply with the Dawes General Allotment Act, register themselves with the Department of the Interior, and apply for their sixty acres of land in trust.[21] The Department of the Interior then prepared to make the remaining reservation lands available for public use or private purchase.[22] The allotment process was meant to guarantee health and prosperity for Native Americans who best conformed to white American norms for American Indians.[23] This was a deeply sardonic guarantee, for it coincided with the Ghost Dance movement, the Wounded Knee massacre, and the lowest population total in the United States for Native American groupings since 1492.[24] This end of the Indian Wars justified an American push for intervention in Cuba, the annexation of Hawaii, and a greater confidence in the possibility of (white) American power over territories and peoples abroad.

Colonel John Gregory Bourke sought to bring this confidence to bear on a reinvigorated conquest of Mexican people living along the Mexican border.[25] The invigorated medical modernity also participated in this imperial redefinition of America's borders.

Public health projects were also central to the practice of national progress in Mexico.[26] In northern Mexico, the cities of Monterrey, Torreon, Saltillo, Coahuila, and Chihuahua passed compulsory vaccination statutes as evidence of their medical modernity.[27] Mexico City and the federal government incurred massive foreign debts to transform the sewage system and drain the swamps and wetlands surrounding Mexico City. In Mexico City, engineers drained two lakes, raised parts of Mexico City, and built a water distribution, sewage, and drainage system that involved digging a vast tunnel through the mountain range surrounding the Valley of Mexico.[28] The National Council of Health installed the Pasteur Institute's most advanced disinfecting ovens and fumigation techniques in Veracruz and Laredo.[29] The National Council of Health brought the American Public Health Association to Mexico City to witness these Mexican monuments to medical progress. The Porfiriato wanted American public health officers to register and absorb the vast modern medical transformation underfoot in Mexico. In the process they turned Mexico City into a temporary medical borderlands.

Others in Mexico did not experience the ties between state formation and public health as evidence of progress, national or otherwise. The decade marked a new phase in the open campaigns to dispossess the Yaqui, the Seri, the Raramuri, and the Apache of their hold over their river valleys and mountain territories in northern Mexico. Railroads and landowners actively expanded their landholdings, dispossessing peasants or incorporating villages into their hacienda holdings.[30] Branches of Gobernación actively recruited workers from Germany, Italy, France, and England to help whiten and Europeanize the Mexican industrial workforce.[31] Gobernación also recruited ostensibly temporary nonwhite, non-European workers from China, Korea, Cuba, Jamaica, and the United States.[32] Many of the architects of these policies used the language of efficiency, modernity, and order to justify these forms of economic growth and public exclusion. Porfirio Díaz's contemporaries sardonically referred to his cabinet as the *científicos* (scientists). Historians of this time period use the term *rifle sanitario* (sanitary rifle) to refer to the military cleanup of political threats to the Porfiriato.[33]

The established orders in Mexico and the United States did not control the language of medical modernity. Men and women outside the medical establishment used their participation in public health projects such as smallpox vaccination to stake their place in the national politics emerging at the Texas-Mexican border. Exiled Mexican journalist Justo Cardenas celebrated compulsory vaccination in Nuevo León.[34] He expanded on the assumption that modern states intervene in their communities to prevent epidemics. Demands by racial minorities and transnational communities for state medical interventions, when the language of germs so easily lent itself to exclusion and expulsion from national body politics, unsettled the idea that public health policies only belonged to *cientificos* or Progressive era reformers.

The overlapping demand for public vaccination by community members and public health officials lay in counterpoint to the debates among North American public health officers over state responsibility—from vaccination to quarantine—for the health of migrants and citizens in border zones. The Texas State Health office catalyzed this debate during the third inaugural for President Porfirio Díaz by demanding that Mexico vaccinate Mexican workers working in Texas, because of smallpox cases in San Antonio in 1891. The Texas government's demand in this international health conference interrupted the mutual embrace of federal inspections, disinfections, and quarantines at key border hubs and ports. The subsequent debate over quarantine and sovereignty between Mexican physicians and Texan health officers made it clear that the medical racialization of Mexicans in Texas as migrant workers had political dimensions in Mexico. Although some participants emphasized that state resources should also go to public health projects away from international borders, American, Mexican, and Texan officials agreed on the primacy of quarantine and detention to the practice of national sovereignty. The quarantine principle implied continued disagreement over any quarantine in a shared border space. Moreover, the debate over public health sovereignty ignored any discussion of the rights and privileges of citizenship. Finally, the cross-border medical agreement on quarantine turned transnational affinities into an ongoing threat to firm boundaries around the body politics in Texas, Mexico, and the United States.

Making a Claim for Modern Citizenship at the Border: Vaccination in Nuevo León, 1891

On May 6, 1891, Laredo journalist Justo Cardenas trumpeted the vanguard modernity of the state of Nuevo León. He reprinted correspondence between

Eduardo Liceaga, the president of the Consejo Superior de Salubridad (National Council of Health) and Governor Bernardo Reyes of Nuevo León. "It is only just to note that the compulsory vaccination law in Nuevo León is the most advanced and fruitful," Liceaga wrote, "[far more] than the policy in the Distrito Federal." Cardenas reminded the readers of *La Colonia Mexicana* that smallpox was "feared in Europe and the United States, but not in Nuevo León, where the appearance has not generated any panic whatsoever."[35] According to Cardenas, the residents of Nuevo León responded more calmly and scientifically than the metropolitan centers that exported their models for progress. In Nuevo León, the case mortality in smallpox epidemics was less than one in one thousand. Liceaga argued, and Cardenas concurred, that this was because Nuevo León authorities made the vaccine compulsory, available to all, and free in the state-run dispensaries. Nuevo León's policy required that everyone register his or her vaccination scar with his or her municipal authority. By "everyone," the policy makers meant only "men eligible for citizenship." The law demanded proof of vaccination for state services. In the absence of an acceptable vaccine take and the proper paperwork, Nuevo León required residents to seek out a certified physician or a *casilla*—a state-certified dispensary—that provided certified vaccinations. The scars on the body were not enough to prevent a fine. For Justo Cardenas, the low smallpox mortality was proof that Nuevo León had transformed the threat of smallpox into a mere reminder of an unscientific past.[36]

Compulsory vaccination also reinscribed a politics of gender that followed the relative household status of everyone in Nuevo León. Every dependent —according to the statute, wives, daughters, and sons—had to name and identify a male household head along with their age, race, and nationality. Even though Nuevo León was extending health benefits to all residents and, by implication, expanding the boundaries of state citizenship, the additional requirements narrowed the bounds of citizenship by demanding official allegiance to idealized gender arrangements and diminished legal autonomy for women and children.[37] Moreover, compulsory vaccination demanded domestic transformation. Justo Cardenas reminded his readers that public health depended on the proper training of women. His essay "Hygienic Methods to Prevent the Spread of Smallpox" turned domestic spaces into a contact zone between public policies and individual bodies. Cardenas emphasized the need for a generous political context because "smallpox is a perfectly avoidable disease, with a little individual initiative. However, authorities have the obligation of helping the less fortunate classes, freely and without obstacles of any kind, following all the means counseled by modern science to avoid its presence and its spread."[38] The presence of smallpox was more than an individual disaster; it revealed "a collective abandonment of hygiene and at the individual level, a complete unawareness of its most elemental principles."[39] The burden of smallpox prevention lay in the proper regulation of domestic spaces: destroying any dried lymph, pus, or material from sores in sulfur-based disinfection baths, periodic revaccination, and, above all, the isolation of the patient and his or her clothes from the rest of the household. This was a good example of the thorough transformation of domestic space that came with the gospel of germs, the burden of which journalists and public health officers reluctantly thrust upon women.[40] Cardenas and Liceaga made this burden clear to readers of *El Progreso* in Laredo and South Texas. Any reluctance on the part of households and policy-making bodies to comply with these ideals demonstrated a near complete abandonment of the minimum standards of civilization.

Throughout the Americas, civilization represented a shifting ideal that helped delineate the boundaries of citizenship. For Frederick Jackson Turner, the frontier was the dividing line "between civilization and savagery," a civilization that never included Mexicans.[41] To Faustino Sarmiento, the well-known Argentine liberal, barbarism represented the threat rural Latin America posed to the civilizing benefits of modern liberalism.[42] Porfirio Díaz and allies like Nuevo León governor Reyes and Liceaga claimed to represent the forces of civilization and order.[43] For Cardenas, vaccination marked a key dividing line between the savagery of Texas and the civilization available in urban Nuevo León. Similarly, in Mexico the rhetoric of civilization seemed to belong to the political establishment, but critics of the Porfiriato used the rhetoric of civilization to condemn the country's "barbaric" economic and political policies.[44]

Cardenas fled the Porfiriato in 1886 after he criticized the political authority accruing to foreign investors and large landowners in northern Mexico. His exile in Laredo followed the recentralization of power that came with Governor Reyes's imposition of martial law in Nuevo León.[45] Catarino Garza and Dr. Ignacio Martinez, a veteran of the Mexican-Texas yellow fever epidemic, mounted an armed insurrection to challenge the unequal distribution of progress in northern Mexico.[46] Governor Reyes later had Martinez killed in Laredo, perhaps for his visible alternative to Reyes's vision of modernity.[47]

For Cardenas, Garza, and Martinez, the emerging rights of modern citizens also included vaccination. Thus the appearance of smallpox could prove to be a reminder of the incomplete promise of modernity.[48] Cardenas and Martinez embedded the rhetoric of medical science and civilization deeply within modernizing Mexican currents at the border. This claim on modernity by Mexicans in the United States challenged the idea that the border was "the American Congo"—a place that required consistent military attention to keep the people in line with American cultural ideals.[49]

Staking a Claim in Mexico: Public Health Matters in Mexico City, 1892

In 1892, nearly a year after Cardenas's essays on vaccination, Dr. Swearingen, the Texas State Health Officer, presented a paper titled "The Sanitary Relations between Texas and Mexico" in Mexico City.[50] He crossed the Rio Grande and took the Mexican Central Railroad south to the capital.[51] Unlike Cardenas and Dr. Martinez, Dr. Swearingen went deep into the heart of the Mexican modern as a guest of Porfirio Díaz. Swearingen may have started his presentation to the joint meeting of the American Public Health Association and the Asociación Médica Mexicana with a note of caution. His larger message to the international audience of public health professionals was that the greatest health threat facing Texas was Mexico, or the presence of Mexicans in Texas. As he stated on the very grounds of Porfirio Díaz's presidential palace, "While the health officials [in Mexico] were as enlightened on sanitation as those of other countries, the masses of the poorer people, the laboring classes along the Rio Grande particularly, were in a state of dense ignorance as to the blessing of sanitation—know nothing of prophylaxis; but on the contrary, hold the primitive views of their early ancestors."[52] Swearingen emphasized the threat of people's culture over national policies in his discussion of smallpox and "internal sanitation" in Mexico. He extended his analogy regarding the perceived absence of disease prevention among "the laboring classes of the Rio Grande." Swearingen stated that some families "will actually expose their children to smallpox infections that they may catch the disease. In this way, in the interior [of Mexico], smallpox is purposely propagated, and has become endemic."[53] Dr. Swearingen referred to inoculation: taking material from one person's dried smallpox blisters and placing the material in someone else's open incision. American and Mexican medical society increasingly stigmatized inoculation, just as they did midwifery and other vernacular health practices. Families used inoculation in places where vaccination was difficult to obtain. Thus Swearingen's reference to inoculation was an intentionally disturbing way to connect his audience's imaginary Indian or Spanish pasts to current family practices. For Swearingen, Mexican families threatened Texas because Texas was connected to Mexico: "With a border-line of hundreds of miles confronting the republic of Mexico, [Texas] is, of course, more exposed to [epidemic] invasions of this kind than are all the other states combined."[54] Swearingen's use of the phrase "purposely propagated" treated Mexican men and women working north of the Rio Grande as the key medical and economic threats to Texas, and he demanded that the Mexican government ensure vaccination among all Mexican workers in Texas.

To justify his political demands on Mexican federal authorities, Swearingen provided an eccentric accounting of the costs to Texas of a nonexistent statewide vaccination policy. His figures were quoted in a report by T. J. Bennett: "Small-pox prevailed in twenty-six counties in Texas last winter, aggregating over two thousand cases, with some five hundred deaths, and in every instance its introduction could be traced primarily to Mexico. To eradicate this epidemic cost Texas over $150,000. In San Antonio alone there were over a thousand cases, and the expense to the city and county, according to Health Officer Braunagel's report to the health officer, cited in Swearingen's paper, approximated nearly $20,000."[55] Given all these outlays, Swearingen could have endorsed state-sponsored vaccination. Instead, Swearingen demanded that Mexico's northern states shoulder the burden of vaccinating ethnic Mexican laborers' resident in Texas. Swearingen refused to shoulder the political and financial risk of mandating vaccination for all men, women, and children in Texas. This refusal meant Swearingen wanted Mexican bodies in Mexico and Texas to bear the individual costs and risks of vaccination that Texas was unwilling to carry. The top state health officer in the state of Texas wanted Mexican states to incur a public burden and implement public health practices for the good of Texas. Swearingen made the transnational dimension of racial subordination in Texas seem eerily colonial.

Swearingen's rhetoric belittled his hosts' modernizing ambitions: "To-day, while the advanced sanitarians of Mexico are in the forefront of sanitary progress and enlightenment, the peasantry of that country are as benighted as though Jenner had never lived, nor Pasteur made a discovery."[56] By referring to these two icons of the germ theory, Texas's state health officer mocked the efforts of the Superior Council to learn French and German clinical techniques. His claims about Mexicans also ignored simple geography because he made claims about Mexicans in Mexico based on his experiences in the United States. He never worked in Mexico. His medical authority on Mexicans came from his experience in South Texas, when Tejano political authorities jailed and quarantined him during the Mexican-Texas yellow fever epidemic. His confidence in his political and clinical experience in South Texas authored his nearly colonial authority over all things Mexican, whether in Texas or Mexico.

His audience at the Palacio Nacional in Mexico City probably rejected his paternalist approach. A good portion of that audience must have been astonished at his open equation of Mexico with an unrepentant prophylactic barbarism. The hosts had meant to use Mexico City's public works as proof of the viability of modernizing public health projects in Mexico.[57] Liceaga, the president of the Consejo Superior de Salubridad, had promised APHA participants a tour of the Grand Sanitary Canal so that they could witness the current Mexican monuments to progress.[58] Liceaga redirected the audience's immediate response to Swearingen. He stated, "As the paper which has just been read treats of a question whose discussion is of the greatest interest to ourselves, I move that the paper, which unfortunately has not been translated for want of time, be held for discussion until the Mexicans have been able to read it."[59] Parts of the audience had taken umbrage with Swearingen's assertions; Texas State Health Officer Bennett recorded the response as "quite indignant."[60] Local Mexican hostility challenged Swearingen's efforts to sell his racially exclusionary understanding of public health to people outside Texas. The racially targeted audience—as well as people like Cardenas in Texas —did not see any reason to buy into the racial subordination and imperial ambition peddled by Dr. Swearingen. The response to Swearingen in Mexico City exposed the parochial and imperial underpinning to Swearingen's claims about Mexican health cultures.

Cardenas and Swearingen linked Mexican citizenship and vaccination at the Texas-Mexico border in parallel ways. Even though both wrote that vaccination was part of the way forward for Mexican communities in Texas, their claims about vaccination among Mexicans are nearly impossible to reconcile. For Cardenas and Liceaga, the citizens and residents of Nuevo León were at the vanguard of public health. Other places, Texas in particular, were implicitly falling behind in their obligation to their citizenry. For Dr.

Swearingen, Mexicans in Texas were prophylactic barbarians who intruded on the ability of the Texas Board of Health to define and protect the modern boundaries of its body politic. Swearingen and Cardenas provide nearly ideal mutual antagonists: Cardenas emphasized that vaccination was a necessary dimension of modern domesticity and symbolically challenged Swearingen's claim of antimodern barbarism among border Mexicans; Swearingen, unlike Cardenas, wanted smallpox vaccination to be a condition of entry and employment for Mexicans—and Mexicans only—in Texas. Both Cardenas and Swearingen upheld the ideal of universal vaccination, but political differences over the place of Mexicans in Texas contributed to differences in the way they understood the role of vaccination in the Mexican border community. Cardenas believed vaccination would protect the vaccinated; Swearingen argued that vaccinated Mexicans would benefit vaccinated and unvaccinated Texan employers and families. Swearingen's understanding of a healthy and modern body politic meant forcing this ideal on "the laboring classes of the Rio Grande border."[61] Cardenas and Swearingen's mutual commitment to vaccination in the Mexican community in Texas and Mexico only accentuated their political differences over the place of Mexicans in Texas. Progress in vaccination connected Mexicans to Mexico; Swearingen left Americans unmarked in Texas as he tied the need for vaccination in Mexico to a specific working population in Texas, neatly proposing a state-mandated racial distinction between Mexicans and Americans.

There was a general conversation among Mexican and American doctors in Texas and northern Mexico about what they called a working-class Mexican relationship to medical authority. This indifference to medical authority became an important marker of difference between doctors and patients. Northern Mexico–based doctor Jesus Chico idealized the way physicians were willing to transform their personal behavior and domestic landscapes in light of new medical information.[62] Dr. Chico drew a stark difference between doctors and others in Mexico: "We physicians, now well aware of the possible danger, take every personal precaution we can, and admonish seriously the families to take the required measures, but in the majority of cases they do not heed our advice, partly on account of their not being sufficiently educated to acknowledge the necessity of the sacrifices expected, and partly because experience has shown them that the danger of contagion is a remote one."[63]

This presentation played well among some Anglo doctors in Texas. Dr. William Yandell, the representative from the El Paso County Medical

Association, used Dr. Chico's assertion to draw an even starker portrait of Mexican attitudes toward epidemic disease. According to Yandell, both "our Mexicans" and "their Mexicans" shared an "utter disregard of all precautions against spreading contagious diseases, except from fear of the law."[64] Therefore, he concluded, "the masses are only to be taught by the strong arm of the law. The laws for the protection of public health, except in our Mexican villages, are more strictly enforced in our country than in Mexico, because the masses in our country fear contagious diseases, while the masses in Mexico do not."[65] For Yandell, mere persuasion or education could not overcome the political will of the Mexican population along the Rio Grande. Mexican attitudes toward smallpox threatened the United States.

Smallpox and vaccination were not the only practice connecting communities in northern Mexico and Texas. Once railroads connected San Antonio and Laredo to Monterrey, Nuevo León, and Saltillo, Coahuila, the towns by the railroad grew explosively. In 1880, Laredo was the county seat for a population of slightly more than 5,000 people. The population tripled to more than 14,000 people by 1890 and quadrupled to 21,851 by 1900. Brownsville and Cameron County, the one-time economic hubs of the Rio Grande border, shrank by nearly a thousand people between 1880 and 1900. Even more striking, the number of people born in Mexico doubled between 1890 and 1900 in Laredo and Webb County but stayed steady in Brownsville and Cameron County.[66] This difference in the Mexican national population reflected the differential impact of railroads on border towns. Some of northern Mexico's aspiring classes moved north as part of their rejection of Porfirio Díaz's continued reelections after 1884. Many of these migrants, including Garza, the Idar family, and Cardenas, helped create a vibrant press along the border.[67] Even the counterinsurgency efforts aimed at forestalling Garza's uprising against Porfirio Díaz brought more U.S citizens to the lower Rio Grande valley.[68] The U.S. Army moved mostly African American troops to forts along the Rio Grande as part of its larger response to Apache, Comanche, Mexican, and American cross-border raids.[69] Monterrey, Nuevo León; Saltillo, Coahuila; and Laredo and Eagle Pass became important labor and transshipment hubs. These hubs provided a national stage for local officials and an organizing center for Mexican and American exiles. The Rio Grande border hubs were becoming a key theater for the consolidation of federal authority.

Dr. Swearingen's presence at the APHA conference in Mexico City was no accident. Liceaga and the Consejo Superior de Salubridad (National Council of Health; NCH) had been pushing to host the annual APHA conference since the late 1880s. In 1890, the APHA elected Dr. Domingo Orvañanos to the presidency. In 1891, the organization agreed to accept the invitation by Liceaga and the NCH and hold a joint conference in Mexico City; the NCH scheduled the conference to overlap with Porfirio Díaz's inaugural. The APHA's secretary, Dr. Irving Watson, encouraged state and territorial health officers across the United States to travel to Mexico City because their presence might interest physicians in Mexico to "become so closely identified with our work as to reap the unlimited benefits that would follow from such an alliance."[70] Watson also wanted state and territorial health officers to witness a national state with a central health authority and a single sanitary code, "the most extensive, comprehensive, and the broadest ever adopted by any government in the world, probably."[71] For many public health advocates, state and territorial health officers were one of the most important obstacles to the reestablishment of a civilian-run National Board of Health. The APHA meeting provided an opportunity to create a shared understanding of public health.

The organizers convened a special forum to discuss and challenge Swearingen's presentation. The forum featured three responses to Swearingen's assertions. In the first, Swearingen reiterated his earlier point that Mexican authorities should conform to the step he proposed to eradicate smallpox. As Bennett near gleefully put it, "He can keep it down in Texas, but not out of Texas without assistance of the other side."[72] The second line of argument involved Mexican authorities. Bennett did not name the authorities, but he said they "did not relish the plain and straightforward presentation of a state of affairs which does not reflect much credit upon them as sanitarians."[73] They emphasized that they had already implemented the policies that Swearingen demanded, and—if they were from Nuevo León—probably argued that their vaccination policies were far more forward-thinking than any in Texas.[74] Dr. Gibson, the medical director of the U.S. Navy, led a third response and sought to use this discussion to create a uniform international authority. He called for a commission of thirteen members drawn from Canada, the United States, and Mexico "to propose a plan of international cooperative action for the protection of the respective countries."[75] Southern public health officers —"delegates who insisted on State's rights, and opposed national participation in State quarantine affairs"—worked actively to challenge the threat to their recently won state sovereignty, by which they meant the power to impose their own quarantines.[76]

Swearingen's presentation and responses to it illustrate that while most of the delegates agreed on the principles behind quarantine and vaccination, it was the politics of quarantine that brought them into conflict. Public health officials shared and debated ways to make their states, their nations, and their most representative publics healthier and more public. The USMHS had already started to implement federal inspection and quarantine authority across the ports and borders of the United States. In this debate, health officers in Texas and other southern states openly challenged the assumption that national territory meant federal authority. Swearingen and his post-Reconstruction generation of southern state health officers consistently resisted federal authority for this medical intervention into the economic life of their ports and railroads.[77] The ambiguous place of state quarantine was also a diplomatic matter between Mexican, American, and Texan governments. Drs. Swearingen and Liceaga had already exchanged hostile correspondence over the yellow fever quarantines the state of Texas had imposed in 1891 on ships arriving from Veracruz and Tampico.[78] For these southern state health officers, state sovereignty was a requirement for the exercise of public health. For American and Mexican federal medical officers, Texas medical sovereignty had become a consistent problem for any international health accord between Mexico and the United States.

In Texas, the governor's office held final authority over public health matters. The Texas legislature mandated that the state health officers had the power to determine "the exact condition of things" in the midst of a threatened epidemic. The governor's office claimed the exclusive political authority to represent the facts of public health matters to and for their particular body politic. The policy stated:

> In all differences and disputes between any such points, contiguous or remote within this state, such differences shall be immediately reported by the local health authorities, if any, and if none, by the inhabitants themselves, reported to the Governor, and on the receipt of such a report he shall forthwith investigate the same and report the exact condition of things, and upon investigation of such report shall issue his proclamation declaring the determination of the issue and by said proclamation the aforesaid difference shall be ignored.[79]

The Texas legislature gave the governor's office—and by extension the state health officer—the authority to determine the facts and then assess the legitimacy of city quarantine. Moreover, the governor's office only took fiscal responsibility if the state health officer declared the quarantine. The financial incentive for each municipality to agree with the state health officer provided another tool to centralize the regulation of commerce and order. This political authority forestalled any "shotgun quarantines" or any other independent action by a municipality, like jailing state health officer Swearingen in Laredo in the midst of a yellow fever epidemic. The Texas State Health Office kept quarantine officers at key entrances into Texas. The officers at El Paso, Laredo, and Eagle Pass worked "to guard against introduction of disease from the west."[80] Texas also placed temporary quarantine stations at the railroad stations in Denison, Gainesville, Texarkana, Paris, Waskom, and Sabine River Crossing, during "the time of threatened danger from cholera [when] Texas quarantined against New York."[81] The state health officer embodied the governor's will and way, especially when quarantines became key tools for the exercise of state medical sovereignty.

Post-Reconstruction governments of southern states used quarantines to push their sovereignty over and against American federal authority. The power to quarantine was important and crucial enough that these governments rebuked Congress for giving the USMHS and the Department of the Treasury the authority to "dictate rules for the government of public health in forty-four sovereign states—and when at one stroke of a pen, he can lock the wheels of commerce in every American port."[82] Bennett emphasized local southern knowledge over and against a surgeon general's northern experience and European medical training, because "a rule that would admit ships infected by yellow fever at northern ports, would be dangerous at ports in the South. . . . The old adage—'a fool knows more of his own house than a wise man outside' is certainly applicable to the subject under consideration."[83] This emphasis on the importance of local knowledge contained a possible challenge to the Texas legislatures' earlier claim of full political authority over any quarantine in towns and cities in Texas. For Bennett, the bill in Congress gave the surgeon general and the Treasury the authority best exercised by the Texas governor and his state health officers. This bill shifted the power Texas exercised over its cities to the federal Treasury Department and left the governor of Texas with wide responsibility and little power. Bennett and Swearingen emphasized that Texas inspection and quarantine maintained a commercial order while containing epidemics that emerged in Mexico, other southern states, and the Gulf of Mexico. They both performed a post-Reconstruction

(Anglo) American southern medical identity against Mexico and the U.S. federal government. The international discussion of border quarantines in Mexico became a useful foil to project a southern medical identity against the United States.

The importance of quarantine to public health and political authority also troubled Bennett and Swearingen. In a presentation to the Texas Medical Association after the debacle in Mexico City, Bennett feared that by attending "to this feature of government alone, to the neglect of internal sanitation, the government, to use a homely expression, is 'saving at the spigot and losing at the burg.' The lives lost, the time lost, and the property values destroyed in time of the most destructive epidemic are as a drop in the bucket to the lives, labor and property being destroyed every day, all over the country, by diseases easily preventable."[84] In this missive, Bennett argued for the creation of the Department of Public Health in Texas, in order to go beyond the judge-appointed city or county health physician.[85] Like Edson and Cardenas, Bennett feared that quarantine and political apathy would prevent simple government action against "easily preventable diseases" inside national boundaries.[86] Bennett endorsed Liceaga's proposal to prevent the marriage of any person diagnosed with tuberculosis. Swearingen conceded that even intelligently imposed quarantines would benefit from U.S.-based bacteriological research. In 1892, he agreed "that our government [must] found and equip a central laboratory for the study of contagia, with experiment stations, and with a staff large enough to work the whole ground, and paid well enough to secure the best scientific talent," especially "if our government ever expects to compete with Germany and France in the discovery of great scientific truths."[87] For Bennett and Swearingen, quarantines were the definition of medical sovereignty. Swearingen's demand for increased vaccination in Mexico for the benefit of the people of Texas was a foreign policy initiative that supplemented the importance of quarantine.

Quarantine was also central to Mexican health authority, but the possibility of political conflict with entrenched economic powers in Mexico shaped the rhetoric of sanitary authority in Mexico. When responding to rumors of epidemics, the Mexican federal government demanded and took full political authority. In this medical situation, according to Liceaga, "the states of the Mexican Union form only one. The ports and frontiers depend only on the federation."[88] The staff in Gobernación took full authority over ports on the Gulf of Mexico and the Pacific Ocean and frontiers, along with the cities adjoining the traffic corridors along the American and Guatemalan border. The sanitary staff in Gobernación expected the state boards of health to follow the directions and use federal resources. In the ideal situation, allegiance bubbled up and authority flowed down, modeling the patronage relationships Porfirio Díaz and the *científicos* hoped to create with local and regional authorities. The staff in Gobernación claimed political distance from local influence—"with entire independence of the states"—in any public health matters with a transnational dimension, any matters that "involved the international sanitary police." When epidemics did emerge, Gobernación replaced local political authority with members of the Sanitary Council and their local allies in the ports and frontiers. Liceaga's presentation repeatedly emphasized the central state's inability to control large commercial enterprises and private corporations, arguing that the "rights of humanity frequently disappear in the face of commerce."[89] Historians Michael Meyer and William Sherman emphasized the way Mexican public policy seemed a reflection of the business-friendly attitude of *científicos* and the Porfirian elite.[90] Complicating this picture of convergent interests, Liceaga's rhetoric highlights the tenuous hold Gobernación and the National Council of Health, and by extension Porfirio Díaz, had in potentially unfriendly regions and international commercial matters.

Quarantine represented a complicated political opportunity for Mexican federal authorities. Rather than inviting conflict over the right to exercise quarantine, Liceaga described quarantine procedures as one part of a complex way station of public health procedures that guaranteed personal and commercial safety. The quarantine was a blueprint for a project with a "sole thought: to prevent communication between the sick and the healthy individual, and the more rigor used in carrying out this principle the more certain are the results."[91] For Liceaga, the quarantine—especially the quarantine stations at the main ports in Mexico—provided an opportunity to display effective Mexican public health interventions. The liminal space of border quarantine opened up the use of disinfection, "the other resource, entirely modern at least in its application.... The object is to destroy, by natural or chemical agents, all germs wherever they may be, which produce contagious diseases."[92] Disinfection with sulphuric acid, chlorine, and carbolic acid would prevent imported germs from taking root in Mexican soil. Liceaga claimed that efficient quarantine directly challenged short-term commercial interests and thus that "a conflict is waged between the preservation of public

health and private wealth."[93] Medical authorities sought to position themselves within this project as the ideal agency to restrain and discipline the
implicitly national costs of private decisions.[94] In Liceaga's vision, larger and
larger numbers of people in Mexico needed to embrace the importance of
public health and national authority. Quarantines at key Mexican ports were
an opportunity for object lessons in public health.

When Texas state health officers argued for Mexican-specific policies because of Mexican-specific population traits, their professional counterparts
in Mexico challenged their racializing and degrading assumptions about
Mexicans. When state health officers discussed Texas in general, Mexican
national policies toward vaccination and sanitation became part of the Texas-
wide discussion. The infrastructure linking New York, Galveston, Veracruz,
New Orleans, Monterrey, and Havana consistently confounded attempts to
separate an analysis of health in Texas from the situation in New York. In
1892 Mexico City, North American public health professionals discussed and
debated their mutual commitments to isolation, disinfection, quarantine, and
disease-specific approaches. Public health officers staked their professional
identities around the prevention of specific diseases like yellow fever, diphtheria, and smallpox. In Mexico City, most presenters agreed on the importance
of disinfection, isolation, quarantine, sanitation, and clinical research. This
agreement on public health measures contributed to political conflicts over
the timing, extent, and cost of quarantine and vaccination in the midst of an
epidemic.

Conclusion

The discussions at the APHA meeting in Mexico City highlighted the ways
state health officers sought to use quarantines to make their nation and body
politic present at the border.[95] Borders and ports provided a stage to persuade
national audiences of the importance of public health. Differences among
public health officers made the political tensions in these national projects
evident in Mexico City in 1892.

The tensions emerged partly from four different ways the public health
officers framed the word "Mexican." For some Mexican meant a territory, for
others a form of citizenship. Still others treated Mexicans as a class subordinate to the Texas body politic, and others found Mexican to represent a troubling or queer relationship to the American body politic. Liceaga and other
Mexican doctors understood Mexican to be a political relationship to the

Mexican Republic. Swearingen's discussion of the "laboring classes along the Rio Grande" highlighted the way he considered Mexican a subordinate ethnic political relationship to the Texas body politic. Liceaga's discussion of the way stations at Mexico's borders clearly assumed that a Mexican could also be a subject connected to a territory with political boundaries subject to Mexican federal authority. Dr. William Yandell, when he claimed that "the masses in our country [the United States] fear contagious diseases, while the masses in Mexico do not," used this unquantifiable lack of fear to emphasize the queer threat Mexicans posed to the United States.[96] The debate over the presence and prevention of smallpox, cholera, and yellow fever at "the Texas border" wrought a curious fusion of the ethnic and the medical at both nations' edge. The presence of four different ways to use the term "Mexican" made the discussion of public health at the Mexican border intellectually and politically unstable. As the discussion fused this unstable mixture into one word, the cross-border dimensions of both Mexican and American contributed to the substantial political and intellectual problems that emerged in attempts to define Mexican and American in subsequent epidemics.

This is an opportunity not to be lost to put the serum therapy
into effect.—Surgeon General Walter Wyman, 1895

THREE

The Appearance of Progress

Black Labor, Smallpox, and the Body Politics of Transnational American Citizenship, 1895

In January 1895, Sam and Emma Claiborne considered a future in Mexico. These two residents of Tuscaloosa, Alabama, read in a handbill that a large agricultural combine in Mexico was recruiting black workers. Part of the offer included food, medicine, and free transportation to Durango, Mexico. The handbill promised that Mexico was a place where "all of its citizens [received] the same treatment—equal rights to all, special privileges to none." These privileges were available to them in exchange for sharecropping on terms ostensibly better than the ones available in central Alabama.[1] The Claibornes and nearly sixty other black families left Alabama for Mapimi (a city in Durango) to work at the Compañía Agricola Tlahualilo, or Tlahualilo Agricultural Company. According to the handbill and labor agent and black Union veteran Ralph "Peg Leg" Williams, this was the "the greatest opportunity ever offered to colored people of the United States to go to Mexico."[2] Looking past the Mexican border, these southerners saw a future in a foreign place where their skills could provide a measure of progress.

The Claibornes were not the only ones who looked to the Mexican borderlands for a measure of progress.[3] Americans of all kinds looked south. Federal health officials hoped to turn America's southern borders into points of progress. The USMHS was eager to apply the latest clinical techniques in bacteriology and immunology to identify germs and create treatments that would roll back the fearsome diseases that still marked the nineteenth century.[4] They were a key part of the public face of quarantine. The USMHS wanted quarantines at key border hubs to combine the skills of the best diagnosticians, sanitarians, and clinical specialists. The 1878 Quarantine Law demanded that American consulates prepare regular reports on the immediate prevalence of key epidemic diseases.[5] The 1893 Immigration Act made the USMHS a key agency regulating the traffic connecting American cities to the U.S. commercial presence abroad.[6] A growing faith in bacteriology and the increased consular reporting of disease turned American ports and railroad hubs into potential laboratories for effective public health interventions.

The appearance of smallpox at the Hacienda Tlahualilo in Mapimi in the summer of 1895 brought the Claiborne family and the majority of the other Tuscaloosa colonists into direct contact with the new trends in quarantine and American immunology. This chapter examines the way the public effort to modernize quarantines interacted with the Tuscaloosa colonists' organized demand that the American federal government intervene in Mexico to protect their right to survival.[7] The final section explores the ways Mexican, Texan, and U.S. officials dealt with smallpox and vaccination among (African) American labor migrants in Mexico. The chapter argues that the experience of the African Americans who became the Tlahualilo colonists exemplifies the ways the American medical border moved across political borders; their medical experience exposed conflicts and changes in the form of citizenship available to African Americans in 1895.

Families like the Claibornes left Alabama with the hopes of permanently settling or—in the vernacular of the time—becoming colonists in Mexico. When it became clear that the work arrangements in Tlahualilo were not going to be conducive to survival, let alone long-term settlement or property ownership, the Tlahualilo colonists—as black and mainstream U.S. press representatives referred to them—rebelled. They mobilized across the Mexican border and demanded American federal intervention into Mexico on their behalf. When the State Department became aware of smallpox among the colonists, the settlers quickly learned that epidemic disease, not the rights of American workers, bound them "like a human chain" to the medical sovereignty asserted by American public health officials.[8] The colonists' bodies became sites where the state of Texas gave the American federal government authority over quarantine and where the USMHS applied their latest research in smallpox (antitoxin serum) treatment. The space around their presence turned into a three-month detention in Eagle Pass in Camp Jenner and became a model USMHS humanitarian intervention. The Tlahualilo colonists experienced a far uglier dimension of Mexican, Texan, and American public health sovereignty. Their detention inside Camp Jenner demonstrates that quarantine authority over foreign nationals at the border also shaped the experience of American citizens coming back to the United States, who found that America's scientific gaze at the border encompassed (black) American citizens as well as immigrants.[9]

The simultaneous deployment of disease-based detention and smallpox antitoxin research on black bodies at the Mexican border confounded the American/Mexican distinction that most people associated with the Rio Grande border. When the Tlahualilo colonists sought to move north, they disturbed the assumption that, unlike immigrants, border-crossing Americans are white, Anglo, and healthy. Their subsequent three-month-long detention was one of the longest single federal interventions into a nineteenth-century smallpox outbreak in the United States.[10] Camp Jenner drew a clear contrast to an established federal apathy toward the recurring presence of smallpox cases among Mexicans in South Texas and northern Mexico. The position of African Americans in Camp Jenner, and inside the margins of American inclusion, exposed the routine—and arbitrary—ways USMHS officers could decide who was and was not American and whose diseases were and were not worthy of close clinical attention.[11]

The Tlahualilo Colonists Trouble the Border Quarantine

American, Texan, and Mexican public health officers drew medical lines and designated medical zones among increasingly mobile and cross-connected border populations. The overlapping points of medical authority over these populations led to increasingly assertive federal demands for a medical line that allowed for distinctions between Mexicans and Americans in Mexico and the United States. Medical authorities invoked "sanitary principles" to police a border zone: to collapse residents of politically separate yet economically connected towns along railroad corridors into what they sought to treat medically as one Mexican or African American population. The racializing of people along national lines at the border separated these targeted populations from other potential publics along the Monterrey/San Antonio railroad corridor. The movement of goods and people across northern Mexico and South Texas helped justify the importance of medical authority at national borders. The establishment of a (moving) medical border preceded the full-fledged immigrant medical inspections at customs houses along the Rio Grande by two decades.[12]

Three years after the APHA meeting in Mexico City, the Compañía Agricola Tlahualilo set off a labor dispute in Mexico that exposed deep fault lines among American, Mexican, and Texan public health authorities. The conflict had deep roots in the forms of commercial development that overtook northern Mexico under President Porfirio Díaz. In 1888, Díaz gave the Compañía Agricola Tlahualilo legal rights to harvest river water from the Río Nazas. Spanish and British investors bought the Compañía Agricola Tlahualilo and invested in a private railroad and a canal to reroute substantial amounts of the Rio Nazas to the arid lake bed. Once the canal and the reserved narrow gauge railroad were near completion, the Compañía Agricola Tlahualilo requested permission to recruit up to twenty thousand workers.[13] The planners then sought to find the ideal workers for cotton production under these capital-intensive conditions. The need for laborers experienced in cotton production framed the decision to import relevant skills, knowledge, and persons. William Ellis convinced Juan Llameda, Mexican president Porfirio Díaz's financial adviser, that southern black labor had the skills, knowledge, and the necessary productivity to transform northern Mexico.[14] He probably added that violence and political disfranchisement in the South made it more likely that black families with property and experience might more willing to leave the South for other tenuous situations.[15] In December 1894, Llameda contracted with Ellis to "fix the labor question with the aid of the Southern Negro."[16] This contract demonstrated that the financial and political elites in Mexico City believed in the profitable possibilities in skilled southern labor migration to Mexico. These relationships highlight the international dimensions of capital-intensive economic development in northern Mexico.[17]

The transformation of the dry Tlahualilo lake bed into an industrial cotton plantation was a key example of modernity at work in the Porfiriato. A consortium of local landowners and British and Spanish investors received the title to the dry lake bed in the early 1880s as part of a larger concession to develop the region for the arrival of the Texas-owned Mexican Central Railroad.[18] The company expelled the residents of the lake bed and the consortium pressed for water rights from the Rio Nazas. The Tlahualilo planners sought to build a system that would maximize efficiency and surveillance in the allocation of water, the distribution of crops and labor, and every other variable involved in cotton cultivation.[19] The company split twenty-six thousand hectares of their lake bed land into fifteen identical cotton ranches with, "absolute uniformity of dimension, both as to ditches and areas of land cultivated."[20] Each division had its own irrigation system, administration buildings, storehouses, stables, reservoirs, and worker's housing.[21] In 1895, the Compañía Agricola Tlahualilo borrowed heavily from British and American investors to build a private narrow-gauge railroad from Mapimi, Durango, to the Tlahualilo plantation.[22] The loan shifted administrative control to Juan Llameda, the director of the Mexico branch of the Bank of London and a high administrator in the Banco Nacional de Mexico.[23] The high level of debt and fixed costs made people the critical variable.

Men and women ultimately challenged the underpinnings of this complex set of financial and industrial relationships called the Compañía Agricola Tlahualilo. The families, the vast majority of whom hailed from Alabama, rejected the unexpectedly difficult working conditions and demanded that the company meet their understanding of terms of contract. The colonists mounted a campaign to defy, challenge, and resist William Ellis within the Tlahualilo plantation. The appearance of smallpox on the Hacienda Tlahualilo complicated this conflict between the black families and William Ellis. The transnational dimensions of the colonists' organizing efforts, the multinational weight of the Compañía Agricola Tlahualilo, and the presence of smallpox made the settlers a key site of interaction between Mexican, Texan, and American public health authorities.[24] Medical historian Keith Wailoo has argued that far too often scholars follow disciplinary "currents—clinical discovery, scientific theorizing and political transformation—without attention to the ways these streams flow together."[25] The combined labor of the Tuscaloosa colonists, the Tlahualilo managers, American consuls in Mexico, and bacteriologists in the USMHS provided a graceful demonstration of the ways clinical developments, medical debates, and political transformation can come together in disturbing ways.

Llameda and Ellis then worked out the kind of laborers, process of recruitment, workplace arrangements, and distribution of risk around the workers and the cotton harvest. The contract spelled out the ways the Compañía Agricola Tlahualilo would cover the costs for furnishing an infrastructure for black American sharecropping on the Tlahualilo plantation. The company agreed to provide water, land, a church, and a monthly wage of six pesos to the migrant households, and to pay for the transportation of nearly one thousand labor passengers. In return, the company planned to garnish the proceeds from Ellis over the next three years to cover the cost of the railroad. For his part, Ellis agreed to weigh the cotton, sell the cotton to the company, and distribute 50 percent of the remaining proceeds to the erstwhile colonists.[26] The company made him responsible for any debts that colonists might leave unpaid. Ellis also took responsibility for the supervision of daily labor. He also managed the rations and the company store and claimed authority over the each laborer's time on the plantation. This hierarchy meant that the Compañía Agricola Tlahualilo's vision of methodical control and reliable productivity depended on William Ellis's whim and his charismatic authority. The arrangement gave Ellis the authority to hire other laborers, have the land "properly worked," and charge the colonists any expenditures relating to the acquisition of this labor. As subsequent events will show, the colonists equated Ellis's judgment with terror, arbitrary authority, and a return to bondage. Ellis came to represent Tlahualilo to the colonists.

In return for half of the revenue generated by black workers at the Tlahualilo plantation, Ellis agreed to provide the Compañía Agricola Tlahualilo with "100 colored families, practical workers in the cultivation of cotton, in good health and in the full enjoyment of their civil rights."[27] Ellis recruited households instead of individuals because a full household would have more hands in the fields and have a higher tolerance for the risks of sharecropping in a strange land. Households would also be more reluctant to leave the plantation than individuals would. For Llameda and perhaps Ellis, the presence of families might also make black workers less likely to spend their leisure time in San Pedro or Torreon. Families might seem more respectable and less dangerous to Mexican audiences who already found the streets to be sites of danger.[28] Ellis's use of the term "practical workers" may have implied workers too pragmatic to strike or to organize.[29] A fear of political organization as well as a desire for workers who had no financial or criminal blemishes on their record likely prompted the final clause of the sentence: "in the full enjoyment of their civil rights." The demand for workers in good health reflected an awareness of the demands of cotton cultivation in the high-desert conditions of the Tlahualilo lake bed and expenses associated with medical care for agricultural workers. The contract terms revealed a mutual agreement on the ideal gender identities, health and familial status, and workplace arrangements for productive agricultural labor in Mexico.

Bringing the workers at the center of the contemporary American southern agricultural renaissance seemed the ideal solution to Ellis and Llameda.

Others in Mexico objected to the exploitation of the American race question to resolve labor problems in northern Mexico. According to *El Tiempo*, "this way of stopping the lynchings and helping get rid of a race which the Yankees detest is very harmful and disquieting to Mexico."[30] For *El Economista Mexicano* the project revealed the difference between private and national interests: "Good results for the company would result, but not for the country, because the Negro element is not acceptable from two points of view: the ethnographic and the social."[31] The article raised fears of intermarriage and miscegenation, reflecting an elite ambivalence toward *mestizaje*. Writers in central and north-central Mexico considered African Americans in northern Mexico to be a political disease, suggesting that "today the Negro cancer is one of the greatest stumbling blocks to the power of the United States." Rather than letting African Americans labor in Mexico, they thought it was "better we continue seeing our fields deserted and living with a small population than to admit North Americans of the Negro race."[32] In central Mexico, racially conservative editors believed it better to keep a northern Mexican desert than face the possibility of a class of settled black tenant farmers and smallholders within a commercial Mexican cotton economy.

The structure of black life in the foothills of Alabama shaped the colonists' anger at their situation in Tlahualilo. In 1890s central Alabama, the majority of African Americans experienced rural life and valued the kind of dignified autonomy and independence that farm ownership or even tenancy might provide. The handbill that coal miner Sam Claiborne read—distributed by Ralph Williams, Ellis's representative in Tuscaloosa—played on this value. The handbill promised each family authority over individual plots of land with the assumption that each household would be free to arrange their time and labor on this land. In return for this independence and the use of this land, the company planned to claim half of the cotton grown on each plot. Williams and the handbill promised "railroad fare, together with clothing, provisions, medicines, and all necessaries until after the cropping year."[33] When the railroad cars did arrive at the Tuscaloosa station, their presence added weight to the promise that there would be food, medicine, shelter, and tools. The railroad cars turned the future sharecroppers into potential colonists (they came from a variety of disciplines: some were farmers, artisans, and small-businesspersons). Moreover, the presence of Ralph "Peg Leg" Williams, a black labor agent and Union veteran, helped make the Tlahualilo experiment in labor seem possible and realistic. His black body and embodied presence as a Civil War veteran added flesh to the promise of "unequaled inducements for agricultural laborers for the growth of cotton and corn."[34] The colonists got on the train expecting land and freedom.[35]

The train ride probably made the rest of the handbill seem more real. The handbill promised five acres of land free to each household for their own gardens, mules, hoes, plows, and seeds. The company guaranteed one church and one schoolhouse for every hundred people and claimed the land around the plantation was full of wild game. Land had already been cleared by the company, and the handbill promised that two years of work would cover the debt incurred by the train ride.[36] Moreover, Mexico guaranteed equal rights and employers in the region valued black farm work over Chinese or Italian immigrant labor. The handbill made Mapimi and Mexico seem far friendlier and hospitable than central Alabama.[37] Peg Leg Williams touched on the hopes emerging among black southerners who experienced three years of economic depression, two years of drought, and heightened political violence. Moreover, black residents in swing counties across central Alabama experienced additional extrapolitical pressure to vote during the national election cycle in October and November 1894.[38] The train ride was a way out.

The handbill connected health, politics, and economics. The fruitful and productive environment, generous infrastructure, and welcoming political situation made Mapimi and Tlahualilo seem like a promising place to families familiar with southern rural life. When the train arrived at the plantation, the snow on the ground, the dry desertlike lake bed (in contrast to the greenery of central Alabama), the houses with no roofs, and the foul-tasting canal water at the Tlahualilo plantation was a serious blow.[39] When Ellis directed the colonists to form industrial gangs to work under his immediate supervision, he broke the fundamental promise of household autonomy encompassed within a sharecropping contract or a tenancy arrangement. Sharecropping offered the possibility that women and children could work outside the immediate gaze of an employer, and Ellis denied that possibility.[40] This was in direct conflict with the colonists' understanding of land, cotton, and freedom. In Alabama, households moved to find sharecropping arrangements with more independence. The arrangement broke the implicit promise of working for a share in the harvest for which each family risked their time, their labor, and even their American citizenship.

Labor agent Williams and other colonists with enough resources rejected the conditions and left immediately. The remaining colonists turned health

issues—the canal water, the food, and the new disease environment in Tlahualilo—into a key front in their battle with Ellis and the Compañía Agricola
Tlahualilo. People who stayed reported shooting pains rising from their feet,
chronic diarrhea, fevers, and muscle pain. "Medicine and other necessities"
became a key point of negotiation between the colonists and the management
of Tlahualilo. Large numbers refused to work until company authorities recognized and treated their illnesses and pain in a professional manner. They
also refused the attention of Francisco Modromo y Gonzalez, the Tlahualilo
company doctor. Ellis's need for their labor in the first months of planting
was so great that he demanded that Modromo y Gonzalez find a specialist in
"southern" medicine. Llameda complied and brought Dr. Henry Trollingen
from San Antonio. The physician diagnosed malaria and, like Dr. Modromo
y Gonzalez, prescribed quinine for the fevers.[41] The company translated their
demand for relevant health care into racially specific services. However, the
colonists wanted a cure, not a long treatment with quinine. Trollingen was
not what they wanted.

The speedy response gave the colonists a sense of power. This led to more
attempts to wrest autonomy from Ellis. Some colonists stopped working. As
this became increasingly popular, Ellis changed the wage structure. He offered immediate credit in the company stores for a day of labor. The colonists
seized this opportunity to work less and earn enough to keep their household alive for the week. They worked for two or three days, using the rest
of the time to tend to their corn and their sick relatives and to publicly deny
their labor to Ellis.[42] He responded violently to this humiliating attack on his
honor. He started withholding food from the company store. In addition,
he had his police force arrest key leaders and had them lassoed and dragged
"through the colony to show the balance of the Negroes the power that Ellis
has in Mexico, and especially over them."[43] Political theorist James Scott,
historian Robin D. G. Kelley, and anthropologist Devon Peña have called
strategies like "voting with your feet" (leaving) and "foot-dragging" (working to rule) important to the survival of politically vulnerable workers. Ellis's
violent and dramatic response to these "weapons of the weak" demonstrated
that these strategies did constitute open resistance.[44]

The colonists added other forms of collective resistance to their immediate refusal to work. They wrote their contacts and their elected officials in
Alabama. The colonists searched for audiences and possible actors for their
situation in Mexico and the United States. Some colonists fled the plantation

and sought federal intervention on behalf of their kin and coworkers who stayed in Tlahualilo. Sam and Emma Claiborne left their two children with trusted kin, joined a group of forty-seven colonists, and headed for Chihuahua City and El Paso.[45] The record shows that, sometime later, Sam Claiborne forced R. M. Burke, the U.S. consul in Chihuahua City, to take his deposition. The coal miner from Tuscaloosa demanded that the Department of State investigate the conditions on the Tlahualilo plantation. Burke reported that the colonists claimed that they "found themselves in the worst form of bondage with [no] hope of ever securing liberty. . . . They were cruelly deceived, the food furnished being insufficient and not fit to eat. [And] notwithstanding that many were ill—due to change of climate, mode of living, etc— they received no proper medical attendance."[46] Burke was impressed with Sam Claiborne's desire that "the story of the wrongs of his people should be presented to the Department of State."[47] They sought out U.S. authorities in Mexico and demanded their active intervention into the plantation. Claiborne effectively translated the situation in Tlahualilo to an American consul and demonstrated an understanding of the American political hierarchy in Mexico. Consul Burke also interviewed Anthony Jones, a man who considered himself the sole survivor of another group of perhaps thirty-nine colonists who had escaped the abuses of Ellis.[48] This story made its way to the *Houston Post* by early July 1895. The *Post* reported that forty-two fleeing colonists were "overtaken, and 32 of the number, including men, women and children were shot down like dogs and left dead on the ground," and that the remaining ten were "subjected to all kinds of harsh punishment and bad treatment."[49] The specific actions by Claiborne and other colonists pushed accounts of the desperate conditions in Tlahualilo across the United States. As these stories circulated through Texas and the rest of the United States, the State Department began to take an interest in the Tlahualilo colonists.

In Alabama, elected officials transformed the colonists' call for solidarity into a request for paternal federal intervention. This process involved the public participation of two elected officials. The most visible effort involved central Alabama representative William Bankhead (a Democrat). First elected in 1892 with strong populist support and some Republican crossover votes, Bankhead had faced a difficult election in 1894. Populists forced the Democrats to court the black Republican vote, despite both of their open racial misgivings. On July 9, 1895, Representative Bankhead requested a full investigation by the State Department into working conditions in Tlahualilo.[50]

He heard that "colored citizens from Alabama were induced to go to Mexico under conditions that were promised to be encouraging . . . but they are now in a destitute condition." Stating that "these poor deluded colored citizens were my constituents and I feel an interest in them," his request for an investigation encapsulated his general resentment and political dependence on word of mouth in central Alabama.[51] Although Bankhead asked for an investigation, he did not demand actual material aid. The Populist Party representative asked for a direct intervention.

The Populist Party openly advocated federal aid to small landholders and tenant farmers in their negotiations with banks, railroads, and merchants. Representative Tom Watson, the Populist Party's vice presidential candidate, went beyond Bankhead's request and demanded federal aid and cooperation to help the colonists return home:

> Late letters from those in Mexico report their condition being extremely bad, and beg their friends in the states to make all effort to get them again home. They report the climate extremely hot, and that deaths occur daily, while many are down with protracted spells, and that great suffering exists throughout the entire colony. In complying with this request to you I feel that I am in discharge of my Christian duty toward the poor (and in this instance) suffering humanity. It is true that they moved there with their eyes open, and there was nothing compulsory on the part of the government or any individual resident in this country, but by Mexican effort they were duped into it.[52]

For Watson, the colonists' desire for freedom, civil rights, dignified labor, a richer sense of citizenship, and access to property in Mexico—something the Democratic victory in the 1894 election in Alabama rendered nearly impossible for African American male residents—was foolish.[53] Since Watson did not consider the black families that left Tuscaloosa to be full adults, the colonists' self-imposed exile from the United States did not separate them from the United States. Their collective demand for federal intervention simply confirmed their second-class membership in the American body politic. Instead, Watson argued, the State Department needed to do the Christian thing and step in to protect these unfortunate black children from their desires for freedom.[54] The colonists' families in Alabama demanded federal intervention to end the daily deaths their friends and family witnessed in Durango. Bankhead and Watson transformed the colonists' call for solidarity into a

general demand for a racially specific American supervision over the Tlahualilo colonists.

The letter seems to have come during the time Tom Watson worked within
a biracial populism in Georgia and Alabama, a format that disappeared after
his experience with antiblack race-baiting and violence in the election of
1896.[55] The tone of Watson's letter to Bankhead on behalf of the colonists
carried a sense of his solidarity with the suffering of farmers as well as his
white supremacy and latent public hostility to the voting aspirations of fellow black American citizens.[56] The Democrat Bankhead and the Populist
Watson expressed tenuous and surprising solidarity for citizens who were no
longer part of their own immediate body politic. They justified cross-border
intervention into a contract and a labor dispute beyond the boundaries of
American law in Mexico.

The State Department responded to congressional pressure in Washington,
rumors in Texas, and the colonists' actions on the ground in Mexico. Edwin
Uhl, the liaison in Washington between the secretary of state and the consul
general, asked Jesse Sparks, the U.S. consul in Piedras Negras (the town opposite Eagle Pass, Texas), to investigate the "terrible stories of murder and
bad treatment of these Negroes, who still claim to be American citizens and
the protection of that government."[57] The State Department investigation of
labor conditions on a Mexican plantation posed a threat to the international
law underpinning Mexican and American sovereignty.[58] This became clear
after the consular investigation.

The investigation had two consequences. The colonists communicated
their anger with Ellis, the other supervisors, and the general working conditions in the plantation. Sparks confirmed the harsh conditions and rebellious feelings of the Tlahualilo colonists but placed the onus of the difficulties on the colonists themselves.[59] He claimed that for the colonists, life "in
a strange country, among a strange people, not speaking or understanding
the language of the country, not used to their laws or customs, and not being
accustomed to the strong alkali water and change of climate and change of
food" caused the difficulties on the Tlahualilo plantation.[60] Sparks claimed
that these environmental differences sickened the colonists and made them
"uncomfortable, uneasy and hard to manage and control."[61] Sparks thought
the weather, "taken in connection with Ellis' tyranny over these deluded Negroes, [brought] about in this colony almost open insurrection and rebellion."[62] Sparks's report transformed the labor exploitation in Tlahualilo into

an argument that the colonists simply should never have been allowed to leave the United States. The Mexican environment (not the politics of the plantation) physically harmed African American southerners. The colonists were not looking for this kind of response by official American authorities, but they were looking for a federal forum.

The consul's presence provided flesh and blood to the colonists' petitions for federal intervention on their behalf. The colonists openly rebelled the day after Sparks's departure. A group of approximately four hundred colonists left the Tlahualilo plantation and started to make their way to Torreon, Durango, twenty miles across the desert lake bed. When he heard the news, Sparks dispatched a hurried telegram to his supervisor in Washington: "Negro Colonists of Tlahualilo have revolted and left the colony."[63] The colonists' open rejection of plantation authority and the legal expectation that they were obliged to complete their side of a breached contract forced the State Department to deal with the colonists' grievances. Due to his knowledge of and possible experience with strikes at coal mines in Alabama, Sam Claiborne seemed an important presence in this collective labor action.

The mass action by the colonists transformed their difficult private relationship with the Compañía Agricola Tlahualilo into a public encounter with Mexican political authorities. This sudden shift from private disputes to a public conflict forced the State Department and the consuls to address the colonists directly, without interlocutors chosen by the company. Initially, the State Department felt no compulsion to share federal resources to guarantee the colonists' survival in Mexico.[64] These black American citizens had publicly rejected a life of sharecropping under the emerging Jim Crow system in Alabama. In addition to a search for better opportunities, they had sought a more evident freedom and equality outside the United States. This time, the cross-border rumors of four hundred openly defiant black colonists threatened the orderly facade that guaranteed capital mobility and peaceful labor in the state of Durango. The specter of a black peasant insurrection close to the Mexican border forced Sparks to request authorization "to arrange with [the Southern Pacific] railroad for their transportation home, to be paid by the government."[65] On July 20, 1895, the consul general Uhl and the secretary of state Olney refused the first request for railroad transportation, perhaps fearing the costs of an activist relationship between federal authorities and working-class U.S. citizens abroad.

Their first decision did not take into account the changes in the relationships the Tlahualilo colonists were establishing with Mexican political authorities. On their arrival to Torreon, the first city to electrify in Mexico, the group of colonists made their way to the Mexican International Railroad station. They continued their translocal campaigns, asking railroad officials and the consul for food and assistance for their return. Their situation was difficult. Torreon residents and city officials offered food and blankets. Consular officials also conveyed individual offers of employment to the colonists. Local employers offered men jobs in the local coal mines, general work for all families in the local haciendas, and domestic placement in local houses. The colonists refused all offers of individual employment and maintained their commitment to the larger group. Local doctors offered their medical assistance and in the process found smallpox. The news of smallpox transformed the colonists' relationship to the city authorities in Torreon.[66]

The authorities in Torreon had no clear way to deal with the challenge of smallpox among a group of people without Mexican citizenship. Texas newspapers reported that authorities in Torreon isolated and detained fifteen cases of smallpox and that S. J. Johnson of the Mexican Central Railroad took on the responsibility for providing food to the colonists.[67] Johnson also offered to remove the colonists to the United States if local authorities made the request. The *Houston Post* raised an alarm at the implications of this private removal for the people in Eagle Pass, for they "cannot take care of them if 800 [colonists] are turned loose on the border."[68] Consul Burke telegraphed rumors that American citizens were going to be shot in broad daylight.[69] Smallpox raised the stakes of the confrontation that linked the migrants, the city authorities, and American consular authorities. The Tlahualilo colonists, rumors of a military standoff, and smallpox made for high drama.

The discussion between the Mexican ambassador and the secretary of state reached the highest office in the United States. In a July 26, 1895, telegram to Adee at Buzzard's Bay, President Grover Cleveland offered to resolve the labor crisis if and only if there were no local resolutions:

War Department will issue rations for one week and in the meantime, if return to the colony is not practicable or consistent with humane considerations, let the consul assure the railroad company that payment for transportation of sufferers to their homes will be strongly recommended to next Congress, and probably allowed, and if such assurance will not accomplish the purpose, every possible effort must be made to pay for such transportation from emergency fund or some other fund in the State or Treasury Department.[70]

Ambassador Adee forwarded this correspondence to Consul General Sparks. The telegram from the mayor of Torreon and the president of the United States provided enough of a financial guarantee to the representatives of the Southern Pacific and its subsidiary, the Mexican International Railroad.[71] On July 26, 1895, Superintendent Comfort cabled T. M. Johnson in Torreon and gave him permission to load the colonists in Torreon and Mapimi onto boxcars to their way to Eagle Pass, Texas. Once the railroad recognized the group's collective demands, the colonists got on the train and left Tlahualilo, Mapimi, and Torreon behind.

Cleveland's memorandum opens the question of the kind of citizenship demanded by the colonists. They demanded American federal intervention into the workplace managed by Ellis based on their status as American citizens. Their demand for a robust transnational American citizenship challenged a consular vision that treated citizenship as the opportunity to enter freely into contracts. Saidiya Hartman has characterized this vision of citizenship as the liberty of contract where "freedom increasingly became defined in terms of the release from constraint."[72] This understanding relieved consular officials from any responsibility to provide a protection against self-exploitation. Yet the United States stepped in even though American citizenship was not enough.

American illness in Mexico allowed American authorities to intervene in a labor conflict in a Mexican workplace without creating a labor precedent. This act of intervention by the American president raised a difficult question for consuls and corporations in Mexico. What would it mean for the State Department to step into workplace disputes in Mexico? The two largest employers in the Laguna region were the Texas-investor-controlled and incredibly powerful Mexican Central Railroad and, in the Mapimi mines, ASARCO.[73] By acting on the migrants' demands against Tlahualilo, the State Department implicitly challenged the international border that protected entities such as the Bank of London from American view. Moreover, if American or Mexican state authorities publicly intervened on behalf of immigrant American laborers in Mexico, Mexican citizens and other nationals might demand similar interventions by their local and international authorities.[74] The possibility of more assertive laborers might jeopardize the labor arrangements that underpinned capital investments in northern Mexico. The threat of smallpox provided a way for the American federal government to respond publicly to the labor conflict without providing a precedent for other interventions into wages and workplace arrangements.

American medical intervention into this private labor dispute in Mexico added to the growing federal public health regulation of private contracts. The Immigration Act of 1893 gave the USMHS authority to inspect and quarantine any traffic across American borders.[75] The 1892 debate among health officials in Mexico City about the responsibility over quarantine demonstrated the willingness of health officials in Texas, Mexico, and the United States in the 1890s to sequester people and communities in the name of public health. The appeal of public health authority was growing across reform sectors in the United States.[76] The successful mass distribution of diphtheria antitoxin in New York City gave added weight to the power and public health interventions. The federal removal and transportation of the colonists from their situation in Torreon, Coahuila, to Eagle Pass was received positively in America. The Associated Press remarked approvingly that Grover Cleveland, "regarding the case as one of the greatest emergencies involving the lives of American citizens," had approved funds and rations for the colonists' arrival in Eagle Pass.[77] The press celebrated the presidential rescue.

The subsequent quarantine also met with American approval. When Texas State Health Officer Jack Evans inspected the first group of forty-seven and "found them all healthy" but still placed them under "quarantine with guards," the call to quarantine the colonists overrode each individual's medical situation.[78] The state of Texas treated all the colonists as possible smallpox threats. Public health overrode civil rights.

Quarantine, the Tlahualilo Colonists, and the Appearance of Modernity

In 1892, Dr. Robert Swearingen in the Palacio Nacional in Mexico City claimed that a state-directed Texas quarantine was the most effective way to protect Texas and the United States from the threat of foreign epidemics. Three years later, the arrival of the colonists at the Texas border provided the ambitious state health officer the opportunity to prove his contention. The Compañía Agricola Tlahualilo's reluctance to provide or coerce vaccination among its black laborers highlighted an indifference to the health of the laborers. In Torreon, the city authorities kept the colonists at the railroad situation, where fifteen members of their group received treatment for smallpox. The Mexican Board of Health did not consider these cases in the middle of the fastest-growing city in Mexico worthy of quarantine. The colonists' actions and militarized response by Torreon authorities forced President

Cleveland to guarantee their return to Tuscaloosa, Alabama. When the Mexican International Railroad Station manager received word that both Torreon authorities and the president of the United States had given permission to remove the colonists, the Mexican National Board of Health did not challenge the USMHS and demand authority over the colonists. The colonists' arrival in Eagle Pass challenged Texas State Health Officer Evans. Despite limited resources, the Texas State Health Office decided to treat all the colonists, not just the people suffering from smallpox, as a class apart. The state of Texas linked the colonists' smallpox and their exploited class status to a specific political identity—"Negro refugees fleeing Mexico"—and placed all the colonists in quarantine.[79]

Evans, the state health officer, could have treated people with smallpox and asked their immediate family and contacts to disinfect their belongings and wait near medical facilities until the threat of infection had passed. The colonists had taken a variety of actions to force their employers and the State Department to recognize and act on the inequities of their situation.[80] The Treasury could have denied entrance to the colonists suffering from smallpox, a situation sanctioned by the 1893 Immigration Act for noncitizens, but the hypervisibility of the colonists' (African) American citizenship in a military town meant that the Customs Office could not prevent the colonists from entering the United States.[81] Instead, Evans took a more "holistic" approach, treating all of the colonists as possible carriers and victims of smallpox and placing every (African) American migrant associated with Tlahualilo under the Eagle Pass quarantine.

The Texas quarantine demonstrated the ways Eagle Pass residents readily crossed boundaries separating healthy and sick people, citizens and residents, and commerce and quarantine. These actions exposed ongoing tensions between the Texas State Health Office, the USMHS, and the Department of the Treasury over the image of medical authority. On July 27, 1895, Consul Sparks led forty-six colonists across the river from Piedras Negras, Coahuila, to Eagle Pass, Texas. Despite the absence of smallpox among this group of colonists, Evans used the rumors of smallpox to place the colonists in the town's "pest house."[82] Within the building, Evans did not attempt to distinguish the healthy from the sick.[83] Two days later, Evans estimated that 170 more members of the settlement arrived at Eagle Pass in three boxcars. This time Fitch requested a medical examination of all boxcar passengers, and the appointed medical inspector found eight cases of smallpox.[84] It must have been obvious to all involved that Customs (part of the Department of the Treasury) and the State Health Office could not confine all 221 colonists to a 1,250-square-foot room in downtown Eagle Pass. Evans appropriated three boxcars in Eagle Pass and, at the request of Fitch, moved the boxcars to a Southern Pacific Railroad sidetrack one and a half miles south of town. After more complaints by Fitch, the boxcars and the colonists moved to a clearing three miles north of Eagle Pass, this time with two armed guards to keep the colonists in the clearing.[85] The decision to move all the arrived colonists—healthy and ill— to the northern clearing demonstrated that a racial logic undercut the medical emphasis on separating the healthy from the ill.

The question of movement between town and camp preoccupied Fitch. As the customs officer, the Treasury employee who had the authority to request the presence of a federal quarantine officer in Eagle Pass, he provided the initial terms through which the Treasury understood medical sovereignty. He was someone who regulated and monitored the movement of goods and people between Eagle Pass and Piedras Negras; his professional responsibility for well-policed boundaries translated into a chronicle of specific preventable transgressions of the boundaries of the camp. Fitch's memoranda demonstrate a concern with clear, firm, and unpenetrated boundaries. As Fitch reported on the first day, "At present there are between fifty and sixty Negroes sick with smallpox, guarded by four guards and visited by a physician once a day. The sick are separated from the well about one hundred yards and the prevailing wind comes from the infected camp. There are no guards to prevent the sick and well from intermingling and intercourse between the two camps is open."[86] For Fitch, the boundaries established by Evans between the town and the camp, between the sick and the well, and between the clearing and the rest of Texas were far too porous for his comfort. The four key points in his discussion of the detention camp buttressed his fear of the consequences of open boundaries. First, "there were no preparations made to receive and care for these Negroes, although it was known several days previous that they were coming."[87] Furthermore, "if the Negroes desired to escape there would have been no difficulty in their so doing, nor would their absence have been detected unless a large number escaped. There was no roster of the Negroes, nor was there any daily inspection and roll call."[88] Local residents interacted with the colonists, as "quite a large number of people visited the camp and were permitted by the guards to mingle with these Negroes when they were in town."[89] Finally, "at the quarantine station the Negroes were permitted to scatter up and down the stream wherever they could find shade and two guards were placed around them to prevent them from escaping. Two additional guards were placed around them when the two camps were consolidated. Peddlers of watermelon [and] vendors of bread have been seen freely mingling in the camp."[90] Fitch placed great faith in racial isolation, but Eagle Pass residents clearly treated the quarantine as a commercial opportunity. The camp was emblematic of a larger Eagle Pass informality toward modern cultural boundaries.

The Texas quarantine's porous boundaries did not draw an acceptably stark line between those who were quarantined and those who wished to sell goods to the quarantined. The clear evidence of local Mexican residents selling bread and watermelons (or *agua de sandía*) unsettled Fitch, as it reminded him that local Mexicans did not respect the same boundaries the state devised. As George Magruder pointed out, bread, bacon, and coffee were inadequate food supplies in the face of smallpox. Fitch's anger regarding transgressed medical boundaries may have been triggered by his son's discovery of ransacked and potentially infected luggage on an early-morning training run for a regional bicycle-racing meet.[91] Fitch used the theft of the belongings of some members of the second boxcar trip to indict Evans's lack of concern with isolation and other precautionary measures. As Fitch stated, "I do not believe the State Health Officer stationed at this place has a proper conception of the importance of isolation and precautionary measures."[92] Fitch made it clear that racial segregation and camp boundary maintenance were far more important than the medical well-being and civil rights of the Tlahualilo colonists.

Medical well-being was on USMHS assistant surgeon George Magruder's mind when he arrived in Eagle Pass. Magruder did not address the simmering tensions between the colonists, Evans, and Fitch. Instead, Magruder's primary emphasis in his report to the surgeon general was the style of medical care given to the detainees in the camp. Magruder wanted to know why Texas did not provide adequate medical supervision of the smallpox patients and their families: "The camp equipment consists solely of two small tents and a few dozen cooking utensils. Practically no attempt was made towards nursing or furnishing medical treatment to the sick, the management of each case is left to the individual fancy of the friends or relations and the burning of sage and drinking of yarb tea and other forms of Negro medication were in progress at the time of my visit."[93]

The patients determined that the management of their kin's disease and the medical care provided by the Tlahualilo colonists inverted the proper relationship between public health surgeon and patient. Magruder used the measures taken by the Tlahualilo colonists to comfort and care for their relatives as evidence of black anachronism. Given that this was a state-sanctioned quarantine clearing, Magruder implied that state quarantine officer Evans approved "the forms of Negro medication" adopted by the Tlahualilo colonists. Magruder was also shocked at the shelter and food provided by the Texas quarantine office. This situation created the most abject image in Assistant Surgeon Magruder's writing: "As the shadows move [the colonists] painfully change their position in a vain attempt to find relief from the burning sun."[94] The blankets brought by the colonists on their excursion back from Tlahualilo provided the only shelter from the sun. Everyone in the camp shared the same bread, bacon, and coffee regardless of their medical condition, and the people with smallpox lay under the stunted mesquite around the camp. These conditions mocked Swearingen and Bennett's earlier claims in Mexico that Texas quarantines modeled ideal health and hygiene for the United States.[95] Instead, the state quarantine became a place where customs officers, state health officers, the USMHS, the colonists, and the surrounding communities played out their various boundary disputes.

Magruder assumed that quarantine officers should provide tents, buildings, shelter, and blankets, water, certified doctors, and nurses to attend to the patients of smallpox. In an age of increasing federal authority over interstate and international commerce, the image of a clearing, blankets, no toilet facilities, and three boxcars was an embarrassment to state quarantines. The use of blankets and local mesquite trees by the colonists to shield themselves from the sun and warm themselves at night was a full abdication of medical responsibility, especially given that this was a state quarantine. The image of black family members making the primary health care decisions and providing the majority of the treatment for their relatives was even further from the contemporary racial hierarchy and modern American ideal embodied by USMHS. Moreover, sage, herb tea, and other unnamed "forms of Negro medication" formed the primary medical treatment to people with smallpox placed under a state quarantine. To Magruder, the camp itself turned the racial order of progressive white medical authority in 1895 upside down.

Magruder dismissed the treatments provided by detained family members. The American Medical Association and the American Public Health

Association had been treating all forms of "Negro medication" as part of the dangerous superstitions that kept African Americans from achieving American civilization.[96] Moreover, state medical associations across the North and South had already started using these rumors to actively exclude black doctors from their associations.[97] Sharla Fett emphasized that this fall in status for African and Native American herbal medicine in American medical cultures accelerated during Reconstruction.[98] Magruder's use of the trope "Negro medication" demonstrated a widely shared and barely voiced rejection of African and Native American herbal medicine. The use of these terms placed the self-care provided by the colonists themselves beyond the pale of the USMHS and outside the immediate reach of written history. The final incongruity in his report is his refusal to explain why the forms, treatments, regimens, and contexts for "other forms of Negro medication" were more harmful than the bread, bacon, and coffee mandated by the state of Texas. For Magruder, African American medical culture, not the immediate consequences of private and public policies, provided a better explanation of the colonists' status.

Magruder was also concerned with the power and the autonomy of the Tlahualilo colonists' actions. He recognized the desperate and unfair conditions: "The destitute condition of the Negroes, their ignorance of the country and the difficulty of crossing the creek will prevent attempts at desertion to some extent, but as soon as deaths increase it is more than likely that the survivors will become frightened and many will desert, if in fact they do not stampede as a body."[99] The acknowledgment of the distressing conditions added to the threat the colonists posed to the United States. His observation acknowledged the immediate history of collective actions taken by the Tlahualilo colonists but framed these actions within terms that tied the Tlahualilo colonists to herd animals, effectively removing references to any shared claim of citizenship. In his indictment of the colonists' self-care, he did not care to mention that there was not—and still is not—an immediate remedy for smallpox, even in official medicine. His fear of the unpoliced boundaries around the camp acknowledged the relative power of the more than two hundred Tlahualilo colonists.

The quarantine by Texas State Health Officer Jack Evans and the response by Magruder and Fitch allow a glimpse of some of their underlying tensions among state and federal agencies at the border. All three thought that the clearest source of danger to Eagle Pass was the pillaged baggage (bedding and surplus clothing) on the railroad tracks.[100] Magruder was outraged that Evans placed no guard over this baggage to protect the property of the Tlahualilo colonists against theft: "The Mexicans and lower class of whites in the vicinity" displayed a violent disregard for private property boundaries, and the baggage "was heavily pillaged to a considerable extent."[101] Eagle Pass residents had little regard for their own health. When the USMHS detained Mrs. Myers, a respectable American citizen, in Eagle Pass because of the quarantine between Eagle Pass and Piedras Negras, she asked State Health Officer Evans if she could stay in Piedras Negras "to get better hotel accommodations as the state only had a tent."[102] There she contracted a horse and wagon, crossed the Rio Grande on a local wagon bridge, and drove to the first rail depot outside Eagle Pass.[103] Respectable white women in Eagle Pass openly defied state authority, federal authority, and medical authority to avoid sharing medical facilities with black colonists and risking their privileged access to white spaces in Eagle Pass. Fitch and Magruder placed the behavior of the majority of Mexican and white residents of Eagle Pass outside the pale of medical respectability, but they never demanded a full quarantine of these non-quarantine-conforming residents of Eagle Pass.

Assistant Surgeon Magruder could not explain why local residents did not demand the widespread distribution of smallpox vaccines even though Tlahualilo colonists moved through the streets of Eagle Pass, shopping, resting, or passing the time of day while they were being held under guard in the quarantine clearings.[104] Magruder speculated that this apathy toward smallpox prevention stemmed from frequent exposure to smallpox. That is, "the frequent smallpox scares occurring across the river cause the citizens to keep themselves well protected by this means at all times."[105] At the same time, the behavior of American citizens toward the Tlahualilo colonists was indistinguishable from the Mexican residents of Eagle Pass—"and it is unusual now from the fact that the Mexican population in this part of the state has little dread of smallpox and rarely call in a physician without a cause."[106] For Magruder, concern with smallpox was a mark of American citizenship; white and Mexican apathy toward isolation in the face of smallpox made Eagle Pass seem horribly foreign.

Both Fitch and Magruder agreed that the underfunded informality of the Texas quarantine probably endangered Eagle Pass and Texas residents. Fitch focused on the traffic between local communities and the quarantine clearing, whereas Magruder measured the distance between the chaos in the clearing, the prominent place of family-based health care, and the absence of well-policed and documented medical techniques. The regional attention wrought by the debate over the Tlahualilo colonists in the Texas press was unfortunate for Evans. Even though the state was limiting emergency funds for the Tlahualilo colonists, the unhealthy and dangerous conditions in the clearing did not reflect well on Texas. Swearingen conveniently declared that Texas had almost exhausted its emergency funds and that an outbreak of yellow fever in Florida required a transfer of medical resources to the Gulf Coast.[107] At this point, Texas begged to shift authority over the Tlahualilo detainees to the USMHS. The transfer of authority allowed for improvement of material conditions and permitted the transformation of people ill with smallpox into subjects of an ambitious experiment in smallpox serum therapy.

Despite overlapping racial assumptions and American quarantine policies among the USMHS and the state of Texas, the agencies did not provide a smooth transition for the detainees. The unhealthy living conditions in the state quarantine camp contradicted the statements of cleanliness and effectiveness made by Texas State Health Officer Swearingen three years earlier in Mexico City. The movement of Eagle Pass residents and camp detainees between town and quarantine highlighted the emptiness of Swearingen's rhetoric regarding the strength of Texas quarantine. Rather than providing a model field hospital in the midst of a smallpox epidemic, the conditions in Eagle Pass demonstrated the state of Texas's refusal to provide healthy conditions for the residents of Eagle Pass as well as the Tlahualilo colonists.

Putting the Serum Therapy into Effect:
From Quarantine to Camp Jenner

The medical terms and military resources that Grover Cleveland authorized led to other, more intrusive forms of federal intervention. On their arrival to Eagle Pass, the Southern Pacific Railroad and the State Department transferred their power over the colonists to the State of Texas and the Department of the Treasury. This authority over people the State Department had labeled "Negro refugees" opened a wider and ultimately more coercive field of action. The colonists' politically isolated and socially vulnerable status on the border made them more dependent on federal largess and action. The USMHS sought to claim authority over the Tlahualilo situation in Eagle Pass through the Department of the Treasury. After Texas abdicated responsibility, Magruder took control. Surgeon General Walter Wyman described the transfer of authority as an opportunity that fell into his hands. When "the Marine Hospital Service was called upon to assume charge of the Negro colonists returning from Mexico," Wyman and J. J. Kinyoun, the director of the National Hygienic Laboratory, considered this "an opportunity not to be lost to put the serum therapy into effect."[108]

For bacteriologists in the United States in 1895, antitoxin research seemed to be the most promising way to find cures and treatment for infectious diseases. The Tlahualilo colonists had great medical value for the USMHS. Kinyoun wanted to demonstrate the general principles that explained empirically why some vaccination and serum application induced a temporary state of immunity in people.[109] Kinyoun moved from the observation that "the blood serum of an immune animal destroys the potency of vaccine lymph" to the proposition that "[the filtered blood serum of an immune animal] could be used in the treatment of smallpox."[110] The establishment of serum treatments in smallpox and vaccination would provide insight into other communicable diseases like typhus and yellow fever.[111] Sternberg, in the introduction to his 1895 monograph in immunology titled *Immunity, Protective Inoculation in Infectious Diseases and Serum Therapy*, made the following argument for smallpox serotherapy:

> We infer that the blood and tissue juices of an individual who has recently suffered an attack of smallpox or scarlet fever contains an antitoxin which would neutralize the active poison of the disease in the circulation of another person immediately after infection. Whether a small quantity of blood drawn from the veins of the protected individual would suffice to arrest the progress of the diseases mentioned, or to modify their course, can only be decided by experiment; but the experiment seems to me a legitimate one. . . . It may be that an antitoxin can be obtained from the blood of vaccinated calves which would have a curative action in smallpox.[112]

The reasoning in this passage is important. Sternberg argued for the application of serum based on an analogy drawn from experimental evidence. He was confident that someone could develop a method to obtain smallpox antitoxin obtained from the blood of vaccinated calves. The "practical application of bacteriological research" meant applying smallpox antitoxins at the earliest convenience.[113] In December 1894, Kinyoun and the USMHS started workshops in his Washington laboratory to train other American health officers in the techniques necessary to create diphtheria antitoxin. By early 1895,

Kinyoun started to apply the techniques for diphtheria antitoxin to smallpox. Newspapers applauded Kinyoun, the antitoxin, and the USMHS dissemination of the knowledge behind the products.[114] Kinyoun must have hoped that their work on smallpox might place the United States on the same stage as Robert Koch or Henri Roux once the USMHS successfully used antitoxin serum to treat smallpox cases. The timeline of events around the colonists' arrival in Eagle Pass could not be more convenient to the ambitions of the USMHS.

Dr. Kinyoun had returned from France in late November 1894 and had been actively engaged in producing Roux's antitoxin serum for diphtheria. Beginning in late February 1895, Kinyoun actively started applying diphtheria antitoxin methods to smallpox, the most visible scourge on North American soil. Kinyoun's clinical experiments with antitoxin production in 1895 built the clinical road map that led the USMHS down the path to create Camp Jenner. Kinyoun prepared his first batch of filtered smallpox serum on New York's vaccine farm on December 23, 1894.[115] He asked Dr. Elliot, the director of New York's smallpox hospital, to find patients in the early stage of smallpox. Dr. Elliot did so and injected 15 ccs of the serum into two "well developed" African American twenty-something men "with strong constitutions," despite their discomfort and fear.[116] The first patient died of a well-developed case of confluent variola. The four-serum injection had no effect on the patient's hemorrhage, his high fevers, pulse, and respiration rate, or his retention of water. The second patient survived and registered his active resistance to the seven 15 cc injections of vaccinated calf serum.[117] The New York Times reported the results, but its editorial board commented "that it was unwise to assume anything based on the improvement in one case."[118] Still, the board hoped that "further experiments" would lead to the production of "antitoxic serum which will reduce the severity of the disease at the early stages, and lower the mortality percentage for those who have failed to protect themselves by vaccination."[119] Dr. E. Wilson, the bacteriologist for the Brooklyn Health Department, completed a second field trial of the smallpox serum on three children in the Brooklyn public hospital. Dr. Wilson perceived a quicker recovery period among these children than among other non-vaccinated cases. Despite the unclear results, the serum must have seemed promising to doctors caring for smallpox patients in public hospitals. Based on the promise and acclaim of these two serotherapy experiments, Kinyoun and Sternberg thought it was time to proceed to a larger field trial.[120]

When the Treasury took authority over the Texas State quarantine in Eagle

Pass, the presence of smallpox among the colonists made Surgeon General Walter Wyman a crucial part of any federal-level conversation about the situation. According to Kinyoun, the results of clinical experiments in serotherapy conducted by him and his peers "were so flattering that belief was then entertained that we had a safe and efficient remedy for the treatment of variola."[121] On August 11, 1895, Wyman and Kinyoun assigned rising young star Dr. Milton Rosenau, the recently appointed assistant director of the National Hygienic Laboratory, to Eagle Pass, Texas.[122] Wyman and Kinyoun instructed him "to institute the treatment in a sufficient number of cases."[123] The heroic dimensions of this assignment were an open secret. The *New Orleans Picayune* celebrated the arrival of their newly adopted local hero: "Dr. Rosenau [was] especially designated to conduct scientific experiments in a new process of inoculating the smallpox virus."[124] A paper in Columbia, South Carolina, mentioned that Rosenau was "detailed to take charge of the medical arrangements at the camp."[125] In anticipation of the historic success of this treatment, the USMHS renamed the Eagle Pass smallpox quarantine site Camp Jenner.[126]

The USMHS had good medical basis to believe it could use a vaccination variant of the smallpox serum as a direct treatment. Kinyoun told the public that "his special study of Roux's methods for the treatment of diphtheria by serum injection" was "one of the great discoveries in medicine, and has passed through the experimental stage and laid a new foundation for preventive medicine."[127] Kinyoun had been hard at work establishing the same protocols for smallpox. This form of vaccination, based on the principles of immunology developed in the facilities of the USMHS, would open large possibilities in the practical applications of "rational therapeutics."[128] The name "Camp Jenner" symbolized American desire for mastery over smallpox.

These hopes for smallpox serum therapy complicated the encounter between the colonists and the USMHS. As the migrants fell under the control of the USMHS, antitoxin research transformed them from citizens to research subjects. Ironically, given their impressive defiance of the politically connected Tlahualilo Agricultural Company and the American president, their voices disappeared from the public just as their bodies' actions grew increasingly well documented. Analogous to the company's visions of industrial productivity among Alabama sharecroppers, "discipline as strict as the circumstances seemed to demand was inaugurated; system and order soon followed the chaotic conditions which had prevailed."[129] Newspapers reported that

Kinyoun was "manufacturing anti-toxine [sic] for diphtheria" and that his partner Rosenau was "hard at work attending the Negro colonists returning from Mexico."[130] The USMHS was invested in demonstrating that conditions in Camp Jenner would be different from those in the state quarantine clearing.

Within three days of transfer of control, the USMHS increased rations, brought 140 tents from Waynesville, Georgia, and placed twenty armed guards around their camps. The USMHS built a two-hundred-bed tent hospital and a fourteen-by-twenty-foot commissary to address the immediate food and medical needs in the camp. Instead of one central camp, the USMHS built four smaller detention camps in the compound and assigned each colonist, after thorough disinfection of their persons and their blankets, to one of these camps. The USMHS built a bridge across Elm Creek to direct and supervise communication between the hospital, the commissary, the detention camps, and the town of Eagle Pass.[131] Camp Jenner had its own bridge and its own borders.

The USMHS strove to document the proper gender and racial order in Camp Jenner. Rosenau photographed the camp's detainees to spotlight the high spirits of the children under detention. He also included the armed guards and the guarded perimeter in his photographs. In the process, Rosenau included local guards policing the chaparral brush around the camp, emphasizing both the professional authority and the local hierarchy of the USMHS.[132] Even the reporter from *Leslie's Weekly* emphasized the importance of this racial and near imperial hierarchy when he included a photo of Magruder in a pith helmet, leaning back on his chair. The caption simply stated, "Camp Jenner: Magruder in Charge."[133]

As a doctor with the USMHS, Rosenau was given two working objectives. The first was to treat people with smallpox to the best of his ability; the second was to test the smallpox antitoxin under field conditions—Rosenau also took the trouble to report on the returns of the federal government's investment in serum therapy research. He tabulated the fatalities that occurred in the quarantine camp run by the state of Texas as well as the illnesses that emerged in Camp Jenner under his care. The medical entries for Camp Jenner demonstrate that Rosenau compared the clinical course of people who received a vaccination to people who did not receive a vaccination. In this sense, Camp Jenner was also a field trial of serum vaccination before and after the onset of smallpox. There were 154 cases of smallpox, 137 of which were treated by the USMHS from onset to survival or death (see table 3.1). There were 52 cases of confluent variola; in these cases, the smallpox blisters

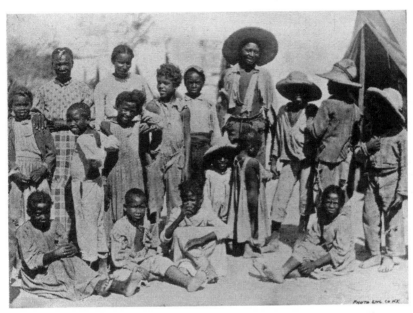

Figure 2. Milton Rosenau, Families in Camp Jenner. Milton Rosenau, "Photos of Camp Jenner" (1895), Folder 15, Series 2: Letter books, in M. J. Rosenau Papers, 1871–1940, University of North Carolina, Chapel Hill.

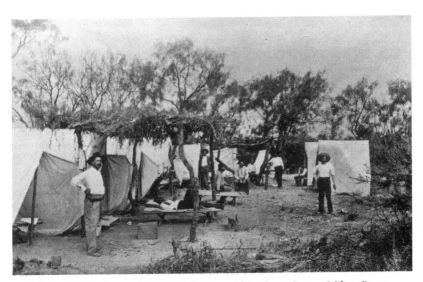

Figure 3. Milton Rosenau, Armed guards surrounding Camp Jenner. Milton Rosenau, "Photos of Camp Jenner" (1895), Folder 15, Series 2: Letter books, in M. J. Rosenau Papers, 1871–1940, University of North Carolina, Chapel Hill.

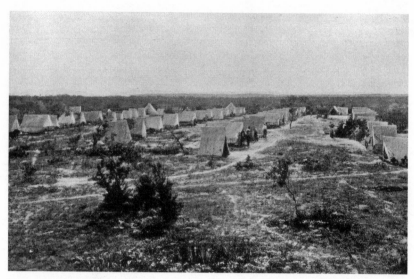

Figure 4. Milton Rosenau, Camp Jenner—an elevated view. Milton Rosenau, "Photos of Camp Jenner" (1895), Folder 15, Series 2: Letter books, in M. J. Rosenau Papers, 1871–1940, University of North Carolina, Chapel Hill.

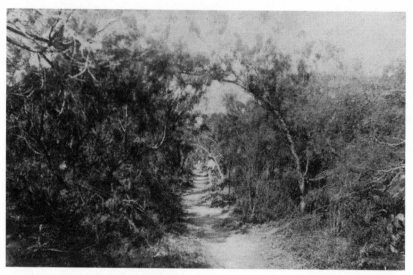

Figure 5. Milton Rosenau, Camp Jenner—guards in residence. Milton Rosenau, "Photos of Camp Jenner" (1895), Folder 15, Series 2: Letter books, in M. J. Rosenau Papers, 1871–1940, University of North Carolina, Chapel Hill.

Table 3.1. Cases of discrete, confluent, and fatal smallpox, Camp Jenner, 1895

Age of Victim	Discrete	Confluent	Fatal
Under 10 Years Old	30	2	3
Between 10 and 20	20	15	9
Between 20 and 30	18	13	6
Between 30 and 40	6	1	2
Over 40	4	4	5
Total	78	35	25

Table 3.2. Fatal cases of smallpox by vaccination status, Camp Jenner, Eagle Pass, Tex., 08/09/1895–10/18/1895

Vaccination Status	Number
Total Cases with Childhood Vaccination	5
Total Unvaccinated Cases	21
Total Successful Vaccinations with Take Recorded	10
Total Unsuccessful Vaccinations	8
Total Vaccinations with No Take Recorded	9
Total	53

Source: Milton Rosenau, "Smallpox—Some Peculiarities of Camp Jenner Epidemic—a Clinical Study of One Hundred and Thirty Seven Cases," edited by Walter Wyman, *Annual Report of the Surgeon General of the United States Marine Hospital Service for the Fiscal Year 1896* (Washington, D.C.: Government Printing Office, 1896), 235.

expanded into each other, creating larger and far more painful bleeding and inflammations. There were 71 cases of discrete variola, in which the smallpox blisters remained separate from each other. In general, a case of discrete variola had a greater chance of survival. There were 53 deaths associated with smallpox in Camp Jenner (see table 3.2).

Rosenau noted that the usMHS did not vaccinate or find any evidence of a previous vaccination among 55 of the people treated for smallpox in Camp Jenner. He also took the time to mention that the usMHS did vaccinate approximately 50 different individuals, mostly before the onset of their case of smallpox (see table 3.3). The report did not mention the vaccination status of the remaining 200 Tlahualilo detainees who did not come down with smallpox. The service probably vaccinated a number of other members of the camp, but those colonists were fortunate enough not to come down with

Table 3.3. Age, sex, and vaccination status of a sample of smallpox fatalities, Camp Jenner, Eagle Pass, Tex., 08/09/1895–10/18/1895

Name	Age	Sex	Vaccination Status
Five Cases with Childhood Vaccination			
Geener Smith	7	Female	Childhood vaccination. Scar. No vaccination status recorded.
Annie Martin	22	Female	Claimed childhood vaccination. No scar. Not vaccinated in camp.
Ella Harris	23	Female	Childhood vaccination. Scar is barely visible. No camp vaccination status recorded.
Henry Thompson	65	Male	Claimed childhood vaccination. Unsuccessfully vaccinated in camp.
Al Rosenbum	66	Male	Claimed childhood vaccination.
Seven Unvaccinated Cases			
Art Wilson	9	Male	Never vaccinated.
Will Merritt	14	Male	Never vaccinated.
Bessie Rosebun	17	Female	Never vaccinated.
Mollie Cardwell	12	Female	Never vaccinated.
W. Ellis	21	Male	Never vaccinated.
B. Wilson	38	Female	Never vaccinated.
E. P. Phillips	46	Male	Never vaccinated.
Eight Successful Vaccinations with Take Recorded			
Suberta Wilson	4	Female	Successfully vaccinated twice. 17 days and 7 days prior to onset.
Aleck Means	14	Male	Successfully vaccinated 14 and 10 days prior to onset.
Lizzie Means	17	Female	Successfully vaccinated twice within 24 days prior to onset.
Ed Hood	22	Male	Successfully vaccinated 17 and 7 days prior.
Lila McAlpin	24	Female	Successfully vaccinated 16 days prior.
Nancy Moore	25	Female	Successfully vaccinated 15 days prior.
Roxey Harris	38	Female	Successfully vaccinated 2 weeks prior to onset.
Tilly Thompson	45	Female	Successfully vaccinated twice within days of taking sick.

Source: Milton Rosenau, "Smallpox—Some Peculiarities of Camp Jenner Epidemic— a Clinical Study of One Hundred and Thirty Seven Cases," edited by Walter Wyman, *Annual Report of the Surgeon General of the United States Marine Hospital Service for the Fiscal Year 1896* (Washington, D.C.: Government Printing Office, 1896), 237–40.

smallpox. He also noted that some people received vaccinations after the onset of their infections. However, successful vaccination did not guarantee inoculation against smallpox.

This decision to vaccinate with the smallpox antitoxin after the onset of smallpox makes clinical sense only if the clinician believed that the serum vaccination might benefit the person fighting smallpox itself. Rosenau noted that there were 8 deaths among the people who were never vaccinated and 17 deaths among the people who had been given a vaccine in camp. The remaining 24 deaths were among people whose vaccination status was unclear. These fatalities were from people who came down with smallpox before the USMHS established Camp Jenner. This cohort was not directly part of the field trial of the vaccination, even though such individuals were part of the population treated in Camp Jenner. Based on the way the USMHS tabulated the medical entries, it is clear that the USMHS officers compared clinical outcomes among the Tlahualilo colonists.

Rosenau and Magruder may have had an indication that the smallpox serum could work to mitigate the harms of a more severe case of the disease, or they may have been trying to treat more severe cases with whatever means they had available. Based on the clinical entries, the USMHS-vaccinated people were slightly older than the cohort average; these individuals were also diagnosed with more advanced cases of the disease. The average age of the people who came down with smallpox in Camp Jenner was 20, while the average age of people vaccinated against smallpox in Camp Jenner was 22.65. The average age of people not vaccinated against smallpox in Camp Jenner was 16.5—a substantial difference. Among the 54 vaccinated people who came down with smallpox, there were 25 cases of confluent variola and 29 cases of discrete variola among the vaccinated.[134] There were 13 incidences of confluent variola and 41 patients of discrete variola among the unvaccinated people.[135] Rosenau referenced difficulties with the serum vaccination obliquely in his report as "some peculiarities of the Camp Jenner epidemic—a clinical study of 137 cases."[136] Of these cases under full USMHS authority, there were 25 deaths, 5 of whom received vaccinations during their illness. The USMHS provided vaccination serum to people who tended to be older and were suffering from confluent smallpox. There were substantial differences between the two cohorts. The discrepancies in the perceptions of the severity of the disease and the age of the patient with smallpox may have affected the physicians' perception of the likelihood of survival of the patient and thus their willingness to vaccinate or use the serum. Rosenau probably engaged in a bit of heroic treatment, over and against the postulates implemented by Koch and his disciples.[137]

There were substantial differences in treatment and outcome among the detainees with smallpox in Camp Jenner, but it is not clear why. Did Rosenau consider older subjects to be more fit for an experimental serum? The record says nothing on this matter. Did he think they were fit to give consent to the new treatment? If he did, why was Rosenau giving vaccinations to detainees far under the age of consent? Did Rosenau use the severity of smallpox as the key calculus for the use of the serum? This is impossible to know, since Rosenau would probably be unable to predict who would come down with smallpox after receiving a vaccination. Maybe the detainees who received vaccinations were in far worse condition than the people who were denied a Camp Jenner vaccination. Rosenau reflected on these alleged peculiarities in Camp Jenner: "Smallpox is supposed to be a more fatal disease in the Negro. The epidemic had favorable soil on which to work on, viz: a number of pure-blooded, unvaccinated negroes with vitality depressed from bad and insufficient food, and exhausted from traveling on crowded freight cars."[138] Yet, given that all the colonists shared the same miserable conditions in Tlahualilo and Eagle Pass, the racial explanation did not explain why some detainees survived and others died. The variety of clinical outcomes could have undercut the racial assumptions about this cohort of detainees. Rosenau's interventions may have been attempts to prevent deaths among the more vulnerable in this cohort. This may have been in line with the perception, echoed in the *New York Times*, that the smallpox serum could mitigate the damage associated with confluent variola among people with no immunity to smallpox or exposure to vaccination.[139] In any case, Camp Jenner was a troubling moment in Rosenau's fine career.[140]

The available Camp Jenner record is silent and unclear on these ethical and clinical matters. Rosenau and Magruder did not explain the reasons why they denied fifty-five people in Camp Jenner a potential lifesaving vaccination. They also did not explain why they were reluctant to test an experimental smallpox serum on fifty-five young people who seemed to be in relatively better health than their elders were. It is possible that these young patients rejected the vaccination, but there is also no record of resistance. In any case, the colonists, detained and dependent on the USMHS for food, shelter, and medical care, were in no condition to give their full and free consent to their treatment. In all scenarios, the record shows that Rosenau and Magruder, and by extension the USMHS, did not live up to their contemporary code of ethics to treat heroically, to observe carefully, or to intervene in a clinical outcome whenever possible. Surgeon General Wyman thought that Camp Jenner would be the place where the United States could prove that they had absorbed and improved upon the clinical principles that created the diphtheria antitoxin. Camp Jenner was at best a mix of failure and success.

Based on the clinical entries, Camp Jenner was not the site of a double-blind clinical study or a place where every patient was treated equally. The USMHS created the Camp Jenner field trial and quarantine under mixed motives: to treat smallpox among American citizens, to contain smallpox among a relatively large (racialized, stigmatized) cohort, and to test the smallpox antitoxin. Unsurprisingly, muddy medical intentions led to mixed outcomes. The effectiveness of USMHS vaccination was also inconsistent—especially for the five people who died even though they had had successful vaccinations before they came down with smallpox. Camp Jenner ended up being a place where the USMHS left American citizens "cooped up" until the State Department found a way to get the colonists back as a group to central Alabama.[141]

Leaving Camp Jenner revealed the detainee's value as workers and their threat as potential citizens to Alabama. The colonists refused to leave individually, and the mayor of Birmingham and the governor of Alabama worked to prevent their return to their home state.[142] The USMHS planned to move the detainees in late September, but the colonists refused to leave without guaranteed train travel to Alabama.[143] When one set of detainees did leave for Alabama, police at the train station in Birmingham forced all the adult males to go work as conscripts in the Campion mine in northern Alabama.[144] The USMHS stopped funding Camp Jenner in mid-October and left the detainees in the hands of people in Eagle Pass.[145] The colonists stayed in Camp Jenner nearly a month and a half after the last case of smallpox.[146] The public perception that the colonists posed a threat to Alabama overrode the USMHS certification that all the colonists were free of smallpox. Every major city between Eagle Pass and Birmingham refused to allow the colonists to disembark in their central train stations. The Southern Pacific ultimately pushed one carload off their trains in the woods between Tuscaloosa and Birmingham.[147] White authorities in Alabama tolerated their presence as long as they maintained an invisible presence as workers, not citizens.

What Is in a Name? Thinking about Race and Citizenship through the Tlahualilo Colonists

Camp Jenner complicates the picture of American citizenship that emerged in the Tlahualilo odyssey. Ostensibly, the return of the Tlahualilo colonists to Alabama reflects the recognition of the extension of American citizenship to a racial minority who had ostensibly placed themselves in exile. The colonists struggled to have the federal government take responsibility for the expenses associated with their return home. Still, the Texas quarantine, the month-long smallpox serum field trial, and the three-month-long detention of American citizens complicates any sense of mutual citizenship. The group of people who left Tuscaloosa for Mexico as U.S. citizens had hoped to become small farmers and property owners in Mexico. They returned as refugees and exiles. Throughout their travails, the colonists acted like a labor collective. They found some traction in the plethora of labels to make consistent and effective demands with the State Department, the Department of the Treasury, and the American presidency in 1895.

In the late nineteenth century, "colonist" was the polite term for families who left their homes in a collective effort to start anew in public lands in the U.S. West, California, Canada, and Mexico. The most common reference to the group of Alabama residents was also "colonists." This term is a key status category for the late nineteenth century. The label assumed that the migrants arrived in Mexico as independent property owners. For African Americans, the "colonist" metaphor also followed from the African Colonization Society (ACS), the national organization that sought to resettle black farmers in Liberia and other English-speaking African territories or West Indian and Caribbean islands. A group with white and black founders, the ACS drew support from black community activists like Henry McNeal Turner, who believed that the antiblack culture of the United States was so ingrained that America was ultimately no place for his community.[148] The ACS drew substantial financial support from white philanthropists who sought to resolve the race question "humanely" by encouraging the emigration of freedmen to places outside the United States.[149] The "colonization" label connoted that they were moved—or colonized—outside of the United States as a politically palatable solution (for white northern liberals) to the problem that working-class black men with political rights posed to the emerging American racial order after the end of slavery. White and black observers used the next label, "laborers," in conjunction with the word "Negro" and applied it in ways that described their efficiency, productivity, and disposition toward supervised labor. This word emerged in reference to contracts, especially to the migrants who wanted a share of the cotton harvest for which they had labored through the spring and summer.

The colonists implicitly or explicitly referred to themselves as citizens in their interactions with official American authorities. They consistently demanded that the "conditions akin to bondage" in Tlahualilo meant that federal authorities had to intervene on behalf of citizens. In their understanding, conditions in Mexico broke their Thirteenth and Fourteenth Amendment rights: their right not to be reenslaved and their right to be treated as Americans in Mexico. The *Houston Post* only applied the label "citizen" to the situation when Mexican political authorities threatened violence.[150] The spectacle of a violent Mexican threat may have heightened a sense of empathy among the readers of Texas newspapers with the colonists in Mexico.

The term "refugees" emerged in USMHS usage and newspaper correspondence after the Mexican Central Railroad agreed to transport the migrants north from Torreon. On July 30, 1895, the USMHS officially referred to the colonists as refugees in the title "Smallpox among Negro Refugees from Mexico."[151] On August 2, the *Los Angeles Times* used the term when it stated that there were "eighteen cases of smallpox among the refugees."[152] Medical authorities used the term "refugee" to name their relationship to and authority over people fleeing or displaced by epidemics. In 1882, Judge Tugwell called the people who fled yellow fever in Brownsville "refugees coming up from Brownsville."[153] In these cases, refugee referred to people displaced by a natural disaster—yellow fever.

The term "refugee" also cast back to the American Civil War, as it referred to the slaves who stole themselves and made way to Union lines as refugees and contraband.[154] This usage highlights the liminal status of the colonists and their dependency on the American officials and authorities for survival.[155] The term also evoked what was colloquially known as the "Freedman's Bureau" but was officially titled the Bureau of Refugees, Freedmen and Abandoned Lands. This bureau was responsible for assisting freedmen displaced by the Civil War, perhaps by helping them look for their lost family members, settle down, and find gainful employment. Congress made the agency responsible for potentially distributing abandoned lands to displaced freedmen in the South. In Tennessee and Alabama, the Freedman's Bureau created hospitals where local residents could get minimal care and vaccinations. Ultimately, the bureau's mandate was to help stateless persons progress into a state of diligent and productive citizenship. Given that the term "refugee" implied a position of dependency toward a federal agency, the addition of "Negro" to "refugee" simply underscored the power the USMHS already held over the colonists.[156] The *Houston Post* made this new power relationship very clear. They reported: "It is intimated that, aside from his going to supervise the sanitary precautions rendered necessary by the presence of a great number of refugees bound for Alabama from Mexico, Dr. Rosenau is especially designated to conduct scientific experiments in a new process of inoculating the smallpox virus."[157] The political effects of the term "refugee" were complex and volatile. USMHS officers Kinyoun, Rosenau, and Wyman referred to the colonists as "refugees" when they planned the experimental use of the migrants' bodies for professional purposes. "Refugee" indicated the colonists' internal and external displacement from the privileges of native-born citizenship promised by the Fourteenth Amendment.

Observers laced the term "Negro" or "Negroes" throughout the written record and used the term to separate the migrants from the shared web of associations, privileges, and autonomies associated with modern personhood. The *Memphis Appeal* editorialized that "the Negroes who attempted to maintain a colony in Mexico are starving and have applied to the United States government for means whereby they may get back to this country. [The situation] is another instance of the inability of the Negro to live without the white man."[158] The USMHS officers' use of the term "Negro" had powerful effects on the conditions of the migrants. Magruder discounted the mutual aid midwives and family members provided for each other in the state of Texas quarantine clearing, calling it "yarb tea."[159] Kinyoun and Rosenau also used the "Negro" label to draw physiological distinctions between the Tlahualilo colonists and the unmarked American body politic. In order to reinforce the possibility of testing vaccine serum, J. J. Kinyoun and Milton Rosenau stated that the patients were not just patients: they were "full-blooded Negroes."[160] Their previous supervisor, Assistant Surgeon General George Miller Sternberg, assumed that black laborers had more immunity to yellow fever and less immunity to smallpox than their normative white American patient.[161] The USMHS sought to develop race-specific remedies to overcome the alleged "Negro" susceptibility to smallpox.

Some African Americans used the term "Negro" as a self-reference.

William Ellis, the African American community activist, businessman, and Tlahualilo labor agent, illustrated the complications that ensued when the term's self-reference obscured an unequal access to power among those who used the term to describe themselves. When Ellis made statements such as "The Negro could not govern himself and had no respect for the authority vested in a Negro [like himself]," he simultaneously placed himself alongside, separated himself from, and placed himself over the colonists in his descriptions.[162] When his black supervisors "attempted to arrest a Negro for a minor offence, they were always surrounded by a mob and forced to release the prisoner."[163] For Ellis, this community solidarity among black workers in Tlahualilo poisoned proper employee hierarchies and led to consistent political mobilization, another drag on labor productivity. Political mobilization was part of a larger tragic flaw that did not augur well for the future of black communities in the United States. The federally sponsored return of the Tlahualilo colonists meant that "Negroes were destined to remain in the United States where increasing race troubles portend ultimately the extinction of the Negro."[164] As someone who styled himself a leader across African American communities, Ellis assumed readers would make the distinction between respectable and unrespectable members in the African American community and place him within the respectable segment. He posited that there was something essentially wrong in African American communities if more than four hundred colonists rebelled against (his) black political authority on a plantation in Mexico. Like Rosenau and Kinyoun, he blamed the failure of his project on the colonists.

For letter writers in the African American national community who were able to place their opinion in the mainstream press, the term "Negro" was a counterpoint to Ellis's criminal actions. In Memphis, a letter writer proclaimed: "Hardly any punishment would be too severe for the deception practiced upon Southern Negroes in the Mexican colonization scheme."[165] Rumors of Ellis's presence brought black communities together in San Antonio when "considerable excitement was created . . . among the colored citizens of San Antonio by the report that Ellis of San Antonio who is said to have gotten the Negro colony to go to Mapimi, Mexico" was passing once again through Texas.[166] William Ellis's callous exploitation of black men, women, and children pushed him beyond the boundaries of decency and solidarity in the African American press.

There were other forms of self-reference when reporters discussed community solidarity across borders. The terms included "colored," "citizens," and "Baptists." For example, "John Clemons, a leading Negro citizen, received a dispatch from John Mitchell, one of the colonists of Mapimi, saying, 'One hundred of us here starving. Can you help us?' Efforts are being made by some of the churches to do something for them."[167] President Abner of the Colored Baptist Association "appeared before the association and explained the condition of the colored people in Mexico. The president talked on the subject of these negroes abroad for about an hour, and their bad condition in Mexico."[168] According to a *Post* reporter in Luling, Texas, "The Negroes all over this region are giving suppers and by other means raising money for the Negro colonists quarantined at Eagle Pass."[169] The labels were part of the networks that linked black, white, and Mexican communities across the nation to Tlahualilo, Eagle Pass, the State Department, and the USMHS. Ellis, the Compañía Agricola Tlahualilo, the State Department, and the USMHS used the terms to justify their interest in skilled cotton labor, their unfair workplace practices, their indifference to the situation in Tlahualilo, their reluctance to negotiate directly with the Tlahualilo colonists, and their intrusive field trial. The dramatic conditions and the use of the terms "Negro," "Colored," and "colonists" also triggered acts of solidarity within African American, Mexican, and American communities with the Tlahualilo colonists.

There remains a question regarding material conditions that maintained the term "colonists." Were the 866 people who signed the railroad manifest in January 1895 in Alabama ever in a position to embody the many meanings of the term "colonists"? Compared to the homesteaders who sought to colonize (settle on) the public lands of the American West, the Tlahualilo colonists did not have access, hope, or the unsupervised time to aim to own land in the general Tlahualilo vicinity (see table 3.4). John Mason Hart, in his analysis of the nineteenth-century movement of American capital and people to Mexico, has argued that American colonists "who had experienced 'marginalization' in the United States became 'Americans' in Mexico."[170] This status depended on a number of contextual variables. The colonists analyzed by Hart arrived with legal titles as property owners to their land. There was no daily oversight of their labor by a supervisor. They received the full amount of the proceeds of the harvest, regardless of how meager or bountiful it may have been. The record of their presence is throughout consular documents, as consuls regularly stepped in to demand the enforcement of title and con-

Table 3.4. Comparison of American colonists to Mexico and African American colonists at Tlahualilo

Category	American Colonists in Mexico	African American Colonists in Tlahualilo
Property	Arrived with land titles	Arrived as sharecroppers
Labor	No daily labor supervision	Placed in supervised gangs
Self-employment	Received the full amount of their proceeds	Had no control over the cotton harvest
Labor Rights	Contracts enforced by the intervention of U.S. consuls	Broke labor law, contract law, and the general rules of respectability
Federal Representation	Most registered with the U.S. consul	Demanded citizenship from the consul in Torreón
Mobility	Free to go, capital allowing	Escorted by city authorities to boxcars

Source: For general colonists, John Mason Hart, *Empire and Revolution: Americans in Mexico since the Civil War* (Berkeley: University of California Press, 2002), 113–14, 117, 166, 183, 188, 237–38, 248–55, 263, 283, 290, 304, 382, 513, 515.

tracts in Mexico.[171] Colonists and the local consul made note of each other's presence upon their arrival. Finally, they were all free to move if they could absorb the cost of abandoning their land and moving.[172]

In contrast, the Tlahualilo colonists arrived as sharecroppers and Ellis placed them in industrial gangs to clear and plant cotton in a dry lake bed. The Tlahualilo colonists depended on the company store for their food and shelter needs, placing an additional financial burden on their situation. Half of their proceeds went to Ellis, even before he would take amounts to cover food, shelter, and the railroad trip to Mexico. The consul in Torreon was openly skeptical of their claims; their activities in Torreon forced the consuls to offer support. Upon their arrival to the United States, the state of Texas, and the states of Louisiana and Alabama, state authorities imposed a quarantine and an embargo on all the Tlahualilo colonists regardless of their smallpox status. The term "colonist" was a point of pride and a category of American status that the Alabama cohort never enjoyed in Mexico.

Observers moved the Tlahualilo colonists and Camp Jenner into a national debate over the future status of citizenship for African American communities. The visibility of federal medical intervention in Camp Jenner provided an ugly medico-racial dimension to the debate over the character and nature of African Americans. Company doctor Francisco Modromo y Gonzalez emphasized the healthy landscape under the Compañía Agricola Tlahualilo's control: "It is certain that the food and usual drink (water) had little or no influence among the colonists; that the causes producing the first disease were change of climate and a wasting moral affliction of the mind."[173] Sparks, the consul who completed the first investigation, emphasized the difference between black southern migrants and a foreign Mexican environment. Rather than discussing the harsh and violent work conditions in the plantation or the absence of vaccination, Sparks drew a hard environmental line between black (and not white) emigrants and the Mexican context. The difference between a brown landscape and black laborers meant that the colonists were "uncomfortable, uneasy and hard to manage and control."[174] Modromo and Sparks concluded that inappropriate labor recruitment, not abusive management and labor mobilization, lay behind the rebellion.

The failure also led to more disturbing claims about the rightful place of African Americans in the Americas. Major Dwyer, the State Department investigator charged with designating responsibility for the costs of the railroad, concluded that "[when people] go as colonists to another country [they] should expect a different food and a certain amount of rough experience."[175] His comment implicitly placed responsibility for adjustment to the new workplace conditions on the migrants themselves. The *San Antonio Express* editorial board extended this argument. African Americans "had been unwilling emigrants to the United States, [but] they have become a part of the life of the nation," and thus the nation has a special paternal relationship to their presence. Further, "even though the colonists forfeited their citizenship by leaving the United States to settle in Mexico, the burden of American responsibility should be extended to rescue the colonists of Tlahualilo from their attempt to establish an independent existence."[176] In this vision of the U.S. political community, it was the responsibility of federal authorities to free the freedmen and freedwomen of their delusions of independence and self-ownership. As the *Birmingham Age Herald* noted, "The press both North and South charged with more triumph than pity, declare Negroes as colonists are and always have been a failure, which is the equivalent that, a Negro is incapable of self-government."[177] As historian Alfred W. Reynolds noted in 1953, "The Tlahualilo project was doomed" because of the "indiscriminate selection of inferior grade emigrants, lack of accustomed southern white supervision, a new and strange environment, cruel treatment, nostalgia, loneliness and despondency."[178] These writers used Tlahualilo as a mandate for racial domination.

Other observers emphasized structural conditions over racial distinctions in the debate over the proper place for African Americans. Knight Render noted the definite power differences between (Mexican) colonists and the Tlahualilo workplace: "You cannot colonize any race of people in Mexico or anywhere else where they are subject to such inconveniences and unsuitable food such as Ellis' colonists."[179] To ascribe the experience of the migrants in Mexico as a process of becoming "citizens abroad" both ignores the terms of the relationships in which they were embedded in the Tlahualilo company and dismisses the extent of the challenge colonists posed to the emerging racial orders in Alabama, Torreon, and Eagle Pass.

The migrants arrived in a region where investors in Mexico City, London, and New York were transforming the land titles and landscapes for their own benefit. The Mexican Central Railroad, an entity created and controlled by James Stillman of Texas between 1880 and 1900, connected mineral and agricultural resources to industrial markets across the South.[180] The migrants' demand for the recognition of their complicated situation endangered the seamless web of inputs envisioned by elite interests in Texas, Mexico City, and New York. The railroad-led movement of citizens and capital involved political resources, political permissions, and local policing. The uprising in Tlahualilo exposed the taken-for-granted nature of these relations within North America.

As the last of the Tlahualilo colonists were finally able to leave Camp Jenner and make their way back to their families in the foothills of central Alabama, the Atlanta Cotton Exposition was inviting the world to celebrate the achievements of the Cotton South. The cotton exposition and the Alabama quarantines against the colonists accentuated the growing confidence state and city governments had about managing and expanding racial segregation within their political territories. When Booker T. Washington exhorted his fellow southerners at the Atlanta Cotton Exposition in 1895, "Cast your bucket where you are, go not into a foreign land," the Tlahualilo colonists may have been his most recent example of the latter. The vivid images and volatile polemics around Tlahualilo must have weighed heavily on his mind.

Camp Jenner Legacies: On Quarantine, Citizenship, and the Appearance of Progress

Quarantines had become a key component of sovereignty in the Americas. The heated debate over quarantines in Mexico City followed from the relatively recent acceptance of isolation as a disease prevention measure in the

United States, Mexico, and Texas. Quarantines gave public health agencies an opportunity to project professional authority at key traffic hubs. As Camp Jenner made very clear, a quarantine was not just a detention site or a way to block traffic between affected and unaffected spaces—it was also a site where public health professionals could implement or test the latest innovations in the prevention and treatment of infectious disease. The previous year, Kinyoun, the director of the National Hygienic Laboratory, had been intimately involved in the successful transfer of diphtheria antitoxin techniques from Germany and France to the United States. The possibility of a smallpox antitoxin serum was a clear priority. The news that there were possibly more than two hundred medical detainees at the Texas border, some of whom had already come down with smallpox, gave the impression of near ideal trial conditions for a highly desired smallpox antitoxin serum. The control over people and the space of a field hospital in the midst of a quarantine allowed public health service officials to tinker more freely with disease prevention and disease treatment options. The Camp Jenner quarantine marked an expansion in the meaning of "quarantine" from temporary detention to a place for experimentation.

This shift in the meaning of "quarantine" is more obvious in the use of the term "vaccination." The record of successful vaccinations in patients who subsequently died of smallpox within a few days challenges our understanding of this medical concept. The public use of the term "vaccination" rather than "serum therapy" or "antitoxin" reflects the way journalists translated germ therapy into lay terms. It also demonstrates a potential professional discomfort around the deployment of untested immunological techniques among USMHS surgeons Kinyoun, Rosenau, and Magruder. The USMHS abandoned the camp on October 21, 1895, weeks before the colonists received presidential approval for their return to Alabama. Camp Jenner did not yield the measure of progress for the antitoxin serum that the service desired. The USMHS exit dramatizes the extent to which resources for the colonists depended on the success of the field trial.

The travails of the colonists across Mexico and the United States exposed the distance between the rhetoric and the practice of quarantine in Mexico, Texas, and the U.S. border. In Mexico City, Swearingen, Bell, and Liceaga defended the quarantines as the frontline of defense against the threat of epidemic disease. Liceaga imported the latest disinfection ovens from France and placed them in quarantine and inspection stations in Veracruz and Nuevo Laredo to stage working demonstrations of a coming medical modernity. The state of Texas built quarantine stations in Galveston, Port Aransas, and Texarkana to demonstrate their commitment to hold Mexican and Cuban yellow fever at bay. The USMHS set up inspection stations in New York City, New Orleans, and San Francisco to intercept typhus and smallpox among Asian and European passengers. When the colonists started actions to hold the Compañía Agricola Tlahualilo responsible for their illnesses, Mexican federal health officers refused to address the conditions in Tlahualilo. The Texas State Health Office only provided food and blankets in their quarantine in Eagle Pass. The Tlahualilo colonists, and not the quarantine officers in Mexico, took the first step to defend against illness. They forced the Compañía Agricola Tlahualilo, the mayor of Torreon, the State Department, the USMHS, and, ultimately, the president of the United States to act on their behalf.

The saga of Camp Jenner also illustrates the way the medical border followed people and did not stop at physical borders. The decision to implement selective vaccination in Camp Jenner demonstrated the medical value accruing to live human bodies under an antitoxin serum regime. The use of quarantined citizens in a field trial at Eagle Pass was what the USMHS practiced in the public smallpox hospitals on the East Coast but on a much larger scale. Similarly, the colonists demanded that the federal government treat their grievances against the Compañía Agricola Tlahualilo collectively. Their collective demands on American federal authorities in Mexico forced the federal government to treat individual colonists as a group, but the USMHS called the group "negro refugees." The use of the quarantined black colonists for the field trial was very distinct from their demand for justice. The USMHS found it difficult to separate the colonists' demands for justice from the opportunity for medical intervention.

The rhetoric of humanitarian intervention shaped the public memories of Camp Jenner. White southern newspapers justified the vast intervention because of what they called the special relationship between African Americans and the South. Black newspapers such as the *Austin Herald* countered that the problem "should concern every citizen," not just African Americans.[181] The USMHS presented Camp Jenner as a humanitarian intervention. Dr. Jerrold Michael repeated this narrative nearly one hundred years later at the graduation ceremony of the Public Health Service Corps when he called Camp Jenner "an episode from the Public Health Service's proud past."[182]

The Tlahualilo colonists and Camp Jenner provided a compelling example of the ways railroads were transforming the relationship between the border, Mexico, and the United States. The colonists knew that there was a contract waiting for them in northern Mexico when a Southern Pacific Railroad car picked them up in Tuscaloosa, Alabama. The colonists took up residence in Torreon around the rail depot for the Mexican International Railroad, a Southern Pacific subsidiary. The direct negotiations for their return to the United States and then to Alabama occurred between the presidential and Southern Pacific Railroad representatives. Agent Johnson would not allow the colonists to board a car without a telegram from the State Department that authorized reimbursement from the federal government. As the colonists refused to leave Eagle Pass in small groups, the Southern Pacific demanded promise of payment from the presidency before they allowed the colonists to get on a train to Alabama. The presence of Camp Jenner gave a vivid illustration of the need to have a medical check on the traffic moving across the Mexican border. Railroads, as much as germs, were binding the human race together. The railroad, by deciding whether the colonists could leave, also created distinctions among passengers and freight. Power flowed along railroad lines.

The political difficulties of quarantine became more evident when the USMHS sought to work with local populations. The detention of friends and neighbors was far more difficult than the detention of black, politically estranged workers. Quarantine transformed the relationship between border residents and the federal government, strengthening the ties between established sectors of border society and tearing at the looser ties connecting the more recent settlers living at the border. Would the presence of quarantine affect all communities at the border equally? In what ways would quarantine affect the federal relationship to black, Mexican, and Mexican American communities at the border? What if the place of medical treatment became a point of contention? Could open resistance strain or facilitate the operation of power at the border? The next chapter examines the growing tensions in the political culture of quarantine in the aftermath of the War of 1898.

Resistance does not refer only to the fight that individuals, or collections of them, put up at any given time against those trying to impose on them. It refers also to the historical outcome of the struggle that has gone before, perhaps long enough before to have been hallowed by custom or formalized in law.—Barbara J. Fields

FOUR

The Power of Progress

Laredo and the Limits of Federal
Quarantines, 1898–1903

Four days into a state-mandated smallpox quarantine on Laredo, Justo Saunders Penn picked up a handbill left at the door of the *Laredo Times*. When he read the handbill's lead, "Protest against Forcible Vaccination," and its first sentence, "We energetically protest against the municipal regulations issued by the mayor of the city on the fourteenth of the present month, commanding that all the inhabitants of whatever age, sex or race be vaccinated," he was shocked.[1] He decided to translate the full handbill for his English-language readers in the *Laredo Times*, prefacing the text with the warning that they were about to read shocking material. Without a shred of irony regarding his unrequested distribution of the contents of the handbill, Justo Saunders Penn demanded that "such a matter at this critical moment should be immediately suppressed, [because] such a paper can only be calculated to occasion dissatisfaction and create serious trouble."[2] The handbill detailed the reasons that the petitioners thought the city vaccination order was personally intrusive, medically inadvisable, openly discriminatory, hostile to a Mexican presence in Laredo, and possibly subject to reform. The petitioners openly called for the Mexico-Texas population to use the vote in the upcoming election to punish the people supporting coercive and racially targeting public health policies. Laredo *Times* editor Penn may have been implicated in the last sentence of the handbill: "We are told that such proceedings on the part of the men in power are for the purpose of pursuing political ends, but we do not wish to believe this, because it is an infamous crime to traffic with the health, the life, with the honor and with the peace of families for political purposes."[3] Maybe this is what was particularly outrageous about the handbill. For Penn, a member of the small but powerful Anglo-American minority population in Laredo, this call for a unified political response by the town's Mexican voters may have been the most powerful dimension of the flyer. The residents of Laredo probably viewed this complicated conflict over the proper care of smallpox in terms alien to the American national press.

The election process continued despite the establishment of a state quarantine and the deaths and injuries that came with the Laredo smallpox riot that came on the heels of the quarantine. The voters in Laredo elected to the office of mayor the opposition candidate—(U.S.-born) rancher, merchant, and council member Antonio M. Vidaurri—instead of reelecting (one-time French national) rancher, merchant, and council member Louis Christen, the mayor initially in charge of the quarantine. The Associated Press reported that only two weeks after the smallpox riot, the voters had the gall to vote in a "Mexican mayor at Laredo."[4] This free-floating Mexican/American binary threatened the ability of American observers to connect with people affected by the epidemic and the quarantine in Laredo.

Between 1898 and 1903, the medical orientation of the ethnic Mexican majorities in Laredo grew in symbolic importance to American national politics. Three days after Penn picked up the antivaccination handbill in the streets of Laredo, the medical demands of the Agapito Herrera family catalyzed a near open battle between the Herrera family and the residents of the Zacate Creek neighborhood against volunteer inspectors, the city police, the Texas Rangers, and the (black) Tenth Cavalry divisions.[5] The ensuing military occupation of Laredo, called either the Smallpox War or the Laredo Smallpox Riot, aimed to guarantee cooperation among all families with the requirements of quarantine. Harrison Gray Otis of the *Los Angeles Times* observed that "Laredo, Tex, as a riot center, appears to be trotting Havana Cuba a close second," a statement that nicely connected the Mexican border to the imperial theaters of the Caribbean and the Pacific.[6] Otis did not stop there. The next day he wrote, "Those Mexicans at Laredo will probably come to the conclusion that it is nicer to be vaccinated in the regular way than with a Gatling gun," another suggestion that quickly bridged the coercive dimensions of state vaccination to the violent subjugation of resistant ethnic cultures in the aftermath of the Spanish-American War and the Indian Wars.[7] The national coverage implied that Mexican families had a hostile relationship to an implicitly American medical modernity.

Four years later, Laredo returned to a prominent position in American public health annals. The new U.S. Public Health and Marine Hospital Service (USPHMHS) sought to implement the first U.S.-based mosquito eradication campaign against yellow fever in Laredo, but local families refused to cooperate with American public health officers. This quiet resistance led a Cuban-born American USPHMHS officer to conclude, "The people endeavor to conceal the fact that any of their family is sick, as they have an antipathy for the American physicians, some of the more ignorant even going so far as to claim that the Americans would give them medicine to poison them."[8] American federal authorities desired full cooperation with modern forms of quarantine and treatment. The power behind this desire contributed to difficult and violent debates over the boundaries of public medical authority and individual household prerogatives in the city. Border quarantines became another example of ethnic resistance to American modernity, a story familiar to readers knowledgeable about the Indian Wars and the American occupation of Cuba, Puerto Rico, and the Philippines.[9]

However, people sought ways to maintain patient autonomy in the face of quarantine, building alternative medical venues for the Mexican majority living in the lower Rio Grande Valley. Both post-1898 American medical projects required Mexican and Mexican American cooperation for their success; a number of Mexican families sought to maintain a measure of independence in the face of these new medical borders. The American need for symbolic Mexican cooperation, to extend Nayan Shah's notion of "queer domesticity," created a powerful state desire to transgress private Mexican household boundaries and punish what the multiethnic authorities perceived to be a dangerous domesticity among working-class Mexican and Texas-Mexican households in Laredo.[10]

The Spanish-American War transformed the place of the 1899 smallpox quarantine and the 1903 yellow fever epidemic in Laredo in American culture. Scholars who have engaged the Laredo Smallpox Riot have emphasized the distance between American national ideals, multicultural Laredo, and Mexican popular culture in Laredo. In his 1935 hagiography of the Texas Rangers, Walter Prescott Webb used the presence of a small contingent of Texas Rangers during the smallpox riot to maintain the "one riot, one ranger" narrative that suffused his monograph, *Texas Rangers: A Century of Frontier*

Defense.[11] Arnoldo de Leon emphasized what he saw as the larger aims of the quarantine; it was "especially directed toward *Mexicanos,* its purpose was to prevent cotton pickers with the disease from migrating into the states from the border region."[12] Emphasizing that the smallpox war "was but one of the many frontier eruptions that dramatized the cultural gulf separating the Mexican majority from the Anglo minority," Robert Utley returned to the way in which the residents of Zacate Creek outnumbered the Texas Rangers, implying a near innate hostility between Mexicans and the Rangers. In James K. Leiker's impressive analysis of African American soldiers' place in the making of the modern Mexican border, the Laredo Smallpox Riot anchors an extended analysis of the social, legal, and military hostilities between black soldiers and their Mexican American neighbors along the Rio Grande. For Leiker, the call by Laredo city authorities for "the Negro soldiers" in the Tenth Cavalry in Fort McIntosh was the paradigmatic example of the ways black soldiers rescued the (white) Texas Rangers from a Mexican (American) threat, after being called by (Anglo and Mexican) city authorities at the border.[13] The Laredo Smallpox Riot underlined the ways African American soldiers with power complicated the binary Anglo-Mexican analyses of the Texas-Mexico border. This was politically different from the Camp Jenner experience in 1895, where the absence of open conflict turned Camp Jenner into "an excellent example of the beneficent influence of the Marine Hospital Service married to its military power."[14] The American victory over Spain in 1898 and the ongoing occupations of Cuba, Puerto Rico, and the Philippines forged an even more intimate link between American military and medical power at the Texas border.

The yellow fever epidemic of 1903 at Laredo drew military and medical authorities even closer together. In 1902, the USMHS was at the height of its public authority. Walter Reed effectively demonstrated that yellow fever had a mosquito vector.[15] William Crawford Gorgas ran a mosquito eradication campaign in Havana, Cuba, that prevented the reappearance of the annual yellow fever epidemic.[16] Margaret Humphreys emphasized the way the fever appeared on the heels of the public health victory against yellow fever in Havana as well as the expansion of USMHS power to include quarantine authority and the gathering of national vital statistics. Humphreys argued that "the newly named Public Health and Marine Hospital Service was soon furnished the opportunity to display its competence in controlling yet another yellow fever epidemic, this time in Laredo, Texas."[17] Humphreys touched on the resistance many locals gave against the USPHMHS, a resistance that enabled Gregorio Guiteras, the quarantine coordinator, to claim that "large parts of the people, particularly the ignorant class, were filled with the idea that the physicians and the authorities were in a conspiracy against them."[18] Mariola Espinosa pointed out how Guiteras used his experience with the astonishing authority wielded by Mexican working classes in Laredo to call for "martial law at the beginning of a disease outbreak."[19] The military dimensions of these interventions brought national identity to the fore. However, as there were ethnic Mexicans on all sides of the official and popular dimensions of public health conflicts in Laredo, the attempt to turn these difficult tensions into American/Mexican conflicts obscures the racial and class complexities that undergirded the American staging of public health in Laredo. Mexicans were on all sides of the American/Mexican split being re-created in these two epidemics.

Bringing the New Public Health Back to the Border

Laredo grew drastically between 1880 and 1900. The Mexican Central Railroad, the Texas-Mexican Railroad, and the International & Great Northern (I&GN) Railroad lines all met in Laredo, making it the key railroad hub between Mexico and the United States at the turn of the twentieth century. The population of the town changed alongside this economic boom, increasing from 15,000 in 1890 to 22,000 in 1900. Laredo's native-born white population grew at a slightly quicker rate (from 6,913 to 10,697) than its mostly Mexican foreign-born population (7,918 to 11,034).[20] Historian Elliott Young connects the presence of the white Anglo population to the commercial establishments associated with the railroads.[21] Although the Villegas de Magnon family is a good example of a Mexican elite establishing a base within Laredo commerce in the 1890s, the vast majority of Mexican settlers in the 1890s settled on the outskirts of town. Many recent settlers cobbled together their houses—their *jacales*—from tin, adobe, tree branches, and local firewood.[22] A visible number settled on the east side of downtown, just past Zacate Creek, living between the tannery and the railroad yards. Fort McIntosh, on the west side of town, housed a variety of American infantries. The Tenth Cavalry had been stationed in Laredo since 1895 and had been employed to ensure that Mexican insurgencies would not disrupt law and order on the American side of the river. The threat of unrest led to the now seemingly permanent presence of black troops at the Laredo border since the 1890s.[23] By 1890, there were

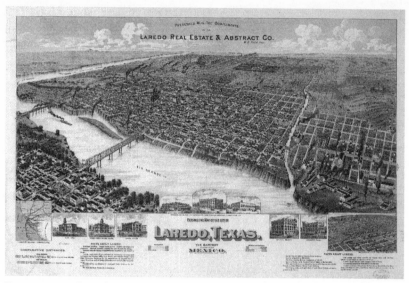

Figure 6. Map of Laredo, 1892, Courtesy of the Maps Division of the Library of Congress. "Perspective Map of Laredo," American Publishing Co. (Milwaukee, Wis.), 1892, g40341 pm009180, hdl.loc.gov/loc.gmd/g40341.pm009180 (accessed March 30, 2011).

slightly more than two hundred African Americans living in Laredo, working in the businesses associated with supporting troops during their leisure time. The eastern and western margins of Laredo were visibly different from the Anglo and Mexican business district. Concern with smallpox connected the margin to the center.

Although Laredo had experience with smallpox cases, the perception in early February 1899 was that there seemed to be substantially more cases than in previous epidemics. The city council passed resolutions that placed more medical authority in the hands of people associated with city hall. On February 1, 1899, the council faced increasing numbers of smallpox cases despite local police enforcement of smallpox detention measures. The council and the Laredo Businessmen's Club also feared that the state of Texas might impose a smallpox quarantine on the full city. In a well-publicized vote, the Laredo City Council decided to change its approach to smallpox prevention, to do unto its residents what it feared the state of Texas might do to Laredo.[24] The council charged the house guards (security for city hall) "to formulate themselves into a corps of health inspectors to make it their personal business to look after the sick and see that requirements are lived up to."[25] These one-time security guards inspected everyone who was rumored to be ill, placed a yellow flag outside the houses of those who were infected with smallpox, and ensured that no one entered any quarantined house. The council also gave volunteers, council members, and city hall employees nearly unquestioned authority to inspect, isolate, and detain Laredo residents under suspicion of smallpox. These public policies relied on a civic-minded and intrusive performance of middle-class respectability.

This middle-class response to smallpox carried along an impulse to contain, segregate, and isolate other people. The key problem for this project was the presence of voters and city employees among the people targeted for inspection and isolation. This enfranchisement complicated the humiliating dimension of the isolation and detention measures. The quarantine looked Mexican-specific outside Laredo, but ethnic Mexican participation on all sides of the quarantine policies challenged the racial logic of quarantine. This dimension of potential political equality complicated the free enforcement of disease measures.

The universal measures centralized authority in the mayor's office. The mayor and city physician — and not the city council — appointed the health inspectors. Public participation and ownership over the power of inspection increased, giving select town residents official authority to enter any house "when they reason to believe a nuisance may exist," thus giving these public-spirited individuals the authority to designate healthy and ill spaces. The definition of nuisance in the city council mandate was also broad: "anything whatever that may be liable or about to become liable, to affect the health and comfort of the city of Laredo."[26] The local press was happy to connect these liabilities to the possibility of smallpox. As the *Chaparral* reported, "There is a case of smallpox on San Bernardo Avenue, near the Corpus Tract, in a house that would make a better summer henhouse."[27] Two weeks later, the *Chaparral* wrote that "authorities have allowed — or not prevented — to become eyesores to the public, beside most proper pest quarantining places for smallpox and anything else. . . . These wooden *jacals* are built way up into the middle of town."[28] The *Chaparral* explicitly connected *jacales* to the threat of smallpox, arguing for the removal of these residences — and implicitly their residents — from the city limits of Laredo. By February 18, the *Laredo Times* and the *Chaparral* published lurid descriptions of working-class residences that transformed the aesthetics of a house into a literal pox on the landscape of Laredo. In this growing town of fifteen thousand people, designation as an inspector confirmed who belonged in the highly visible circles of power in a small town. The transfer of authority gave volunteers and security guards the ability to humiliate or exclude people from the fully enfranchised community of Laredo on allegedly medical grounds. The policies associated with smallpox containment became an ideal stage to assert a medically certified, public-spirited, and potentially coercive identity over others in Laredo.

These medically certified public identities started appearing in the *Laredo Times*. The smallpox epidemic increased the level of scrutiny of domestic matters among people whose public lives normally made the local paper. This scrutiny gave some private responses to the threat of smallpox a patriotic sheen and identity. Some residents may have registered their discomfort with the threatening intrusion of inspectors by openly taking on the responsibility of fumigation and vaccination in their households. The local press turned these decisions to withdraw and self-medicate into evidence of public participation. The *Chaparral* reported that Reverend Mcmurry was fumigating his home, a private event suddenly turned public. The *Laredo Times* reported the cancellation of the Casino Mexicano's Fancy Dress Ball, as well as the Cecilian Club Musical and Valentine Day's Party, and expressed the feared that "this social lethargy will continue for weeks at a time."[29] The Sociedad Josefa Ortiz de Dominguez held its annual ball, but only in the residence of Mrs. Dominguez, with a very limited number of guests, "on account of the fear of spreading smallpox."[30] The Improved Society of Red Men rescheduled its secret meetings, declaring, "The members of the Yaqui Tribe No. 6, Improved Order of the Red Men, are hereby notified that we, as good American citizens with the general good of the community at heart, will not meet in our wigwam until the present epidemic of smallpox existing in our city is under control."[31]

The Society of Red Men's declaration equated a sense of American belonging with a visible withdrawal from public life, implicitly stigmatizing people whose work and household arrangements forced them into Laredo's shared public spaces. Even the side effects of vaccination became evidence of public commitment as the *Times* reported on its gossip page that "Mrs. Ellis reported that she was suffering from the ill effects of vaccination."[32] Smallpox's social and symbolic constraint on the privileges of Laredo's multiethnic high society became evidence of patriotic American citizenship.

Public discussion of the physical and symbolic constraint of smallpox on Laredo's poorer residents did not become evidence of an implicitly American identity. Rather, the discussion turned individuals in smallpox detention into people who publicly failed to take advantage of compliance with the city's prevention measures. The city established a temporary hospital built in an abandoned mill and tannery by the Zacate Creek neighborhood. The *Laredo Times* published the names of the people detained in the hospital—"Agapito Samudio, Ruperta Ruiz, Miguel Samudio, Francisco Rios, Nicolasa Tanguma, Francisco Santos, Ignacio Nuncio, Pablo Nuncio, Genoveva Ramirez, Plutarco Salazar, Lupe Alviar, Margaret Jaramio, Esebio Alviar, and Pablo Lucio"—and thus permanently associated them with smallpox.[33] The "pesthouse" was meant to contain the public disorder of smallpox. The space also became a site that trumpeted the failure of individuals to comply with Laredo's isolation measures.

The public scrutiny of the pesthouse transformed individual acts of defiance into acts of collective resistance. This was particularly true for black residents after the return of the Tenth Cavalry to the Laredo border. The *Times* reported that after the night city physician John Hamilton placed Mary Porter and Cynthia Colman in the pesthouse, they both escaped and fled "down to the river." This action prompted the first arrest warrants in this epidemic, charged with the criminal rejection of the conditions in the city hospital. This small action received the prurient headline "Patients Escape from Pest House. Two Colored Girls."[34] Colman and Porter were the only two people whose exit from the smallpox hospital merited an arrest warrant. Their mere presence in an increasingly Mexican medical space made them more visible. Perhaps the treatment they received at the hands of Tejano, Anglo, and Mexicano volunteers at the pesthouse reminded Mary and Cynthia of the lack of federal protection they enjoyed relative to the men enlisted in the Tenth Cavalry. Soldiers, and in this case African American soldiers, used Laredo and Nuevo Laredo as an escape from the discipline of military life. Many working-class Mexican, Mexican American, and American locals were hostile to their federally mandated presence at the border, as well as their informal presence in the neighborhoods and bars in both cities. Many probably translated this resentment into hostility toward black women in Laredo. Their female presence in town and outside of the fort was an indication to their fellow Laredo residents that black families could become a permanent part of Laredo, and—by extension—the black federal military presence would continue to buffer the ongoing encounter between working and propertied classes in Laredo. The conditions of an abandoned mill and tannery cum smallpox hospital challenged Cynthia Coleman's sense and working knowledge of proper cleanliness, especially given Coleman's work as a laundress in Laredo.[35] The headline "Two Colored Girls" pointed out how African American women did not fit in a triracial gender order where African American men embodied the face of federal authority, the majority of young women were ethnic Mexicans, and Anglo women seemed linked to already established propertied households.[36] The article exemplified Justo Saunders's ongoing disaffection with Laredo's dependence on the presence of black troops and associated black professionals in Laredo for its civil order.[37] Rather than containing disorder, the pesthouse in the old mill had become a public site of medical transgression and racial anxiety, a place of disorder within the increasingly self-surveilled and policed urban spaces of Laredo.

Even though increased inspection also heightened working-class dis-content, city officials and local merchants believed more inspection would eventually overcome local resistance. The city and the Businessmen's Club demanded more medical police, more public participation, and more state and federal resources. Mayor Christen reported that Governor Guadalupe Mainero of Tamaulipas was going to come through Laredo and asked Gov-ernor Sayers for additional soldiers to protect the Tamaulipas governor from smallpox.[38] President Villegas and the Public Health Committee of the Lar-edo Businessmen's Club wired Governor Sayers with the following message: "Local authorities are incompetent and unable to cope with smallpox situa-tion and we request that you take charge of same at once."[39] The club probably made this demand on the State Health Office resources in order to prevent a statewide quarantine on Laredo.[40] Perhaps most damning, J. M. McKnight, the state health officer stationed in Laredo, wired Texas State Health Officer Walter Fraser Blunt stating, "There are at least 150 cases here. Situation very serious."[41] These calls for outside intervention wrought a shift in local tactics.

The call for public participation ended the reaffirmation of Mayor Louis Christen's public authority. The Businessmen's Club decided to call for state-level intervention and had Mayor Christen bring this agenda to the open city council meeting in Market Hall. During discussion, some city council mem-bers, such as Brewster and Ugarte, refused to pass the suggested increasingly stringent measures like compulsory vaccination. The mayor and the city physician, after discussing the city health code, realized that "a liberal inter-pretation" could allow the city to place compulsory vaccination within the already established emergency measures.[42] Rather than airing the discussion and coming to a final vote in city council, some of Laredo's best men—a few elected aldermen, members of the Businessmen's Club, U.S. Army officers, and the editors of the *Chaparral* and the *Laredo Times*—agreed to Mayor Christen's expansion of public health authority under a generous reading of the existing emergency measures.

The generous reading enabled measures that were more personally invasive and far more damaging financially to anyone who failed to comply. The city now required vaccination or revaccination of anyone who had not received a successful vaccine in the last two years. They required that every parent vaccinate their children. Furthermore, the mayor had to certify everyone who claimed to have suffered from smallpox. This gave Mayor Christen final authority to determine who might be subject to compulsory vaccination. The measures centralized medical and juridical authority into the body of the mayor.

Mayoral authority expanded to the designation of the inspectors. Appointed by the mayor and accompanied by peace officers, inspectors started their work at eight o'clock each morning. The inside of each house would come under inspection, whether or not anyone was present at the door. If anyone refused to comply with the inspection order, the police brought the protesting party directly to city hall to be fined or perhaps jailed for refusing to comply with the city health code. The measure also converted disagreement with the suspension of due process into a civil offense. If, during a household inspection, someone refused to allow the examination of any part of the body, the code demanded that the peace officer move the person to city hall, detain them, and fine them for refusing to permit a physical inspection. If the inspector and peace officer met no resistance, the inspector was to vaccinate every member of the household; upon completion, "he shall make a note of the name, age, sex, nationality and place of residence of the person vaccinated or re-vaccinated, upon a blank for that purpose as of the sanitary condition of the premises." The measures created a map of stigmatized households within Laredo. If someone was to be found ill with smallpox, they were to be transferred to the Zacate Creek pesthouse (if possible). If the city-appointed volunteer inspector deemed their house a danger to the public health or a source of contamination, the inspector had the fearsome authority to destroy the house and belongings. If an individual, whether healthy or ill, moved back into a house after the inspection determined that the house was a danger to the public, they would be charged with illegally occupying a building.[43] In addition, the city asked every resident to comply and share relevant information with the inspectors. In return, the inspectors promised to proceed "treating everyone fairly" after they forced their way past domestic and personal boundaries that established a respectable gateway between public and private life.[44] The inspectors brought a threatening air into each home visit, especially those that violated an inspector's sense of order.

The city's new measures turned compliance into a matter of public discipline. Everyone who received a city vaccination had to return to the physician's office within two weeks for another inspection to confirm whether the vaccination "took" successfully.[45] Shared public spaces became another casualty of public medical scrutiny in Laredo. The mayor closed all churches, schools, and places of public entertainment and banned all beggars, peddlers, and dogs from city streets, regardless of their actual contact with smallpox patients. The measure banned all gatherings of crowds in the plaza or elsewhere. This decision turned everyday assembly into a criminal act. Of course, this demand complicated any attempt to organize an alternative slate for the coming April 4 election for city council, let alone debate these antismallpox measures. The quarantine measures banned the American act of petitioning city hall and a local Mexican tradition of open assembly. Public dissent threatened a new quarantine social order.

Moreover, the possibility of dissent gave inspectors—both employed deputies and "representative citizens"—the authority to punish potential transgressors. Doctors Davila, Kross, Gongora, and Valdez began "at the Arroyo Zacate and are coming west, inspecting every house and everybody from the Texas-Mexican track to the river."[46] They reported that they faced considerable resistance, but "after perseverance and a considerable amount of talking," they vaccinated "those who needed vaccination."[47] Despite the resistance overcome, the inspectors had Espirideon Hernandez arrested and fined for refusing vaccination by the city at the bridge crossing.[48] The city also arrested Herlinda Hernandez for entering her house after the city declared the place a public danger.[49] The city and the *Laredo Times* used Mr. Hernandez and Ms. Hernandez to publicize the costs of defiance. Their noncompliance was now more commensurate with Colman and Porter's defiant escape. Laredo was becoming a place where Mexicans seemed to resist vaccination, even though Mexicans were also doing the vaccinating.

The public discussion in Market Hall, the arrests, and the wide declaration in the city newspapers set a promising stage for a spectacle of Mexican incompliance, American order, and African American invisibility. When Texas

State Health Officer Blunt asked Governor Sayers to impose quarantine on Webb County because "the annual exodus of Mexicans threatens Texas," he effectively equated Mexican labor migration with smallpox.[50] Blunt's framing obscured the ways ranches, farm owners, and small merchants benefited from the movement of workers into Central Texas. J. O. Nicholson, the secretary of the Businessmen's Club, implied a similar failure of American political authority close to the Mexican border when he demanded that the governor take control of Laredo because "of the inability of local authorities."[51] Governor Sayers linked the situation in Laredo to federal health authorities when he wired Surgeon General George Sternberg requesting five hundred tents to house people diagnosed with smallpox.[52] The next day, March 15, 1899, Blunt declared a statewide quarantine on Laredo. This announcement resonated across a country still testing the new professional boundaries of American identity after the seeming military victory in Cuba, Puerto Rico, and the Philippines.

Physicians on the margin in Texas sought to use the statewide smallpox quarantine on Laredo to confirm their contribution to the future of the United States. Dr. Pugh, an applicant for the position of quarantine officer at the East Texas port of Sabine Pass, telegraphed Governor Sayers offering his services as an immune physician for the smallpox quarantine. Pugh was an American, professionally and immunologically prepared to step into the medical breach for Texas. Another East Texas physician, Dr. Gilliam of Edna, made the medical and national stakes in the quarantine very clear, telling the governor, "If you are in need of physicians to treat smallpox at Laredo or elsewhere command me. I am an immigrant having had it."[53] Dr. Alfred Abdelal expanded on this argument when he volunteered his services. By saying, "Texas is my adoptive state, I was naturalized in Brownsville in 1867. Have read in the papers of the epidemic affecting Laredo," Abdelal declared his loyalty to Brownsville, Texas, and the United States.[54] Perhaps doctors Pugh, Abdelal, and Gilliam must have seen the value of declaring their biological fitness and cultural commitment to the United States through service to Texas. However, their appeal from the margins of medical authority did not persuade Governor Sayers or Dr. Blunt to include them in the struggle against smallpox on the Mexican border. The quarantine, this spectacle of state medical power, belonged to professionals who did not need to show their papers in order to lead the state of Texas to the Mexican border.

The Laredo smallpox quarantine also became a spectacle of Texas police authority. Texas State Health Officer Blunt demanded a citywide meeting in Market Hall, right next to the central plaza. This state-mandated meeting was in direct violation of the emergency medical regulation that banned all local assemblies to prevent the spread of smallpox. He also treated Laredo like a foreign city under military occupation and demanded a properly certified translator to make sure that "the Mexican masses" understood his proclamation. This demand unconsciously and erroneously implied that Americans (Anglo and otherwise) and Anglo-Texans were not the primary medical threat to Texas and that Spanish—as it merely followed English—was a subordinate language, not worth a printed proclamation.[55] This demand turned a civil association—the Businessmen's Club—into an arm of the state of Texas, inducing a capillary relationship to the Texas State Board of Health. C. C. Pierce translated for Dr. Blunt and became the embodied voice that declared the consequences of any failure to comply with the proclamation. Pierce voiced the open threat that the inspectors would tear down each house where they identified smallpox. The people diagnosed with the disease would be placed in the tent city built with USMHS materials that had seen service in Cuba and Puerto Rico. The Texas state quarantine transformed the hospital for people with smallpox—the wooden mill on the away side of the Zacate Bridge—into a detention hall for everyone exposed to smallpox. This form of collective isolation spatially branded the detainees as people with smallpox; it also guaranteed exposure to any remaining smallpox viruses. Until the tent city was finished, the old tannery—and its remaining odors— became housing for the victims of smallpox. Dr. Blunt also made an anticipatory call for armed reinforcement from the Texas Rangers, since rumors floated among authorities that families "will die before they allow any family to be moved."[56] Even in translation, the promised movement of federal and state resources buttressing the call for house destruction, compulsory vaccination, and involuntary detention must have seemed quite threatening to Laredo residents. Saunders reported a widespread perception that when the Tenth Cavalry exercised their horses close to Laredo, many people "thought the colored soldiers were called out to assist in forcing vaccinations on those who refused."[57] Local sanitary inspectors reported "trouble with only a few, who are very persistent in their refusal to be vaccinated."[58] Saunders even mentioned that these resistant individuals "were brought before the mayor this morning on charges of resisting the inspectors and refusing to be vaccinated" but that they yielded and consented to vaccination after meeting with the mayor.[59] Based on these precautions and preparations, the *Laredo Times* definitely gave its readers the impression that the Texas State Health Office was prepared to invade and turn Laredo into it's own private Havana.

Although Laredo could metaphorically be an American Havana, the colonial metaphor aptly describes the Texas Health Office's dependence on local knowledge, local cooperation, and local labor. Since Dr. Blunt required every state-employed physician to reside in the field hospital to treat patients, Mayor Christen and Businessmen's Club leader Villegas appointed people they could trust as health inspectors. In this case, three of the inspectors were local physicians, two of whom had been born in Mexico. Members of the Businessmen's Club were the remaining health inspectors. The use of the Businessmen's Club meant that probably half of the inspectors either were born in Mexico, were Texas-Mexican, or were Spanish (from Spain). In addition to this American/Mexican presence in the quarantine, the majority of the men doing the administrative work for the quarantine—the purchasing agent, the hospital cook, the detention camp guards, the fumigators, the drivers of the removal wagons, and the people attending to the people in the removal wagons—were Texas-Mexicans or simply ethnic Mexicans.[60] This ethnic dimension added a difficult class component to the city's quarantine, as key employers and storekeepers in downtown Laredo comprised the majority of the city inspectors. This embedded the intimate humiliations associated with home inspection into already complicated workplace and credit relationships. Laredo's Tejano and ethnic Mexican residents completed the majority of everyday tasks inside the smallpox quarantine. The Tenth Cavalry, recently arrived from Havana and San Juan Hill, provided the local federal presence and military experience necessary to turn five hundred field tents into a viable hospital. This federal relationship probably added to the sense of American belonging among the people carrying out the quarantine. Although Blunt made it clear that he ran the inside of the quarantine as a military occupation, the quarantine was far more diverse than Blunt's monolingual assertion of Texas authority. This spectacular medical assertion of Texas identity through the quarantine obscured the cooperative labor of Tejanos, Mexicans, and African Americans on the border.

The sudden medical occupation of streets and the open threat to burn suspect residences occasioned a creative use of the existing public sphere. A group of residents petitioned either the Idar family or Justo Cardenas to publish a public protest in handbill form against the violent compulsory vaccination and involuntary detention measures promulgated by the state of Texas and enforced by their neighbors and employers. The loose group of petitioners distributed the handbill across Laredo. Judge Rodriguez forwarded a copy of the petition to Governor Sayers with the following preface: "I enclose you a protest from citizens of Mexican origin which is incendiary and will likely bring out serious results."[61] In the *Laredo Times*, Justo Saunders Penn warned his readers that the petition should be immediately suppressed.[62] The original handbill seems to have disappeared, perhaps because newspaper owners Justo Cardenas and Idar were among the people arrested for inciting a riot. Both Saunders Penn and Judge Rodriguez implied that the arguments were not only beyond the boundaries of acceptable political debate, the medical proposals threatened the very survival of Laredo during the smallpox epidemic. This logic turned the petitioners into internal subversives.

The text itself, however, follows the lines of argument that Justo Cardenas laid out in his 1890 piece on smallpox vaccination: vaccination was important but should be undertaken in consultation with a family physician; smallpox epidemics are familiar to long-term residents; and people are perfectly willing to go get a vaccination from their doctors or their dispensaries. Moreover, the petition pointed out that the vaccination campaign would be an issue in the coming election and was not an issue over which to start a war. The vaccination campaign threatened working-class Texas-Mexican neighborhoods, and these residents would exercise their political power and implement more equal and less class-driven vaccination campaigns. The full text follows:

Protest against Forcible Vaccination

The undersigned residents of Laredo Texas wish to manifest that we energetically protest against the municipal regulations issued by the Mayor of the city on the fourteenth of the present month, commanding that all the inhabitants of whatever age, sex or race be vaccinated, and conferring absolute power on the doctors and sanitary inspectors to profane home and perpetrate all kinds of abuses against the persons who may [have] most rigidly complied with without respecting any other than the Americans. Indeed instead of commencing vaccination in precinct no. 4 or in no. 1 or with the people at the Heights, it began at the Arroyo-Zacate with the Mexico-Texas population against whom it appears all rigor is used and who must pay all the misfortunes which befall Laredo, because this population is defenceless, does not complain and suffers everything in silence. We do not oppose vaccination at the proper time and under proper conditions, but we do oppose it now for the reasons which must be studied by all the inhabitants and the authorities as well so that they may understand the justice that is with us:

1st. That the doctor is not content in going alone, profaning the home, and compelling our children, our wives and our mothers to expose to them their persons, but it must also be done in the presence of three or four other officers that they may laugh at the expense of the families.

2nd. That vaccination during an epidemic is most dangerous as has been demonstrated by experience and the opinions of the most eminent doctors. For this reason in places where smallpox is a frequent visitor vaccination is suspended as soon as the first case is discovered in order to prevent the spread of the disease and to prevent its complication with other maladies.

3rd. Because vaccination cannot be applied to all persons, or under all conditions. Indeed it may result fatally, and it is necessary that the family physician cognizant of the state of the patient's health, should order it so that it may not be injurious. But to administer vaccination to all persons, at any time, and under any conditions is to send the Mexico-Texas people to the graveyard; and this we cannot, we must not permit, without protesting energetically in order that the responsibility may be rendered effective in every unfortunate case.

We are told that such proceedings on the part of the men in power are for the purpose of pursuing political ends, but we do not wish to believe this, because it is an infamous crime to traffic with the health, the life, with the honor and with the peace of families for political purposes. But in any event the people have enough energy and will know how to use its rights in the coming elections.

We protest with full right in due form and with the energy which we possess against the regulations which order compulsory vaccination and against the manner of administering it.

Librado González	A. B. Vela	Miguel Machardi
Carlos Díaz	Jesús María Salinas	Policarpo Caballero
Teodosio Cerda	J. Kerckholp	B. S. López
Joaquín V. de León	Nicanor Zurita[63]	

The handbill laid a claim to belonging in Laredo in its first sentence: "We the undersigned residents of Laredo." They merely requested the end of city-mandated compulsory vaccination. This petition challenged the form, the personnel, and the medical logic behind the demand for one-size-fits-all vaccinations. Moreover, the petitioners sought to challenge the way quarantine measures had become embedded in the spatial politics of Laredo. The mayor's transformation of the local merchant class into sanitary inspectors turned an already coercively intimate act of medical inspection into a public spectacle. His decisions—and the policies voiced by C. C. Pierce and mandated by Dr. Blunt—gave the inspectors pushing their way through the doors a hard medical edge. The city health officer's decision to inspect the houses in Zacate Creek first reminded people living between the railroad yards and Zacate Creek that their housing stock was already under siege and their sense of dignity immaterial to Laredo's welfare. The petition named the conjoining of medical, political, and class privilege; the petitioners challenged the way these privileges and a universalizing call for vaccination wreaked havoc, seemingly working to "send the Mexico-Texas population to the graveyard." The use of handbills with only a small number of petitioners underlined the way the medical ban on assemblies turned public dissent into a criminal act. The petitioners' decision to sign their names to a potentially illegal act of democratic dissent highlighted either a faith in the democratic process or a sense of marginality and tragic martyrdom.

The petitioners presented an existing alternative to the medicalization of class inequality in Laredo. They demanded smallpox prevention measures that took the consent of individuals and households seriously. They touched on common local medical knowledge gained from their hard experience with prior smallpox outbreaks. They referenced shared public memory on both sides of the Rio Grande and evoked earlier moments when doctors ceased vaccinating people because of the challenge weakened vaccine lymph posed to a person's health in the midst of an epidemic. The language of the petition, "to prevent its complication with other maladies," highlighted public and professional knowledge of the damaging effects of vaccinations. The petitioners demonstrated that they knew vaccination was exposure to a weaker illness, recovery from which also granted immunity against smallpox. The complications of the effort were known "in places where smallpox is a frequent visitor." The petition charged that elected officials and council members foolhardily ignored the hard-won common sense on the compulsory vaccination matter. Ultimately, the petitioners hoped for a public health politics that recognized their presence and their stake in this epidemic.

In addition to demonstrating their ability to open a debate regarding the wisdom of universally requiring the vaccination, the petitioners touched upon recent forms of resistance and counterinsurgency in the Laredo region. The petitioners drew on perceptions that resonated with other late nineteenth-century forms of dissent with medical authority. The local police accompanied recently appointed inspectors into residences to identify and detain people suffering from specific communicable diseases. Many families with people threatened with detention considered this uninvited and police-escorted entrance into each household part of a continuum of continued intrusion into their communities.[64] The city repeatedly targeted the railway yards and the Zacate Creek neighborhood for detention and house destruction. The petitioners claimed, rightfully, that this confirmed the disdain the established Laredo citizens may have felt toward them.[65] Forced detention vividly reminded them of their subordinate relationship with state police power.[66] Moreover, recent memories of counterinsurgency in South Texas and Nuevo León heightened their awareness of their precarious hold on life in the United States. The statement "to administer vaccination to all persons, at any time, and under any conditions is to send the Mexico-Texas people to the graveyard" highlighted their anxieties about the future of Tejanos in Texas and their uneasiness with the promise of American progress in Laredo.[67] However, the petition made it quite clear that the advocates preferred to use the ballot, not the bullet, to prevent extermination by expedient vaccination.

The city of Laredo treated the call to the ballots as if it were direct resistance. Neighborhood residents and police authorities used the petition to solidify lines of exclusion and humiliation in Laredo. Like Espirideon and Herlinda Hernandez, some Laredo residents were arrested and brought before the judge for refusing to be vaccinated. Many others acted on their reluctance to relinquish control of their immediate family members and refused to turn them over to an institution run by people hostile to their needs. As a result, sheriffs and other law officers started accompanying the volunteer inspectors in their inspection of Laredo houses and households.[68] Dr. Blunt supplemented this police presence with the request for a division of the Texas Rangers. The presence of the Rangers was meant to strike enough fear in

Laredo households to preclude the need for sanitary inspectors and sheriff deputies to force their way into each house and overcome this troublesome (and implicitly Mexican) recalcitrance.

Apparently, the Texas Rangers were unable to listen to the concerns of Zacate Creek residents. When city physician Hamilton crossed the bridge into the Zacate Creek neighborhood on March 19, 1899, he faced an assembly— according to the *New York Times*, a group of five hundred Mexicans—voicing demands outlined in the petition. The Herrera family demanded the presence of a trustworthy physician before they would approve the removal of their sister to the local pesthouse. Neither the medical nor police authorities acceded to this demand. The assembly refused to relinquish the sister and used rocks to communicate this sentiment to the city marshal and the health officer. John Hamilton claimed that someone in the crowd shot a rifle in the direction of the city marshal.[69]

These rocks catalyzed the violent response promised by Justo Saunders Penn and Judge Rodriguez. The city deputies started shooting; Zacate Creek residents responded in kind. They mocked the Rangers' inability to force the neighborhood to conform to their will. Newspapers recorded the following taunts: "Down with authorities" and, potentially as insulting to City Marshal Nicasio Idar, "Bring out your Negro soldiers."[70] A number of "community-minded" businessmen grabbed their guns and ran five blocks east to help City Marshal Idar put down a potential class uprising.[71] The *San Antonio Express* reported three deaths, and the first two were Agapito Herrera and his sister. The rifle battles at Zacate Creek in Laredo overwhelmed any news coverage of the welfare of the Herrera family, especially after the death of Agapito Herrera. The rifle shots silenced a wider political spectrum.

This resistance to medical police authority forced the Texas State Board of Health and the city of Laredo to literally call in the cavalry. The Tenth Cavalry rode in, confirming Zacate Creek residents' prediction that "Negro soldiers" would rescue middle-class Laredenses.[72] The *Express* reported, "The colored troopers of the Tenth Cavalry, 'the Black Demons of San Juan Hill,' appeared on the scene with orders from their commander to 'shoot, and shoot to kill,' after which resistance was only spasmodic."[73] According to the Associated Press, a crowd in Market Plaza greeted the Tenth Cavalry cheering, "Hurrah for San Juan Hill," and lined up behind the cavalry men. There was no more room for discussion in this militarized, near imperial public health campaign. The next death made this very clear to the witnesses and participants in a newly armed mob of soldiers. The AP reporter stated, "The leader of the first crowd encountered by the military undertook to talk instead of obeying orders to clear out, and was promptly knocked down with a butt of the carbine and was so badly hurt that he died within a short time after being carried away. His followers took the hint and rapidly faded away."[74] The Tenth Cavalry provided visible federal support for the city's demand to inspect, disinfect, and vaccinate the residents. In the minor skirmishes that followed the riot, the local residents probably sought to avoid direct fire against the Gatling gun the Tenth Cavalry brought into the Zacate Creek neighborhood. The military dimensions of the intervention carried over into Nuevo Laredo. Colonel O'Horan in Nuevo Laredo acquiesced to Mayor Christen's demand that the Mexican federal cavalry place troops along the bridge and the southern bank of the river to prevent anyone fleeing this quarantine. The reporter stressed that the "several hundreds of Mexicans driven out of the disturbed district were refuging under the bank" cheered, thinking the troops were there "to assist them against the colored United States cavalry men."[75] The presence of the Gatling gun and the Tenth Cavalry in Laredo exposed the multitiered dependence of Anglo and Mexican border authorities on Tejano police officers, state-level (Anglo) Texas Rangers, the Mexican Federal Army, and the Tenth Cavalry. The Mexican and American inspectors and the city physicians became the point of contact between the newly minted medical threats and the multiethnic and nearly multinational military machinery backing Texas medical police authority. In Laredo, this multiethnic coalition of the powerful waged a military counterinsurgency effort against the Mexican majority living by Zacate Creek and the railroad yards.

These public health policies, when enforced by the Tenth Cavalry, the Texas Rangers, local Tejano deputies, and downtown merchants did little to guarantee the quality of the relationship between city health officers and the working-class ethnic Mexican residents of Laredo. The frequent presence of Tejanos, Mexicanos, Mexican Americans, and Mexican immigrants as sheriffs, elected officials, volunteer inspectors, and local health officers present the most important challenge to the American/Mexican dyad into which most scholars have placed the Laredo Smallpox Riot.[76] Walter Prescott Webb and Robert Utley drew up the smallpox riot as if it were another contest between legitimate American authority and illegitimate Mexican authority, a simple case of "vaccination with a six shooter."[77] Tejanos like Sheriff Solis and Marshall Idar on one side of the debate and petitioners like Mr. Kercholp and Carlos Diaz all exercised their right as American citizens to demand city policies that reflected their values and their commitment to public health. These ethnic Mexicans deserve "an illustration of the great cultural distance between Mexican and American culture."[78] David Gutierrez has argued that immigration has been a point of contention and community formation for Mexican communities in the United States.[79] The Laredo smallpox riot highlights the way public health provided a flashpoint and a point of contention shaping Mexican communities' relationship to emerging forms of public state power.

The question of vaccination at the turn of the century helps illustrate a longer debate over the proper relationship between public health policies and private household boundaries at the border between Texas and Mexico. In 1890, Justo Cardenas emphasized the porousness of the boundary separating the proper care of individual citizen bodies through vaccination from the feminized burden of maintaining a properly hygienic household. In 1892, public health officers at the joint APHA/Asociacion Medica Mexicana meeting discussed the difficulties they faced enforcing compliance among their national publics, establishing disinfection stations at key trade hubs and port towns, and establishing sole authority over quarantine matters. The Laredo quarantine became a place where the city of Laredo and the Texas Board of Health sought to establish their version of a properly muscular quarantine.

The petitioners' challenge and the standoff at Zacate Creek forced the muscular state of Texas to reveal its dependence on local and federal police authority. Local federal cavalry, the Texas Rangers, armed businessmen, and local Tejano elected officials and city hall staff came together to suppress the threat posed by an ex–sheriff's deputy and his family's neighborhood friends.[80] Economic development in Central Texas and northern Mexico was still dependent on the labor power and lower reproduction costs of seasonal migrants. The neighborhood of Zacate Creek probably had long-term residents as well as a number of workers who used Laredo and Zacate as a central hub between Monterrey, Nuevo León, and San Antonio, Texas. The conflicts between the Tejano police authority and this Mexican neighborhood indicate that the boundaries around Laredo's political community included factors other than ethnicity.[81]

The violence of the vaccination campaign highlighted different emphases in a relatively similar understanding of smallpox. Walter Blunt acted as if the only way to deliver vaccinations and smallpox disinfection in border areas like Zacate Creek and Laredo was at the end of a gun barrel because he believed Mexicans did not trust American medicine. The petitioners and the residents of Zacate Creek emphasized the importance of individual consultation for vaccination. They also placed the destruction of households within a larger continuum of assaults on ethnic Mexican homes in South Texas. The unauthorized inspections, the compulsory vaccinations, and the fumigation and incarceration of household goods lay far outside what the petitioners considered legitimate state authority. The political debate and intellectual conflict over the location and consultation over the treatment and prevention of smallpox had important actions. Police actions caused the death of one individual. Police and community actions in the riot injured seventeen people; the Laredo police arrested twenty-five people in the aftermath of the riot.[82] The actions taken after the smallpox riot confirmed that Zacate Creek's residents were not part of Laredo's inner circle.

In three days, the actions taken to register discontent with the forced vaccination and removal of families reached national audiences. The *New York Times* reported that in the establishment of a smallpox quarantine in Laredo, there was a "clash against Mexicans: 500 armed men interfere with Americans in removing smallpox patients."[83] The *Los Angeles Times* wrote that "Laredo seemed to be "a riot center, trotting Havana Cuba a close second."[84] The *Times* reporter's headline transformed Sheriff Solis, Marshall Idar, and their deputies into "Americans" and at the same time dissolved Agapito Herrera, Laredo's one-time police deputy, his daughter, and their neighbors into an armed Mexican mob. Two days later, Harrison Gray Otis of the *Times* again observed, "Those Mexicans at Laredo will probably come to the conclusion that it is nicer to be vaccinated in the regular way than with a Gatling gun."[85] The coverage effectively implied that "Mexicans" had a hostile relationship to an implicitly national medical modernity and that the U.S. military—even the (black) Tenth Cavalry—had the right to treat "Mexican" residents in a violently paternalistic fashion. The parallel that journalists drew with the occupation of Cuba and the Philippines continued to imply that violent means were necessary to incorporate "those Mexicans" into the modern culture of the United States. By the end of the riots, every ethnic Mexican resident of Laredo, regardless of their individual relationship to the conflict in the Zacate Creek subdivision, had a more tenuous claim over the administration of public health in their own city.[86] News coverage in the Anglo-American press took a difficult and multilayered debate over coercion and medical authority in the city of Laredo and transformed it into a Mexican spectacle on American territory.[87]

The smallpox riot stained subsequent American depictions of Laredo. The Associated Press reported that a mere two weeks after the smallpox riot, there was now a "Mexican mayor at Laredo."[88] Headlines like these made it clear to readers outside South Texas that ethnic Mexicans threatened American public health and safety in the United States. Readers could easily draw a variety of parallels with news of violent dissatisfaction with American pacification efforts in Cuba and the Philippines.[89] Even Justo Saunders Penn, the vitriolic editor of the *Laredo Times*, who complained about the working-class Mexican and black military dimensions of Laredo, felt threatened by the implications of A. M. Vidaurri not being American.

The *Washington Bee*, a prominent African American newspaper in the District of Columbia, presented another cause for the discontent in Laredo. In Calvin Chase's summary of events, the conditions at the border changed when Dr. John Hamilton arrived in Laredo, because that was when the "trouble grew out of the discovery that smallpox was south of the river." Calvin Chase emphasized that American authorities and Mexican families on both sides of the river took the appearance of smallpox in the spring for granted and that the doctor's declaration of quarantine surprised everyone. Chase added that when "some joker tipped that troublesome doctor off to the fact that there was a case or two of the disease in Laredo . . . [and made] him think it was something new and extraordinary," Hamilton transformed Laredo by turning an abandoned wool warehouse and cotton mill into detention facilities. The doctor stunned the community, probably including African American communities in Laredo and Fort McIntosh, when he refused to allow visitors at the pesthouse. As Chase put it, "This was an undreamed of outrage and a section of board fence [surrounding the warehouse] was torn down." When the house-to-house inspections were met with resistance, "he sent the obstreperous to the detention hospital."[90] When the obstreperous person's relatives organized an assembly to confront this new form of medical police, the city and the doctor called on the Tenth Cavalry. Chase inverted a racial metaphor to emphasize the strength and power of this black regiment, stating that the doctor "drew a handful of spades and had the Tenth Cavalry beat everything in sight." Chase mocked the doctor's working analysis that the presence of smallpox among Mexican American (native Texan) families was a threat to the nation. First of all, the annual appearance of smallpox in Mexican communities at the border was as much part of the Texan cultural landscape as the fandangos, danza, bullfights, and fiestas that marked Laredo. The disruption came "when a short-horn doctor from the effete East comes to the Rio Grande loaded down with quills, claims the right to enter your jacal, and proceeds to tear a piece of hide off your arm just because he does not like your looks or your liver—when these things happen, then there's sure to be a little unpleasantness and a funeral or two."[91] Chase was the only American writer who tried to empathize with the ways native Texas-Mexican families may have felt about this uninvited state medical authority. In the process of empathizing with local Texas-Mexicans, he created two others. The first was a feminized white geographically foreign medical authority that threatened the manly accommodation between the (black) U.S. Army and various communities at the Texas border. The second was a region whose throat-cuttings and smallpox outbreaks were beyond political intervention. Black troops provided the necessary force to keep peace between an ambitious and intrusive East Coast middle-class attitude and the near-foreign cultural landscape at the border. The smallpox riot confirmed this dependence.

The quarantine against Laredo lasted another two months. The state of Texas policed the railroad traffic between Laredo and San Antonio. Fundraising drives around Texas aimed to send clothes and funds for food. The epidemic still drained Laredo's finances. Local authorities, including the Laredo *Chaparral*, started a campaign "asking that Webb County be released from paying state taxes because of the ruination brought on by smallpox."[92] After three months of quarantine, all the residents of Laredo probably sighed in relief when they read in the *San Antonio Express* that "the epidemic has dried up in Laredo."[93] This news gave State Health Officer Blunt the opportunity to end his three-and-a-half-month-long quarantine. Residents could now make their way north to seek work in the railroads and cotton fields of Central Texas. The I&GN and the Texas-Mexican Railroad resumed service, and steel ore, wool, and cotton started moving north from Mexico. In August, the U.S. Army redeployed the Tenth Cavalry to the Moros province of the Philippines.[94] Occupying had its burdens.

Making Laredo the Next Havana

The American military encounter with yellow fever in Havana changed the stakes for federal control over quarantine at the Mexican border. Carlos Finlay and Walter Reed successfully demonstrated that the *Stegomyia* mosquito was a vector for the transmission of yellow fever.[95] William Crawford Gorgas translated this epidemiological insight into a massive disease prevention campaign, turning Havana into a disinfection, mosquito eradication, patient isolation, and mosquito netting field trial.[96] Using the martial authority provided by the occupation government in Cuba, Gorgas and the U.S. Army demonstrated to the world that mosquito nets, larvae eradication, fumigation, disinfection, and patient isolation could prevent the spread of yellow fever in Havana. The USMHS used its medical victory in Havana to increase its political authority in the United States.

Walter Wyman seized the developments in Havana to push Congress for USMHS authority over any national quarantine. The subsequent Perkins-Hepburn bill called for a name change to the U.S. Public Health and Marine Hospital Service (USPHMHS), gave this service the authority to call quarantine over state boards of health, provided for additional staff in the hygienic laboratory, and directed the agency to collect and publish vital statistics. The successful containment of yellow fever in Havana helped convince some southern legislators to support this centralization of federal authority.[97] As Henry Clayton of Alabama stated, "This bill will unite, harmonize, and rationalize the work of the state and federal health officers in the interests of public health and commerce in our country."[98] The bill passed, effectively placing authority over yellow fever quarantine fully under the authority of the surgeon general and the newly renamed USPHMHS.

This administrative coup raised the stakes for the USPHMHS. One of the central claims for this expansion of administrative authority was that the service would "destroy the opportunity for the fearful and frightful panics and the prostration of public business that take place in many sections of this country on the first announcement that yellow fever has appeared in a given place."[99] When news reached Walter Wyman that yellow fever had reached epidemic proportions in Monterrey, Nuevo León, and that there were four cases in Laredo, Texas, the general confidence in mosquito eradication turned the Laredo border into a political opportunity. In his telegram to surgeons R. D. Murray and Gregorio Guiteras, Wyman again turned the urban Texas-Mexico border into a staging ground for American medical progress: "Believed here good opportunity for demonstrating possibility of restricting spread of fever by new methods, as at Havana, screening patients and destroying mosquitoes."[100] Wyman's disease prevention campaign gave the local dynamics of public health measures in Laredo a national audience.

The federal presence in Laredo depended on Texas State Health Officer George Tabor. On September 2, 1903, the state of Texas declared quarantine on Monterrey and all other rumored infected points in Mexico. Dr. Tabor asked city and county officials across Texas to initiate mosquito eradication projects. He also directly warned all residents of Laredo that the penal clauses of quarantine were in full force and would be enforced against anyone evading quarantine regulations. Laredo authorities placed three employees under State Health Officer John McKnight's guidance to help guard the bridge and the riverbank in Laredo. In Mexico, public health declarations also carried an echo of violence. Governor Reyes placed a quarantine with "a strong military force around Monterrey with orders to shoot anyone who undertakes to enter that city from yellow fever points."[101] The threat of yellow fever to local economies led to a military enforcement of medical boundaries around both cities. These decisions resonated with the 1899 quarantine at the border.

The threat of fever in Laredo and the military dimension of epidemic yellow fever in Monterrey meant drastic changes to their immediate situation. *Laredo Times* editor Justo Penn "feared that this spread of yellow fever in Mexico may force the border officials to enforce an absolute quarantine against that country. In that event no trains of any kind will be permitted to cross and the entire border will be guarded to keep out travelers."[102] Tabor's declaration confirmed this fear. Penn also worried that the conditions in Laredo looked favorable to the explosive growth of yellow fever: "Now that fresh rains have fallen and sultry vegetation will grow luxuriously on vacant lots and in the streets, the growth of weeds is a cause of sickness and they should not be permitted to stand. The entire city needs a general cleaning up and the city fathers should take energetic measures to bring about better sanitation."[103] Penn concluded that "should an epidemic strike us with the city in such an unsanitary condition the loss of life would be great."[104] He also postulated, "Unless the authorities take the most energetic measures to stamp it out, the inhabitants of that city are in grave danger and the Texas border will also be menaced by the scourge."[105] The threat of yellow fever to their immediate person and their loved ones was the most dreaded possibility. Some may have remembered the economic devastation that followed the 1899 Laredo smallpox quarantine around Laredo, and others may have remembered the

1882 Mexican-Texas yellow fever epidemic. For Penn, the commercial connection to Monterrey and the general aesthetics of the border town endangered all of Laredo's residents.

When reports of two cases in Nuevo Laredo arrived in Laredo, the situation changed. Alonzo Garrett, the U.S. consul at Nuevo Laredo, was the first case in Laredo, and "an exodus of Laredo residents" immediately followed. The state of Texas declared "a quarantine against New Laredo so rigid that it will be almost a physical impossibility for any one get into this city. Both the railroad bridges and tram bridges are heavily guarded and guards are standing up and down the river for miles."[106] People started fleeing in fear of the yellow fever cases in Nuevo Laredo, and the mounted guard started reporting "people from Laredo, Mexico, attempting to cross at various points."[107] That people attempted to cross the medical quarantine line should have been expected, as the USMHPHS and the state of Texas drew another three-hundred-mile medical line to intercept all traffic across the Rio Grande. On September 23, 1903, Dr. Murray and Dr. Guiteras confirmed two more cases of yellow fever in Laredo, after the initial fumigation and inspection work.[108] James Whitaker, an employee in the office of the Electric Light and Street Railway Company, was the first fatality.[109] The other case was J. H. McKnight, the Texas state health officer in charge of the quarantine. All three initial cases openly contradicted the assumption that the first incidents in the United States would be among Mexican seasonal laborers.[110] Certainly, the border-crossing mobility that Consul Garrett, Texas State Health Officer J. H. McKnight, and James Whitaker had to do for their work exposed them to the mosquitoes in Monterrey and Nuevo Laredo, respectively. However, their close ties with the federal quarantine effort prevented a public panic over border-crossing white American professionals.

The public anxiety spread from the possible connections between the American professional class in Laredo, the large Mexican working-class in Laredo, and the difficult economic conditions that came with the state yellow fever quarantine. Laredo mayor Dr. Amador Sanchez, recalling the disastrous economic impact of the 1899 quarantine, asked his fellow mayors in Central Texas to help Laredo avoid the human and economic devastation of yellow fever. Sanchez and Tabor arranged to have oil companies in Beaumont and Central Texas ship gasoline to Laredo on a regular basis.[111] Sanchez also asked for direct fiscal aid: "Fever had been mostly confined to the well-to-do class citizens. Now that it is invading the ranks of the poorer people it is necessary that the city bestir itself for their relief."[112] Observers turned this plea into something else. In Dallas, the paper reported that Mayor Sanchez claimed "the conditions of this city have greatly reduced the poorer classes, and hundreds of Mexicans are in want."[113] The *Morning News* turned this call for empathy into an appeal on behalf of Mexicans, not Americans. The public emphasis on poorer Mexicans in Laredo haunted subsequent accounts of the epidemic.

The potential medical attitudes and actions of poorer Mexicans haunted the preparations for the quarantine and the mosquito eradication project. Dr. Tabor and Dr. Guiteras were aware that they had to explain the mosquito vector theory of yellow fever to everybody in Laredo. Compliance with the order to put kerosene in still water to kill the *Stegomyia* larvae was hard to come by in Havana, and even less likely in Laredo. People relied on water companies (horse-drawn wagons carrying barrels full of water) for their household water, so water storage was a key part of each working-class household. The dry weather, the general scarcity of water among the poorer classes, and the tasks of oiling this water and cutting off the breeze with mosquito netting during the hot summer made eradication more difficult. The campaign had to make the proposal to place a layer of oil on each household's valuable source of water had to seem obvious and necessary to every affected household.

There were degrees of discomfort with the application of the mosquito vector to yellow fever prevention. Justo Saunders Penn, editor of the *Laredo Times*, the only paper being published in Laredo during the yellow fever epidemic, could not resist reprinting "the latest mosquito joke." This joke spoke to a latent discomfort with the mosquito and germ theory behind yellow fever. As William Nesbitt wrote,

> They've found the bug that eats the bug that fights the bug that bites us. They traced the germ that kills the germ that chews the germ that smites us. They know the bug that knifes the bug that stabs the bug that jabs us. They've seen the germ that hates the germ that biffs the germ that nabs us. They've struck the bug that slays the bug that flays the bug that sticks us. They've jailed the germ that guides the germ that taught the germ to fix us. But still these bugs—microbic thugs in spite of drugs—combat us. And still these germs—described in terms inspiring—get at us.[114]

Laredo witnessed the fumigating, screening, and netting of households with people suffering from yellow fever. Penn, through Nesbitt, gently mocked the near criminal persecution of anthropomorphized germs and bugs. On the other hand, Penn heartily endorsed the persecution of potential yellow fever miscreants. This witticism probably marked the boundaries of official ambivalence regarding the implications of the mosquito theory to yellow fever prevention.

City authorities were not patient when other forms of public ambivalence combined with a local history of public grassroots dissent. Laredo authorities moved to eliminate the possibility of official dissent once the USMHPHS established the federal quarantine in Laredo. The *Dallas Morning News* reported that "F. V. Marquez, of a Spanish sheet named 1810, was arrested today under an affidavit charging him with libel. This sheet appeared yesterday, and contained an article treating of the yellow fever situation in which the physicians and officials are ridiculed. It also declares that there is no yellow fever in Laredo, and urges its readers to resist the authorities who are doing the disinfecting, etc."[115] Jailing Marquez for mocking American medical professionals communicated two messages: first, elected officials feared the power of the Spanish-language press among Laredo's Mexican residents; second, American medical professionals were not confident that local Laredo residents would agree with the need to eradicate the conditions that allowed *Stegomyia* mosquito larvae to thrive. Marquez's arrest also implied that city and health authorities were anxious about the cooperation of local (Mexican) families with the quarantine and the mosquito eradication project.

This open American political concern with general Mexican medical cooperation amplified any note of dissent uttered by Mexican families in general and Mexican women in particular. Penn reported locally that "the physicians continue to meet with rebuffs from the poor and ignorant class of the people. Some of them are possessed by the remarkable hallucination that they will be poisoned if they take a 'doctor's medicine.'"[116] The *Morning News* reported that after "one of the officers placed oil in a barrel of water in the yard of an old Mexican woman of the poorer class, and immediately upon their leaving, the old lady dumped the barrel of water over, remarking to one of her neighbors that it was a preconcerted plan on the part of the Americans to do away with the Mexicans."[117] Edward Butler, a *Los Angeles Times* reporter, implied that this hostility was a centuries-old pathology within Mexican folk culture: "The Mexican people, in their ignorance, imagine that the old time methods of treating the yellow fever epidemic are today in vogue viz. that of poisoning those who are so unfortunate as to contract the disease in order to kill them, and thus stamp out the epidemic. It is characteristic of the Latin race to hand down 'dichos' ('sayings') from family to family for centuries, and from father to son for years and years have been passed along the unwritten history of measures taken to stamp put epidemics in olden times."[118] Moreover, Butler added, Mexican physicians believed there was substantial antagonism toward medical authority among the working classes in northern Mexico. An unnamed physician stated, "There is a belief among the people that the doctors have been ordered to kill the sick ones. This is absurd and is the greatest proof of their ignorance. The poor ones give the physicians enough to do during their lifetime."[119] These anecdotes dramatically outline the general lack of authority these middle-class professionals felt they exercised over Mexican families in Laredo.

This fear of the power of Mexican families flowed into a public discussion of concealed cases in Laredo. Under the yellow fever prevention guidelines established in Havana, each person with yellow fever needed to be treated in a place safe from mosquitoes. Penn described the process in Laredo: "Every house where a fever patient is found must be fumigated and screened and all the surrounding houses disinfected and the mosquitoes killed."[120] This isolation prevented mosquitoes from inadvertently carrying the yellow fever virus from one person to another, and screens, mosquito netting, and double doors were some of the most visible ways to prevent mosquito access. Thus concealed cases meant families who independently assumed the burden of treating the muscle pain, vomiting, internal bleeding, fevers, and potential infections that came with yellow fever. Most families were overwhelmed when patients entered the more intense phase of suffering; this is the point when inspectors or family members decided to seek aid from public authorities. For example, Consul Alonzo Garrett and Dr. McKnight received their care at home when they came down with the disease. As Dr. Murray and Dr. Tabor supervised both cases, the press and public health officers did not treat them like concealed cases. When observers referred to the problem of concealed cases, they meant cases concealed from the eyes of the USPHMHS medical officers or other medical authorities.

Making each case available to American medical oversight was crucial to the form of yellow fever prevention that the USPHMHS sought to implement in Laredo. Each yellow fever case was a potential source of another case of yellow fever. The USMHPHS sought patient isolation to break the chain of infection; they also sought to place people in their field hospital to physically remove them from mosquito conditions beyond immediate USMHPHS control. Each day a case went unsupervised by the medical authorities, the authorities assumed that more cases would follow. Contact with the medical gaze was needed to assuage the general anxiety over the spread of disease across different neighborhoods. For this reason, each case the inspectors identified was, by definition, always concealed from American medical authority because it had previously gone unidentified and contained. The anxiety over concealed cases was more an anxiety over controlled medical cases.

This anxiety over the process of medical discovery complemented the earlier anxiety over Mexican medical attitudes. Reporters placed responsibility for the absence of medical authority on the families with yellow fever victims. The *Morning News* reported:

> The house-to-house canvass was continued today by the physicians and will be continued until every house in the city and surrounding country has been visited, examined and put in a sanitary condition. The work of the physicians is made necessary because of a lack of confidence among the poorer class of Mexicans. In many cases the people endeavor to conceal the fact that any of their family is sick, as they have an antipathy for the American physicians, some of the more ignorant even going so far as to claim that the Americans would give them medicine to poison them.[121]

Saunders Penn wrote,

> The physicians continue to meet with rebuffs from the poor and ignorant class of the people. Some of them are possessed by the remarkable hallucination that they will be poisoned if they take a "doctor's medicine." Whence comes this fear it would be hard to say. It works a great hardship on these poor people. It causes them to conceal their sick and even when the sick can be found, they sometimes refuse to take treatment but depend on teas made from roots and herbs to cure them. This usually results in their death if they have a severe case.[122]

In both of these Anglo-American accounts, a Mexican fear of physicians—not the experience or the memory or the knowledge of the political power of physicians to call for the destruction of their homes—led to wariness around the inspections and guaranteed the early deaths of some of the more severe cases. The *Morning News* offered a succinct explanation: "These deaths are among the poorer classes of Mexicans, who conceal their sickness until it is too late to save them."[123] In these accounts, the independence of Mexican families guaranteed their early deaths.

Both federal and state medical authorities lifted these sardonic anxieties to the level of policy. Dr. Tabor told the *Morning News* that "in fully 75 percent of the cases which terminated fatally it has been discovered that the patients, Mexicans of the lower class were in a dying condition when found by the physicians. Most of them were averse to taking treatment from educated and experienced physicians and to following the regime imposed by those who know how to grapple with the disease, preferring the old methods which have long obtained among the Mexicans of the lower classes."[124] For Tabor, this attitude toward contemporary treatment placed the local victims of yellow fever beyond public redemption, an unfortunate attitude toward Texas-Mexicans. His colleague Dr. Robert D. Murray had managed the Mexico-Texas quarantine twenty years before and experienced near full cooperation by using local Spanish-speaking attendants, treating people inside their own houses, and providing general medical supplies through the USMHS grocery and dispensary.[125] There had been medical, if not political, cooperation with the USMHS quarantine in Brownsville. Dr. Tabor and Dr. Guiteras had no use for this memory of cooperation between local families and federal authorities at the border.

Quarantine authorities desired cooperation from local Mexican families, and Mexican women assumed a symbolic prominence among the people resisting medical authorities. The economic conditions of the quarantine also brought women into the public sphere. Penn reported on the petition presented to the city council by fifty-seven Spanish-surnamed women. They placed full responsibility for their situation on American medical authorities:

We, the undersigned, being mostly widows with families to support with our own hands, would represent that on account of the pest which has most unfortunately attacked our city, most of the well-to-do families that have given us employment in doing their washing, ironing, sewing and etc., have left the city; that since then we have been unable to find any work and we have been thrown suddenly wholly on our own feeble resources, with large families to support and no means of doing so. Hence we humbly petition the Honorable Mayor and the Board of Aldermen either to aid us in obtaining work or to furnish us means with which to support ourselves and our families while this epidemic lasts.[126]

The petitioners moved into the public sphere, openly demanding that the well-to-do members of city council do something to address their economic situation. This demand reflected earlier demands for economic assistance in the midst of quarantines. The petitioners brought the often hidden class relationships that connected the supposedly well-to-do and working class into public view. They touched on the mobility and access to political information that members of Laredo's merchant class enjoyed relative to their domestic workers. For these widows, the dislocations forced them to bring their vulnerabilities and their identities as head of households into the public view. The quarantine required these working women in Laredo to use their identity as widows and family members to demand cooperation from the public.

The appearance of unexpected petitioners probably catalyzed public memories of the petitions, tensions, and violence over patient care in the Laredo Smallpox Riot. When Guiteras expressed the need for "a mosquito proof hospital," city officials refused to cooperate. Guiteras expressed his intense frustration with the mayor, the sheriff, and the local Businessmen's Club: "It was impressed upon me that the very class of cases I wished to remove to a hospital would absolutely refuse to go, and that there was no authority to force them to do so."[127] He did not see the need to entertain this local ambivalence toward the removal of people suffering from yellow fever when the United States faced a potential medical crisis. As he stated, "Doubtless the necessary authority could have been assumed, legally or otherwise, (as had been done before in Laredo during a smallpox epidemic in 1895 [sic]). There is every reason to suppose that, as in the instance cited above, this would have led to some bloodshed, but the situation would have been controlled. There was no one in authority, however, ready to take the necessary risk, and the sheriff of Webb County, who could have been of great assistance in such a case, was lukewarm in his efforts to aid us."[128] Guiteras wanted the shadow of federal military violence to coerce enhanced local cooperation with the yellow fever prevention effort.

The shadow of military violence was dimmer in Laredo four years after the declaration of victory over Spain in 1898. In 1899, the Tenth Cavalry left for the Philippines, having established its authority in colonial conflicts in San Juan Hill, Havana, and the Laredo Smallpox Riot. Two years later, Governor William Howard Taft started the expulsion of the African American regiments from the pacification efforts in the Philippines, emphasizing "the incompatibility of the Malay and the Negro."[129] On August 16, 1903, the Tenth

Cavalry left San Francisco for Laredo.[130] On September 17, the garrison at Fort McIntosh started building mosquito cages to detain any soldier who came down with yellow fever. These isolation cages implicitly rejected full African American immunity to yellow fever.[131] On October 10, Lieutenant Osborne imposed an absolute quarantine on any traffic between Fort McIntosh and Laredo.[132] This military quarantine order complicated any attempt by American medical authorities to call in African American troops for a show of military medical force. The experience with fevers and disease in Cuba and the Philippines probably gave military surgeons pause. In November, following the order to expel black troops from southern states, the army found a way to bring troops through the quarantine and protect the state of Texas. As Penn bluntly stated, "The train will be in charge of a Marine Hospital Service and a guard of State Rangers and will be run through the state, doors and windows being securely closed while passing through the towns and cities of the state."[133] The quarantined, yet mobile, railcar demonstrated that federal authorities were more committed to moving black troops out of South Texas than to keeping quarantine.

On November 30, 1903, the state of Texas lifted the quarantine around Laredo.[134] Guiteras continued his disinfection work in Laredo through December, seeking the places where mosquito larvae might survive a winter.[135] Dr. Edmond Souchon used the difficult experience in containing yellow fever in Laredo to argue that mosquitoes were not the origin, the source, or the vector for yellow fever.[136] This, however, slowly became a minority opinion among state health officers. Four years later, Dr. Trueheart placed mosquito eradication and patient isolation at the center of quarantine methods against yellow fever.[137] Laredo marked the beginning of the end of absolute quarantine at the border. Modified quarantines emerged in its wake.

A Border Crucible: Mixing and Melting
National Identities into Public Health

Six months later, Guiteras reflected on his experience containing the yellow fever epidemic in Laredo at the Texas-Mexico border. The USPHMHS considered their efforts in the Laredo epidemic a success, although nearly one out of every seventeen of the border city's residents came down with yellow fever: 1,050 cases and 103 deaths in a town of 18,000 people. The Laredo campaign was the first federally coordinated mass public health effort in the United States to prevent the transmission of yellow fever by mosquitoes. Under

Guiteras's guidance, the state of Texas and the USPHMHS were able to keep the epidemic in Laredo, mostly through mosquito eradication projects. The USPHMHS experience in Laredo confirmed two key principles in a newly prominent American public health practice: First, Walter Reed was still correct in his observation that *Stegomyia* mosquitoes transmitted yellow fever between people. Second, crucial parts of Surgeon Gorgas's mosquito eradication efforts in Havana, Cuba, during the American occupation could be duplicated in the United States. The USPHMHS transformed the yellow fever epidemic in Laredo, Texas, into a useful federal staging ground for grander claims for American medical expertise and political authority.

The USPHMHS's on-the-ground experience with the complexities of the Texas-Mexico borderlands frustrated this triumph over disease. According to Guiteras's report, the biggest challenge he faced was eliciting full cooperation from individuals and city authorities. He first had to explain the three-year-old mosquito vector theory of yellow fever transmission to his fellow professionals, reporting that, "with one or two exceptions, the Laredo physicians were unacquainted with yellow fever, and at that time, when there were still many persons who denied the existence of the disease, they were lukewarm in reporting cases."[138] Moreover, local residents seemed to be skeptical of public medical authority throughout the epidemic. Guiteras reported that "the ignorant class of the population seldom called in a physician, fearful that they might be quarantined or sent to a hospital."[139] Laredo residents' fear of the power of state medical professionals to isolate and quarantine irked Guiteras as he sought to build a field hospital where he could isolate, house, and treat anyone suspected of having yellow fever. As he noted, "After consultation with the mayor and other prominent citizens I was dissuaded from carrying out my intentions respecting the establishment of a hospital."[140] Guiteras gave the impression that the majority of Laredo's working-class residents forced this popular consensus regarding medical authority on the city, the state, and the federal authorities. Working-class authority frustrated Dr. Guiteras, but he found the Laredo political and military authorities' acquiescence to working-class fears far more troubling.

For Guiteras, this popular consensus was a direct medical threat to the United States. Laredo's political indifference challenged the new common sense required by yellow fever prevention efforts. According to Guiteras, "The lack of authority to carry out the sanitary measures was, as may be seen from what has gone before, the most important obstacle to our success in dominating the epidemic. It interfered with the house-to-house inspection, with the oiling of barrels and cisterns, with the screening and disinfection of houses and premises, and prevented the establishment of a yellow fever hospital."[141] The local political culture in the border town constituted a direct threat to the kind of political power Dr. Guiteras wished the USPHMHS could yield in the United States during epidemics. The recent American experience with yellow fever in Havana during the occupation supplied Dr. Guiteras with an alternative political model for disease prevention in the continental United States: "The Laredo epidemic has shown conclusively to my mind that results such as were obtained in Habana in the suppression of yellow fever during the American occupation cannot be obtained elsewhere, where the disease is widely spread, without the undisputed authority and the means that were at the command of the government of intervention in Cuba. These powers in reality amounted to martial law."[142]

At one level, Laredo's residents seemed to be the obstacle to the export of medical progress and unilateral political authority back to the United States from its colonies abroad. Even Nuevo Laredo—the sister city on the other side of the Rio Grande—seemed to be a more productive alternative to the paralyzing fear of medical intervention held by Laredo's officials. The two towns shared two bridges, a ferry, three railroads, and a yellow fever epidemic but did not share a joint political authority. In direct contrast with Laredo, Governor Reyes of Nuevo León declared martial law to enforce cooperation with health officer Dr. de la Garza's efforts in Nuevo Laredo. Guiteras observed that "the Mexican authorities, indeed, had the advantage of power, which we lacked. They were not confronted by the good citizens insisting that 'his house is his castle' and that they would shoot the first one who attempted an entrance, but on the other hand, they lacked the 'sinews of war' to make their power effective."[143] For Dr. Guiteras and the USPHMHS, the relative autonomy that Laredo's working-class and ethnic Mexican residents wielded at the border during a yellow fever epidemic was a cautionary lesson and a vivid justification for the expansion of American state capacity and federal public health authority across the United States. For the residents, forcing the USPHMHS doctors to provide them with medical treatment for yellow fever within their own houses gave them a substantial measure of control and personal authority. Conflicts over yellow fever quarantine efforts were part of the experience of citizenship at this American medical border.

Dr. Guiteras's report left out the complex dimensions of the thorough medical transformation of Laredo that the USPHMHS achieved with the co-operation of residents. All of Laredo had to internalize the placement of oil in standing water to kill mosquito larvae, even in the barrels of drinking water maintained by *colonia* residents. The mosquito eradication projects compromised their drinking water, and the state of Texas and the U.S. Army established a modified quarantine around Laredo. This cut the town off from the railroads and the surrounding countryside. Despite the claims of a universal quarantine, the U.S. Army still moved the troops in the Tenth Cavalry division stationed at Fort McIntosh—mostly black cavalry who had recently arrived to recover from their counterinsurgency efforts in the American occupation of the Philippines—out of Laredo in a railcar during the height of the quarantine.[144] Other residents confronted the possible destruction of their houses (*jacales* and "huts," in the parlance of the USPHMHS) when Dr. Guiteras or others identified yellow fever among residents. The report registered little empathy for the difficulties working-class men and women faced finding enough food while negotiating two months of a state quarantine and a federal mosquito eradication project in Laredo.

Empathy aside, Gregorio Guiteras took the time to describe Laredo's residents using neat racial criteria: "The population of Nuevo Laredo, of course, consists almost entirely of Mexicans, there being few Americans. In a measure the same about Laredo, TX [sic]. It is estimated that there are but 3,000 Americans in the place. Moreover, the Mexican populations consist almost entirely of the lower class, ignorant and superstitious."[145] Guiteras's statement turned Laredo into a working-class "Mexican" town. His description omitted the Anglos and African Americans at the border from the report and transformed Laredo's diverse and cosmopolitan Mexican and Mexican American population into Mexicans.[146] His medical report placed Laredo far outside an American consensus around yellow fever, a national medical consensus that he was imposing on Laredo. He drew a stark and incorrect contrast between American medical values and Laredo's "ignorant, and superstitious" Mexican residents. Guiteras—a Cuban physician once in exile whose medical expertise and revolutionary activities helped him become a medical officer with the U.S. Army during the American occupation of Cuba—made the Laredo quarantine into a stage to project his professional belonging and newly adopted American identity.[147] The medical border he helped establish around Laredo also shaped a variety of Mexican and American identities.

Medical borders clearly did not follow political borders. This chapter explored the conceptual and political difficulties public health officials faced when forcing public health practices to conform to political borders after 1898. Though people outside Laredo used the Texas quarantines to stage an alleged conflict between American modernity and Mexican atavism, the political situation around Laredo in the 1890s was already upsetting the assumption that American federal health authorities controlled the practice and privilege of modern public health. American public health policies provided a point of ethnic and racial conflict that helped stage divisions between ethnic others and modern middle-class (white) American identities.

But modern medical policies were under discussion in Laredo. The political debate over the importance of vaccination in the midst of the Laredo smallpox epidemic made this very clear. The ethnic Mexican presence on all sides of the conflicts in 1899 demonstrated that vaccination upset any easy equation between medical technologies and national identities. Local Mexicans and Americans debated the merits of vaccination, isolation, and quarantine just as they debated whether mosquitoes were the most important vector for yellow fever. Life under the quarantines simply raised the political stakes of these medical debates. Establishing easily discernable national identities in a shared territory when Mexico, the United States, and Texas were themselves undergoing vast political and cultural transformations was already a difficult regional, national, and international task. Public health at the border became a key flashpoint in this larger international process.

Smallpox and yellow fever in Laredo became sites of tension over the many definitions of the term "Mexican" in the context of national borders and modern public health. The political tensions in the smallpox quarantine exposed competing identities within American and Mexican communities, issues subsumed under the terms "Mexican" and "American." These issues emerged even as national coverage sought to reestablish a contrast between "orderly America" and "dangerous Mexico." In 1903 as in 1899, there was substantial cooperation and a variety of medical and cultural tensions among Texas, Mexico, and U.S. health officers. In this epidemic, key federal players used the general autonomy demanded by working-class Norteños (northern Mexicans) and Tejanos (Texas Mexicans) to place Laredo outside the borders of a civilized and modern United States. This American medical stance on Mexican border culture sidestepped significant political differences with Texas health officers, in particular State Health Officer Tabor's commitment to the environmental origins of yellow fever. The yellow fever quarantine gave the USPHMHS a place to put to work in the continental United States the national identity they had forged in the military occupation of Cuba, Puerto Rico, and the Philippines. The aftermath provided a stark counterpoint between Mexican and American culture.

After the yellow fever epidemic in Laredo subsided, local and national public health officials came to very different conclusions regarding cooperation with national public health measures. Dr. Amador Sanchez, the mayor of Laredo, called for a cooperative and well-funded federal public health authority for epidemic disease prevention at the border. Dr. Guiteras, a one-time Cuban *insurgente* and the USPHMHS surgeon in charge of the federal yellow fever quarantine in Laredo, reacted very differently. He labeled the majority of residents of Laredo—"the Mexican populations," that is—"almost entirely of the lower class, ignorant and superstitious" and used his experience in Laredo to call for martial law in any future domestic epidemic.[148] Dr. Tabor, the Texas state health officer, held that the quarantine along the railroad lines kept yellow fever in Laredo. He maintained this position, holding to a belief that yellow fever had atmospheric and organic origins and calling quarantine against any yellow fever outbreak in Mexico. The actions placed him in direct political conflict with the USPHMHS. Moreover, Milton Rosenau, the director of the National Hygienic Laboratory, and four other assistant surgeon generals stood in direct opposition to Tabor's muscular assertions: "A quarantine directed against the whole of a large country, certain limited portions of which are known to have been infected with yellow fever within the last twelve months is unscientific and a retrograde step."[149] They thought mosquito eradication eliminated any need for state quarantines against yellow fever. At the federal level, Tabor's formulations and Laredo's indifferences led the USPHMHS to treat both Mexico and Texas as unscientific and retrograde counterpoints to modern American public health practice. These two binaries (Texas/America; Mexican/American) obscured the visible presence of African Americans, a variety of ethnic Mexican populations, different professional medical opinions, and the local Anglo-American accommodation to Texas-Mexico border cultures at Laredo. The American medical border effectively obscured the Mexican border's diversity as the border grew increasingly diverse and complicated.

People in South Texas publicly sought other forms of medical authority. Some pursued the care provided by *curandero* Don Pedrito Jaramillo. In stories told in the 1920s about the turn of the twentieth century, Don Pedrito Jaramillo and the water and airs of South Texas emerge as active healing forces. He told one woman to "take a bath at sunset for three days." He asked a man suffering from migraines to "drink glass of water with left hand. To take three pills, and walk by a hill with cenizo. The day after arrival, boil cenizo, reduce to half; let cool; filter; take a bath in the cenizo water; wear a coat to sweat; take one pill, wait 1 hour, pill, wait an hour." For an unknown heart ailment, he suggested that for five nights someone should "take the lady a glass of water drawn from a nearby river. *El costo de la receta era 10 centavos. El costo de los doctores era 100 pesos.* [The prescription costs 10 cents. The doctors cost one hundred dollars]." For sunstroke, one must "take baths outside for 9 days straight." When Anglo cattle rancher Zachary Gorbett suffered a severe case of measles, Doña Catarina remembered, Don Pedrito recommended that he "put water in a barrel and bathe after sunset." Mrs. Armstrong of San Antonio remembered she "ate a raw onion and took baths in water left out at night" for her chronic fatigue. To avoid chills, Jaramillo told Soto to "drink black coffee and whisky and then bathe in a pond at night. For five days."[150] The memories emphasized the patient's initial initiative, the importance of standing water, and—through the exposure to the night air—the healing power of the South Texas landscape. Cultural studies scholar Jose Limón argues that Don Pedrito Jaramillo poses an alternative form of power to American and Mexican state authority, being "a figure of critical difference, beset as [Mexican Americans] are by a new form of postmodern domination."[151] His prescriptions had power in the 1900s, where, to create a boundary between air and water, authorities "poisoned" with oil the very water Mexicanos held so dear. Water, among Don Pedrito Jaramillo's patients, had to maintain contact with the night. Patients had to feel a connection with the surrounding air. This ethos was a vivid counterweight to the liquid containment that came with the drastic imposition of (Cuban) American state medical authority during the Laredo quarantine.

Other men and women in Laredo found ways to construct a different relationship to state medical authority after 1903. They helped create a new state. When Venustiano Carranza declared his refusal to support Porfirio Díaz's reelection and instead threw his considerable military power behind Francisco I. Madero's reelection bid, many people in Laredo's Mexican elite embraced this liberal and revolutionary cause. Leonor Villegas de Magnon, a regular of the Pansy social club, the club Josefa Ortiz de Dominguez, and the Casino Mexicano's Fancy Dress Ball, established, organized, fund-raised, and

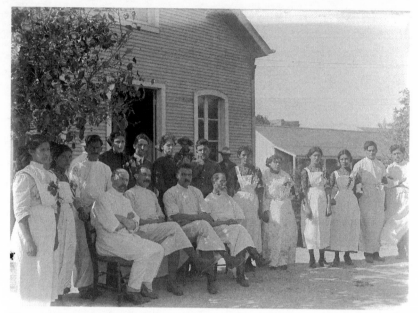

Figure 7. Robert Runyon, "Nurses and Carranza." Courtesy of the Robert Runyon Collection, "run00169," Center for American History, The University of Texas at Austin.

coordinated the Cruz Blanca. The nurses of the Cruz Blanca became known for their fierce defense of Mexican soldiers against Red Cross authority. Leonor Villegas de Magnon remembered using her status as a nurse to help smuggle healthy revolutionary soldiers back into battle. As she retold this story in serial form, "The hospital was surrounded by American soldiers. But as the days went on and the wounded got better, the problem had to be faced. The men could not leave the hospital and go about on American soil; they would be arrested. General González sent word that every man should return to his post the minute he was able to stand. So it was planned to spirit them out."[152] Villegas de Magnon covered the healthier soldiers with a white sheet and told the American authorities they were dead. Their exit from American medical scrutiny resuscitated them, and they returned to the revolution. Leonor Villegas and the Cruz Blanca reshaped medical authority to trouble the firm medical borders demanded by the Red Cross and the U.S. Army. Mexican popular culture and modern medical authority could come together against other medical borders.

There are many types of force, my friend, and
many types of intervention.—Pancho Villa,
El Paso Morning Times, October 9, 1915

FIVE

Domestic Tensions at an American Crossroads

Bordering on Gender, Labor, and Typhus Control, 1910–1920

"Thank god I had been able to wash. My boy and I looked clean as we walked into America,"[1] Nellie Oaxaca Quinn remembered when she recounted her 1915 sojourn in El Paso, Texas. After waiting for months in Ciudad Chihuahua, for her husband to return from his service with Pancho Villa's División del Norte, Mrs. Quinn and her son Anthony hopped a train north to the relative safety of Ciudad Juárez and El Paso, Texas. Once in El Paso, Quinn relied on informal networks other Mexican women had created in the streets of El Paso. After spending the night in the closest church, the Quinns walked out into downtown, where a friendly female pushcart vendor provided directions to affordable residences: "Go down the street till you come to a canal, then turn to right. Go along the canal 'till you come to some huts. You'll know when you get there. There are many poor people living there who will gladly take you and your son in for a few pennies a day."[2] Mrs. Quinn became a laundress and washed clothes in the canal. When she earned enough money to feed herself and her child and to cover the rent, she carried her son back over the bridge to search for her richer in-laws in Ciudad Juárez. Anthony Quinn's memoirs sketched the many spaces of his mother's domestic labor: commercial Ciudad Juárez, the bridge connecting Ciudad Juárez and El Paso, her work washing other people's clothes in El Paso, and their daily efforts to survive along the El Paso irrigation canal. Mrs. Quinn's movements across the bridge in 1915 brought her into informal contact with the men and women responsible for another form of domestic cleanliness: the inspectors of the U.S. Public Health Service (USPHS). The officers, however, were not involved in the arduous physical labor associated with cleaning the households, canals, and streets of El Paso. Instead, USPHS inspectors had the far more abstract task: finding ways to ensure that epidemic disease would not broach the domestic boundaries of the United States.[3] Rumors of typhus and smallpox outbreaks in the battlegrounds and cities of northern Mexico prompted Surgeon General Rupert Blue to assign key health officers and surgeons the task of ensuring "domestic" cleanliness through an unprecedented typhus quarantine along the Mexican border.[4] Recent arrivals to El Paso, like the Quinn household and many of the USPHS inspectors, took on the task of keeping the city clean. Inspectors, domestics, and laundry workers shared the streets and cleaned public and private spaces in El Paso: USPHS health officer C. C. Pierce in a disinfecting station on the north side of the Santa Fe Bridge and Mrs. Quinn on the north side of the irrigation canal in South El Paso. Both domestic workers and health officers cleaned, laundered, and disinfected clothes for people and households other than their own.[5] Nevertheless, residents of El Paso, commuters to El Paso, and Los Angeles–bound southerners and *norteños* applied very different meanings to laundry work and medical disinfection. The unequal distribution of labor and public credit for cleaning and disease prevention in El Paso added to the existing tensions and conflicts in the streets of Ciudad Juárez and El Paso.

The conflicts over public and private "domestic" labors made ongoing contacts between Mexican and American El Paso more visible. People in El Paso responded to these contacts in at least two ways. Many emphasized the contribution that all residents and arrivals could make to the city of El Paso.[6] The second response—a push to define and separate Mexican and American spaces in the households, streets, streetcars, and leisure spaces of Ciudad Juárez and El Paso—is a more familiar part of American historiography.[7] Although the regional origins of people in Ciudad Juárez and El Paso grew more diverse, the typhus campaign strengthened a Mexican/American distinction in a place where migration and urban settlement were already transforming the internal meaning of Mexican and American in El Paso. This city was already the most diverse American border town in 1910, with visible African American, Chinese, and Native American communities. Moreover, internal American migration was also redefining the term "Mexican." Most visibly,

Felix Martinez, a member of New Mexico's Hispano elite, moved south from Las Vegas, New Mexico, and built working ties with elite Mexican exiles in Sunset Heights.[8] The city of El Paso doubled in population between 1910 and 1920 to 77,560 people, drawing more white and black residents from Iowa, Kansas, Louisiana, and Texas, as well as the Mexican states of Jalisco, Michoacán, Zacatecas, Durango, and Chihuahua.[9] Migration from across the Americas transformed El Paso.

El Paso was almost the quintessential greater American crossroads. For black and white southerners bound west, the cities of Anthony, New Mexico, and El Paso, Texas, marked the end of the road for legal railroad car segregation.[10] For people going east from the West Coast, El Paso marked the transition back to segregated railcars. The northern rail hub of Ciudad Juárez and El Paso, moreover, played a key role in the Mexican Revolution. Francisco I. Madero, Victoriano Huerta, Francisco Villa, and Venustiano Carranza turned both cities into supply centers, battlegrounds, places of refuge, gun depots, hostile enemy camps, resting places, and shopping centers at key points during the revolution. As the politics and demographics in El Paso and Ciudad Juárez grew more complex, the public tensions over disease prevention and domestic labor in El Paso provided a medical vocabulary to separate this complex binational urban fabric into Mexican and American spaces.

A Difficult Crossroads: Typhus and Medical Progress, 1893–1917

The election of Surgeon General Rupert Blue to the presidency of the American Medical Association in 1916 marked a peak in the popularity and power of the USPHS. Along the border, twenty years of medical and intellectual change had transpired since the failed experiment in smallpox serotherapy in Camp Jenner. In 1896, U.S.-based advocates of disease-specific theories in public health could only point to rabies and the 1894 diphtheria antitoxin campaign to justify their continued investment in laboratory-based remedies for epidemic diseases.[11] By 1916, the U.S. Army had a typhoid vaccine that yielded temporary immunity.[12] Walter Reed and the USMHS had identified a mosquito vector for yellow fever.[13] Dr. Guiteras and the USMHS had successfully contained a yellow fever outbreak to Laredo, Texas, in 1903. Major William Crawford Gorgas used this insight to keep white American workers alive long enough to finish the Panama Canal by 1915. Public health campaigns in Puerto Rico, Cuba, and the Philippines demonstrated that the U.S. Army could coordinate campaigns against native hosts and native diseases.[14]

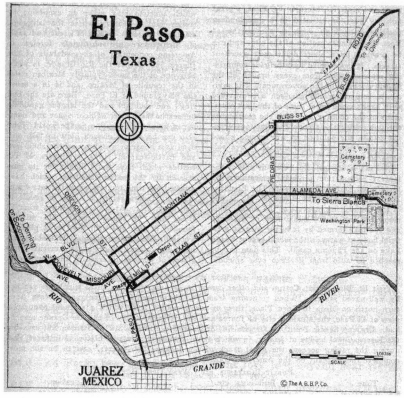

Figure 8. Map of El Paso, 1920. Courtesy of the Perry-Castañeda Map Collection, The University of Texas at Austin.

Internationally, Paul Ehrlich's arsenic dye stain, Salvarsan, bonded with and killed syphilis spirochetes and provided what he called a "magic bullet" against syphilis.[15] The examples were persuasive enough that many audiences in the United States were prepared to accept public health campaigns that coordinated various institutions to target specific diseases.

The Immigration Act of 1893 gave this public health push toward disease-specific intervention a wider legal latitude.[16] Although there were precedents in the Chinese Exclusion Acts, the Immigration Act of 1893 expanded the grounds for exclusion and narrowed the means through which arriving passengers, both U.S. citizens and foreign nationals could use due process and equal protection claims to challenge their exclusion orders.[17] Medical opinion came to intersect with local debates over the boundaries of citizenship, due process, and the legal status of domestic racial minorities and colonial subjects.[18] The act added medical authority to conflicts of police power and individual autonomy.[19] The increasing cultural authority of laboratory-based, disease-specific public health campaigns justified a wider field of discretion for public health officers. Popular opinion gave doctors a wide leeway when compulsory public health measures were necessary to ensure the survival of local, regional, and national communities.

These public health measures also conflicted with important strands in American law, such as the common law belief in personal autonomy and the constitutional principles of due process, equal protection, and liberty of contract. These legal principles challenged medical authority over the medical decision-making process. The courts and the public gave doctors the legal authority over the interpretation of disease, but they also gave citizens the authority to determine the legal boundaries of any medical treatment.[20]

Moreover, innovation and change in the field of public health complicated the boundary separating authority over the diagnosis and the treatment of disease. A scientific innovation—Walter Reed and Carlos Finlay's identification of the mosquito vector for yellow fever—led public health authorities to place gasoline on standing water, mosquito nets over water supplies, and mosquito nets over patients in full isolation.[21] Mosquito prevention redefined individual privacy. The success of these measures also led the USPHS to end their annual quarantines against Cuba and Veracruz and helped American authorities believe they could build a canal across Panama. These were drastic changes in public boundaries. When health departments started using laboratory tests to diagnose typhoid, they found that a number of ostensibly healthy people also had typhoid bacteria. In New York, the conflict between a laboratory culture of typhoid bacteria and the personal experience of health led to an open conflict between private chef Mary Mallon and the New York City Health Department. The publicity about her escapades led to her nickname, "Typhoid Mary," and likely to her subsequent twenty-three years in medical detention on North Brother Island.[22] The New York Board of Health drew up guidelines to lower the costs of permanent medical incarceration and establish due process rights for this new class of citizens: healthy carriers.[23]

Disease-specific innovations and the desire to prevent further epidemics also led to the federal and municipal distribution of disease-specific remedies. In 1894, the New York City Board of Health decided to make the diphtheria serum treatment widely available to everybody suffering from the disease.[24] The subsequent faith in antitoxin serum therapy contributed to the flawed field trial of a smallpox antitoxin on African (American) refugees in Eagle Pass, Texas, in 1895.[25] The USPHS started illegally producing Salvarsan in World War I and made the six- to nine-month syphilis treatment regimen available and financially accessible to men and women through a wide network of federally subsidized community clinics.[26] These three cases illustrate the potentially fraught process through which changing laboratory tests and industrial production methods interacted with the growing faith in medical authority to paradoxically narrow the goals and expand the field of urban public health.[27]

Oddly, typhus had been comparatively resistant to disease-specific approaches in the nineteenth century. Typhus epidemics accompanied crop failures, cold winters, wars, and rising food prices. This link made it clear that social forces shaped the appearance of typhus, and, unsurprisingly, the discipline of social medicine developed around typhus. In Germany, the premier diagnostician and epidemiologist Rudolf Virchow investigated an outbreak of typhus in the Polish borderlands with Germany. He concluded that the people who suffered the most from typhus in Silesia were the ethnic Polish peasants, a caste blocked from participating in politics. It was his medical opinion that typhus epidemics would continue to appear as long as regional politics denied local Polish residents voice and power in the decisions that shaped their lives.[28] For Virchow, voice and power meant universal suffrage, bilingual education, strong labor unions, adequate sanitation, and industrial investment throughout Germany; he prescribed social democracy as the best remedy for typhus.[29] Virchow believed his research in Silesia proved that the prevalence of typhus followed from political conditions and thus political reform was the most effective public health intervention. However, this was a minority point of view. German medical opinion associated the absence of typhus with cleanliness, industry, whiteness, and civilization, while the presence of typhus was due to filth, Jewish cultural practices, the Roma in general, or traditional cultural practices.[30] Medical historian Paul Weindling has argued that the majority of German physicians throughout the twentieth century held people suffering from typhus responsible for their condition. These two approaches placed typhus at the center of a large debate over the role of public health in bridging the presence of disease to the experience of citizenship.

On the whole, interest groups and emerging states used the fear and stigma associated with filth, labor mobility, and outsider status to exclude, disinfect, or expel ethnic migrants or minorities as part of nation-building efforts in industrializing regions in Europe, Africa, Mexico, Canada, and the United States.[31] The typhus epidemic among Eastern European residents of New York City's Lower East Side prompted the U.S. Congress to write the Immigration Act of 1893, in which they defined typhus as a "loathsome and communicable disease" and mandated the detention or exclusion of any immigrant alien with symptoms of typhus.[32] American consuls and port authorities pressured German authorities and shipping lines to contain the movement of Russian Jews, Polish Jews, and other migrants through German borders into the United States.[33] Despite the lack of medical consensus around the social origins of typhus, border stations across northern Europe carried out the punitive cleansing of many Jewish, Polish, and Slavic passengers in Baltic passenger lines. In West Texas and El Paso, medical authorities followed rumors of typhus in Mexico closely. In 1892, Dr. Bennett of the Texas State Health Office published rumors of a typhus outbreak in Zacatecas along the Mexican Central Railroad.[34] In 1894, Dr. Warfield added some terrifying images to accompany the rumors of typhus. Like Dr. Pope in his 1882 survey of housing in South Texas, Warfield argued that the overcrowded housing, the lack of water, and the family refusal to isolate a disease sufferer "all tend to encourage sickness of every sort."[35] In his professional opinion, "the mode of living of the Mexicans of the lower class is so contrary to the laws of nature that the wonder is that they live at all."[36] Despite the implied housing reforms that came with his emphasis on "mode of living," Warfield also called for more enthusiastic policing of Mexican workers crossing the border, since "the quarantine borders at the border do not seem strict enough for as carried out at the present time, anyone with typhus, not in the delirious stage and with strength enough to sit up, can pass across the line from Mexico into the United States without being subjected to any direct examination."[37] The general stigma and fear of the intense muscular pain, the high fevers (104–5 degrees), the visions, the internal bleeding, the presence of blood splotches, the death of one out of five cases, and the ongoing threat of relapses from the initial infection outweighed the lack of medical consensus regarding the source of typhus.[38] Instead of improving housing conditions to prevent typhus, doctors across the United States called for the inspection and expulsion of ethnic migrants.

The public success bacteriologists enjoyed in identifying the key vector for yellow fever, syphilis, tuberculosis, and malaria did not lead to a medical consensus regarding typhus.[39] For advocates of disease-specific approaches to public health, the loose association between typhus and unequal social conditions was theoretically inadequate and clinically unacceptable. This perception changed after 1910, when researchers started applying the insect vector model to patients with typhus. An American researcher in Mexico City and a French researcher in Algeria isolated the body louse as a vector that transmitted typhus from one chimpanzee to another. Charles Nicolle published his findings from his base in the Pasteur Institute in Algeria.[40] Howard Ricketts, working independently on the same transmission model in Mexico City, confirmed that the louse was a vector and that rats were the main host. Two USPHS researchers, John Anderson and Joseph Goldberger, confirmed similar immune reactions to typhus in Poland, Brill's disease in New York City, and *tabardillo* (Mexican typhus) in northern Mexico.[41] With the vector in hand, clinical researchers started searching for the presence of a germ in the body louse. Within four years USPHS bacteriologist Harry Plotz had cultured a bacterial colony of a possible typhus pathogen—the spirochete ultimately named *Rickettsia prowazeki*.[42] In the space of five years, laboratory research had moved a medical debate on the etiology of typhus from filth and famine to consensus regarding a potential germ in an insect vector. The state practice of typhus prevention was about to change.

These discoveries changed the clinical diagnosis but not the treatment of typhus. German and Polish clinicians started using the Widal test to eliminate and differentially diagnose typhus to aid in their clinical research. These improved laboratory techniques did not change the 70 percent mortality rate among adults over forty years old (as reported by the USPHS in 1917 along the Texas-Mexico border).[43] Although the diagnosis of typhus shifted drastically in five years, the treatment still revolved around maintaining the strength of the patient and minimizing the damage from the fevers, attacks on the nervous system, hallucinations, and the internal bleeding and muscle damage. Clinical progress did not match laboratory progress. Typhus had been emblematic of the promise of social medicine; it was now a good example of how the germ theory of disease failed to deliver. The USPHS faced problems explaining why the progress in diagnosis far surpassed advances in treatment.

The medical consensus on louse-based transmission shaped state practices of typhus prevention. Before 1910, USPHS border inspectors indiscriminately applied soap and water to immigrant European bodies associated with typhus. After 1915, prevention efforts focused on separating lice from the same suspect human bodies. C. C. Pierce—the USPHS assistant surgeon whom Surgeon General Blue assigned to coordinate typhus quarantine—emphasized clothing fumigation, residential whitewashing, and the use of kerosene and vinegar baths to eliminate lice and their eggs from human bodies.[44] Recent success in the Panama Canal Zone helped the USPHS assert expertise and temporary control over potentially louse-ridden terrain: clothing, residences, and bodies. The typhus-carrying louse embedded itself in the fuzzy association of filthy conditions and dangerously retrograde cultures. There was now no need to improve other people's hazardous cultural practices, inadequate sanitation, or meager salaries. The destruction of the louse on people crossing through key gateways replaced the expulsion of people or the expensive reform of inadequate housing. The new bacteriological understanding of a vector-based typhus shifted the public health contact zone between patient and inspector from housing to the clothes, hair, and armpits of suspect bodies. Migrants, *colonia* residents, and local minorities had to learn to adapt to this drastic change.

The regional context and outcomes of previous struggles shaped the public health contact zone between public health officers, local residents, and migrants. Some American citizens challenged this expanding authority on constitutional grounds. In *Jacobson v. Massachusetts*, the U.S. Supreme Court ruled that the state of Massachusetts could detain, fine, or use other measures to force compliance with compulsory vaccination measures; inconsistently, the same court ruled that the act of vaccination required explicit consent from each citizen.[45] The New York Supreme Court provided a more robust definition of consent. In *Schloendorff v. Society of New York Hospital*, the court agreed with Mary Schloendorff that any operation completed without the willful consent of the patient constituted assault and battery—although the court did not require damages from the Society of New York Hospital.[46] Both cases showed that state and federal courts were uncomfortable allowing state medical power to extend past the boundary of the human body. Skin provided the point of contact between state and citizen. The existence of this individual border zone depended on the state recognition of each citizen's authority.

Legal authority enforcing this contact zone was in flux on both sides of the Texas-Mexico border. For example, in Chihuahua the mobilization of workers, peasants, and local Indian nations against Porfirio Díaz shattered the ability of state authorities to coerce consent. First, local military mobilization for Francisco I. Madero threatened conservative hacienda owners in Chihuahua.[47] Subsequent conflicts after Victoriano Huerta's coup d'état led the more liberal sectors of the landowning elite in Chihuahua to leave for El Paso and San Antonio.[48] The conflict between the Constitutionalist Convention and Venustiano Carranza led to direct attacks on Pancho Villa's Division del Norte, a struggle that lasted into the 1920s. Public health interventions relied on the relative ability of a local government to coerce, persuade, and coordinate the activities of residents and migrants. The competition among revolutionary factions for the support of the urban residents of the state of Chihuahua broke this form of police power in the state.

El Paso itself was wrestling with the activities of its residents and migrants, half of whom were not around in 1910. The city quadrupled in size between 1900 and 1920; it contained 24,886 people in 1900, 52,599 in 1910, and 101,877 by 1920. The U.S.-born population held steady—there were 39,279 U.S.-born white residents in 1910 and 42,000 in 1920—but the foreign-born population more than doubled, to 42,305, in the space of ten years.[49] The change in the foreign- and U.S.-born ratio created political opportunities for white American newcomers. Tom Lea, a local lawyer and a migrant from Missouri, beat incumbent Mayor Charles Kelly by "advocating the removal of undesirable Mexicans from El Paso" and trumpeting his independence from long-standing machine politicians involved in the Kelly ring.[50] The rumors of typhus from Mexico fell nicely into Lea's reform trajectory and campaign promises against the Mexican presence in El Paso. The political and demographic changes in El Paso and the revolution in the state of Chihuahua provided the local frame for the new typhus prevention techniques the USPHS wanted to implement in El Paso and Laredo.

Moving Responsibilities: Typhus and the El Paso City Jail Firestorm, 1916

As El Paso and Ciudad Juárez grew in population and in diversity, the Santa Fe Bridge forced different sectors of society to come together to cross the Rio Bravo. From 1903 on, inspectors from the U.S. Marine Hospital and Public Health Service (USMHPHS) provided professional weight to the ways people distinguished between locals and outsiders. Between 1903 and 1915, both medical and immigration inspectors worked the Santa Fe Bridge and the railroad passenger cars, making distinctions between upper- and lower-class Mexican nationals; between Chinese nationals, Chinese Mexicans, and Chinese Americans; and between Syrian nationals and Syrian Mexicans. Inspectors forbade entry the people they identified as Chinese nationals and forced lower-class Mexican and Syrian nationals to submit to humiliating medical inspections and certifications. Moreover, inspectors could deny foreign nationalities entry because of trachoma or other medical conditions. The most common exclusion was economic—"Likely to Become a Public Charge" (LPC)—and authorities usually singled out women accompanied by children.[51] American nationals, already concerned about the "bodies out of place" migrating to the United States, wanted to be sure that certified medical authorities regulated this cross-border traffic.[52]

Illness and death among the inspectors in the Santa Fe Bridge inspection station broke the American fantasy that a medical inspection station physically separated the living conditions of Anglo professional households from the living conditions that fostered rats and lice among working commuters in El Paso and Ciudad Juárez. On February 27, 1916, Inspector Morris Buttner passed away from the fevers, internal bleeding, and overwhelming physical stress associated with typhus. His death left his wife and daughter bereft and alone in El Paso. The visibility of Buttner's suffering catalyzed migrant American households in El Paso into action.[53] For some southern and midwestern settlers, Buttner's death underlined the precariousness of American settlement in "border" El Paso; these anxieties conveniently ignored the near doubling of U.S.-born, out-of-state residents in El Paso over the previous five years.[54] His death transformed the inspection station from a place that separated Mexicans from Americans to a place that connected American families to Mexican conditions.[55]

Buttner's death and the presence of domestic workers added to the general sense that the American standard of living was far shakier than they expected. Charities and concerned citizens responded by trying to give the Buttner household "an American standard of living."[56] The *El Paso Times* and the USPHS mounted a public campaign to raise funds for his surviving daughter. Churches, schools, and courthouses rang with appeals for these funds.[57] Through this campaign, boosters for the city of El Paso strengthened their resolve to make El Paso an urban place where American sojourners could profitably settle. The term "American standard of living" was no accident. White workers in El Paso resented the steady wages Mexican Smeltertown workers received. They also feared the possibility that local growers would import Japanese labor from California and Hawaii. There was a concern that these new workers would start competing for other jobs or would start their own farms, as Japanese laborers had done in California.[58] The Buttner household probably was one of the houses that contributed to the rising numbers of Mexican women doing domestic work in El Paso's Anglo households. In order to prevent more deaths associated with challenges to the American standard of illness, city and federal authorities moved their focus from the bridge to domestic laborers.

The subsequent public tensions around this cleansing highlight the role of Mexican women in the germ control campaign and help expose "the complex ways in which the relationship between women and the public terrain is specific to class, ethnic/racial identity and the historic moment."[59] The revolution and social discontent in Mexico, suffrage movements across the United States, and the national debate regarding preparedness for the war in Europe provided a heady historical moment. El Paso authorities called for a visible change in typhus eradication measures in the wake of Buttner's death. Health officers W. C. Kluttz, C. C. Pierce, and J. W. Tappan implemented kerosene and vinegar baths in facilities under their immediate control: the hospital and the city jail.[60] Public health authorities assumed that unattached Mexican male laborers were the vector for typhus. Typhus prevention work also brought health officials into intensive contact with Mexican women who were workers, mothers, daughters, and El Paso residents.

The decision to use kerosene and vinegar mixtures on men detained in the city hospital and the city jail backfired on El Paso's medical authorities. On March 6, 1916, Dr. George Cainan and Frank Scotte ordered fifty of their male prisoners to move into the central courtyard, remove their clothing, and prepare for dousing in a kerosene-vinegar mixture.[61] A spark ignited the kerosene-vinegar vapor above the vats, causing a tremendous explosion. The flames engulfed everyone who was in the prison courtyard close to the baths. The explosion blew out the windows of the prison and placed the patients inside at risk but provided an exit for the people still alive in the prison courtyard.[62] Prisoners and patients ran to safety.[63] A public health decision had become a public safety risk.

El Paso residents responded to the open jailhouse doors in various ways. Some prisoners and some patients escaped. Other residents forced their way into the prison in an attempt to tend to anyone who was unable to leave. The *San Antonio Express* reporter assigned to the story wrote, "The odor of gasoline mingled with that of human flesh and clothing became so stifling that it was impossible for rescuers to approach the doors to unlock them until oxygen helmets were provided."[64] Seventeen-year-old Carmen Alonzo, "the heroine of the rescue work," applied the first aid techniques she learned on the battlefields of Mexico to men suffering severe burns.[65] News of the deaths, burns, and damage within the prison courtyard caused some to call on other El Paso residents to expand their sense of community. In the shadow of the initial deaths, Fred Fisher called on his lay missionary audience to empathize with prisoners, as "the day is out when we look upon prisoners as prisoners. We must regard them as men. Had we not better advantages ourselves, we too might have been in that very prison Monday afternoon."[66] Even Mayor Tom Lea celebrated individuals who acted in ways that treated patients and prisoner as equals by featuring Carmen Alonzo and El Paso fire chief Jim Wray for their heroic work.[67] This expanded sense of community in El Paso openly challenged the federal and city public health authorities' seemingly callous regard for the victims.

Reporters and observers also focused on the actions of authorities and detainees after their escape from the courtyard. The *El Paso Times*, the *San Antonio Express*, and the *El Paso Herald* reported on the effort to find the prisoners who fled the flames in pain. There were fifty men slated for disinfection, but the rescuers counted eleven deaths and placed thirty-eight others in the local hospital. One prisoner was missing from the official count. According to the *San Antonio Express*, two Mexican laborers still on fire managed to cross the river and told residents of Ciudad Juárez that El Paso city authorities had rounded up Mexican men, poured gasoline over them, locked the doors, and lit a match in the immediate vicinity.[68] The USPHS and the city of El Paso had taken a major risk establishing kerosene-vinegar baths within criminal detention facilities.

One reporter surmised that the many people living in Ciudad Juárez gave the prisoners' report "real credit, [due to] ill feeling in [Ciudad] Juarez for several days because of the precautions taken against typhus fever being brought over by Mexicans from the interior."[69] Some residents in Ciudad Juárez made their anger clear over the American conflation of public health practices and punitive facilities in El Paso. Crowds attacked the everyday signs of U.S. intrusion. One streetcar driver, Charles Phelps, was shot through a streetcar window on his way back from the racetrack, and his passengers trampled him in their attempt to flee. Drivers with American passengers in Ciudad Juárez made their way to El Paso.[70] U.S. reporters noted attacks on Americans, mostly race fans, in the commercial and entertainment districts in Ciudad Juárez. According to the report, people in Ciudad Juárez resented being placed in kerosene-vinegar baths and being stigmatized as typhus vectors, especially when they too may have felt threatened by epidemics and disorder to the south of them in Chihuahua, Durango, and central Mexico. Americans expected a response from authorities in Ciudad Juárez, but municipal authorities under the Carranza government declined to prevent the uprising.

The Customs Office closed automobile and streetcar traffic over the Santa Fe Bridge into Ciudad Juárez that very day. Over the next two days reporters linked attacks on U.S. nationals and property to continued anger about *el holocaust* (the firestorm). The U.S. Army continued demanding that General Francisco Murguía use armed troops to protect the circuit between El Paso and the racetrack in Ciudad Juárez. The firestorm in the courtyard shared by the city hospital and prison made the journey to racetracks and ballrooms in "sporting" Ciudad Juárez a visibly military venture.[71]

The firestorm also challenged El Paso's reputation for sunshine, public health, and progress, an image promoted by the city's civic boosters. As the *El Paso Morning Times* remarked, "Not only El Paso but the whole country is convinced that someone has been criminally negligent.... We owe it to ourselves to explain just how it came about that two score of unfortunates under our care were allowed to be cremated."[72] Mayor Tom Lea and El Paso judge Dan Jackson responded to this pressure and convened a grand jury to determine which member of the Sanitation Commission or Public Safety Commission was responsible for the El Paso firestorm and the streetcar riots in Ciudad Juárez. The *El Paso Times* called on Judge Jackson to "disclose something to place the city in a less unenviable position than it occupies in the mind of the people" and thus separated El Paso's public authority from the individuals responsible for the antityphus campaign.[73] Judge Jackson demanded that USPHS surgeon J. W. Tappan and C. C. Pierce appear before a grand jury to account for their use of kerosene and vinegar.[74]

A large crowd gathered at the courtroom door to hear the grand jury's indictment and got even more news than they expected. This group became the first assembly of people in El Paso to hear of Pancho Villa's attack on Columbus, New Mexico.[75] Local oral histories claim that Villa held the United States responsible for *el holocaust* when he heard of the injuries to and murders of twenty Mexican nationals in the El Paso city jail.[76] His troops attacked Columbus, and 110 of his men died while killing thirteen men Villa associated with the gun trade and the U.S. military effort. This battle prompted President Woodrow Wilson to commission General Pershing's pursuit of Villa.[77] This invasion also stalled Wilson's negotiations with the Carrancista government. Alexandra Stern argued, "reading these events through the lens of biopower," that Pancho Villa regained legitimacy among the working-class urban residents of Chihuahua and Ciudad Juárez because he punished the United States for the firestorm that engulfed soldiers of his who had been imprisoned in the El Paso city jail.[78] Perhaps Chihuahua residents resented the norms and discipline that would reshape working-class households in urban Chihuahua under a typhus eradication regime.

News of the Columbus raid transformed the community members gathered at the court house into a crowd. The community outside the courthouse walls read the Columbus attack through the lens of race: they assumed working-class Mexicans supported Pancho Villa and they shifted their attention to the Mexican neighborhoods surrounding downtown El Paso. Spectators stopped waiting to hear which city official was responsible for the deaths in the firestorm and turned their attention to the Mexican residents of El Paso, blaming them for the deaths in Columbus. The assembly turned into a mob and moved five blocks down to Chihuahuita, the "Mexican" neighborhood closest to downtown El Paso, and attacked any person that looked Mexican.[79] The newly American mob took Villa's raid as an illegitimate reprisal for the firestorm in the city jail; the mob demanded immediate retribution against the closest Mexicans in the United States.[80]

Federal authorities responded quickly to the news of an American mob making its way to Mexican El Paso. General Bell moved his troops off their posts on streetcars and the Santa Fe Bridge, transferring them to Chihuahuita. The troops protected the community of public health officers from the threat of Mexican reprisal on the bridge; in Chihuahuita and South El Paso, the troops contained an American crowd seeking to damage what they considered a Mexican neighborhood. The mob's violent redefinition of ethnic Mexican El Paso's community into foreigners challenged General Bell's claim on the legitimate exercise of violence at the border. The mob's violent push to enforce a Mexican/American boundary in El Paso forced the U.S. military to abandon their policing of Mexicans on the Santa Fe Bridge and to begin policing Americans on the streets of South El Paso.[81]

The firestorm and the Columbus raid shifted the terms of discussion for prisons and kerosene-vinegar baths. Susanna Houghton, a British resident of

Ciudad Chihuahua, confirmed the punitive aspect of the kerosene-vinegar baths when she told reporters, "The lower classes of Mexicans report that Villa raided Columbus because of his belief that the El Paso City Jail horror was deliberately planned by Americans."[82] In the immediate aftermath of the jail fire, officials such as Pierce searched for antilouse substances that were safer and less painful than the flammable baths. By March 18, the *El Paso Times* touted the public health authorities' use of staphysagria tincture to rid hair of lice.[83] The USPHS adopted the homeopathic mixture because "since the recent city jail horror, in which 25 persons lost their lives while being given a sanitary bath, health officers have had considerable difficulty administering the old solution."[84] In border stations, too, the horror of the prison deaths meant little to no cooperation with kerosene-vinegar baths.

Pancho Villa's surprise raid on Columbus, New Mexico, changed the political context of the kerosene-vinegar baths. The *El Paso Times* editorial board highlighted an obvious tension between prison management and public health management when they circulated a sardonic rumor "that police throughout the country are threatening prisoners with a gasoline bath in lieu of the third degree."[85] The mutual violence that emerged in the aftermath of *el holocausto* and the Columbus raid transformed the initial vaguely empathetic community-building reaction in El Paso. The kerosene-vinegar baths catalyzed two separate and mutually opposed Mexican and American communities that inhabited both Ciudad Juárez and El Paso. The USPHS pushed this Mexican/American division across El Paso as well as the Santa Fe Bridge.

City and federal authorities then moved typhus prevention from bridges and jails to the streets of El Paso. Paralleling his earlier appropriation of Mexican homeopathic measures for American disinfection measures, Pierce "appropriated" at least twenty Mexican residents from the Chihuahuita neighborhood for suspicion of harboring typhus and moved them to the county hospital. Assistant Surgeon Tappan pioneered automobile raids in the name of typhus prevention. The USPHS drove around South El Paso looking for people who looked like they would have lice and brought them to the disinfecting baths at the Santa Fe Bridge, stripped them of their clothing, and bathed them. While a family might have been fighting over the baths at the bridge, public health authorities disinfected their residence by burning or fumigating their belongings. Pierce reported, "While we did not pretend to clean up all of the lousy persons in that part of town, that fact that we were doing this, made others bathe and disinfect themselves, so that the change in the lower part of the town was noticeable."[86] The city of El Paso and the USPHS used the spectacle of terror and disinfection to create a culture of fear among the Mexican residents of El Paso.

Nellie Quinn, a resident of the Mexican part of town, remembered the 1916 public health campaign and the changes imposed on her family: "Some inspectors came to the neighborhood and started boarding up a lot of the shacks as unsanitary and unsafe. The women and children began crying as they were literally put out on the streets, but the inspectors said there was a terrible epidemic of smallpox further up the canal and all the area had to be cleaned up or burned down."[87]

The decision to condemn and destroy housing in working-class Mexican sections of El Paso challenges the idea that the germ theory of illness would lead to more targeted interventions. Rather than focus on the rats in El Paso, the city destroyed the housing for poor people. Landlords and tenants responded to the public stigma of the cleanup campaign by refusing to rent to anyone associated with the destruction of Chihuahuita. For women who depended on the streets to walk to the more prosperous sections of town to jobs as domestics or to get work laundering clothes in the river, a direct attack to working conditions came in the form of auto raids, public disinfections, and housing destruction. The city cleanup campaign targeted the working and living conditions for independent laundresses and domestic servants and left the poorer Chihuahuita residents homeless but in closer contact with El Paso's public spaces. Mrs. Quinn remembered, "The bloc[k] we were living in was condemned. . . . There was no house to be had anywhere. Everyone in El Paso was afraid to take anyone in from the contaminated neighborhood. I took [the] children and went to live under a tree in the outskirts of town. It was nice weather at the time. Thank God there were a lot of trees because other people got the same idea. Families just went out and found a tree to live under. I would say we lived there three or four months."[88]

As El Paso moved to define, contain, and disinfect the threat of typhus, families in the suspected neighborhoods bore the burden of this destruction. The auto raids and house destruction amplified the semimilitarized dimensions of the USPHS's approach toward epidemic disease. The militarization of public health tactics deepened the contradiction between neighborhood cleansing, cleaning labor, and the cleaning that typhus prevention required from the USPHS. As American men in official uniforms moved to cleanse the people in these spaces, many other American households in the city of

El Paso called on the domestic labor provided by Mexican women to live up to the newly established standards of cleanliness. By working in middle-class households or cleaning clothes in the neighborhood laundries, families from South El Paso and Chihuahuita provided much of the labor necessary to keep a clean and medically certified look. The disinfection measures that targeted Mexican neighborhoods attacked the ability of working-class families to survive on a daily basis. However, more prosperous and stable households in El Paso, whether they were Anglo or Mexican, still required daily labor to keep their domestic space and public face properly burnished. The typhus eradication campaign hindered the daily survival and everyday reproduction of domestic spaces inside and outside El Paso's homes.

Moving Spectacles: Women, Streetcars, and the Typhus Bath Riots

Even after the firestorm and subsequent riots, the USPHS maintained an inspection regime for the people who walked across the bridge. Inspectors subjected select male and female pedestrians to full body inspections; moreover, they hired (ethnic) Mexican male and female bath operators to help move selected immigrants and commuters into the sex-designated baths and to assist in placing their clothes in chemical baths designed to kill any insects among their clothes and belongings.[89] Day laborers and recent arrivals—men and women like Nellie Quinn who could not afford a streetcar—braved both inspection and forced bathing when they walked over the bridge into El Paso, Texas. In contrast, those men and women moving past the inspection station in their streetcars and automobiles witnessed an instructive spectacle in the unwritten benefits of their wheeled transportation. The streetcar ride insulated passengers from the perils of an unwanted inspection, and a simple glance out the window made the benefits of this privilege obvious.

The campaigns against typhus in El Paso's poorer Mexican neighborhoods raised the local profile for city authority and the USPHS health officers. The campaign cemented the contrast between now-suspect Mexican neighborhoods and (white) Anglo health inspectors: This also brought public health officials into close contact, or made them part of, the local disease environment. When the inspectors, city health authorities, and USPHS officers reviewed the cases of typhus among the people they detained in Chihuahuita and South El Paso, they invented a hidden trend. The majority of the cases were in South El Paso and Smeltertown—exactly where they looked for cases.

Patients were all recent arrivals from Mexico; however, they came down with typhus more than a month after their stated arrival to El Paso.[90] Most USPHS officers knew that the incubation period lasted between one and two weeks and that onset was marked by a severe headache, high fever, and a cough as well as possible muscle pain, sensitivity to light, and delirium. The onset of typhus after a month of settlement provided a solid argument for improving living and work conditions for people living in these two Mexican neighborhoods. USPHS assistant surgeon Pierce ignored this argument and stressed national origin over epidemiology, stating that all of these cases had spent a good portion of their lives in Mexico prior to their residence in South El Paso or Smeltertown. When city health officer Kluttz died from typhus fever on January 4, 1917, his death highlighted the seeming futility of auto raids, home destruction, and individual medical detention.[91] Pierce pushed for more aggressive USPHS disinfection policies that suggested stronger connections between ethnic Mexicans in El Paso and ethnic Mexicans living in Mexico on the other side of the bridge.[92] Mayor Tom Lea demanded the end of any contact between El Paso and Ciudad Juárez. After more pressure, President Wilson approved a full quarantine on traffic between the two cities. This quarantine led to inspections of everything crossing over the bridge.

The decision to enforce full disinfection on the Santa Fe Bridge required USPHS officers to act as if there were no overlapping households, communities, and workspaces in El Paso and Ciudad Juárez. Moreover, the decision to expand the reach of the typhus baths struck directly at key class distinctions among working commuters to El Paso. The USPHS did not expect the level of resistance they confronted on the streets when they began bathing all commuting laborers on Monday, January 28, 1917.

On that morning, a streetcar full of working commuters crossed the Santa Fe Bridge. Pierce stopped the streetcar at the end of the bridge and requested that everyone, including women, enter the disinfecting plant. Most observers reported that "the greater part of them refused to go along."[93] According to one observer, "Their indignation increased once they were ordered off the streetcars, after having paid their fares and could not have their nickels refunded."[94] Pierce insisted again; observers reported that Carmela Torres pushed back, hard.

The press coverage of women's actions reinforced what Irene Ledesma called an "implicitly Anglo, 'American,' and male criteria [that] touched only peripherally on the women's experience."[95] The El Paso Times presented the commuters' response as a surprising and violent reaction to a reasonable request: "When women were ordered to get off the streetcars and submit to being bathed and disinfected before passing to the American side," it started a "near riot among Juárez women."[96] The *New York Times* emphasized the directly insubordinate mood of the crowd through its headline: "Quarantine Riots in Juárez: Women Lead Demonstration against American Regulation."[97] The term "quarantine riot" reinforced images of antimodern Mexican city residents resisting attempts to eradicate the threat of contagion by USPHS quarantine facilities.[98] The coverage contrasted disorderly Mexican women with orderly American public health practices.

The spectacle of Mexican women publically resisting American authority in El Paso became the central object of the coverage.[99] The *San Antonio Express* headline escalated the *New York Times*'s contrast between American reason and feminine Mexican female resistance with the headline "Anti-American Riot Led by Red Haired Chief of Woman Mob."[100] The polemic reached its peak in *El Paso Times* bullet points: "Auburn haired Amazon at Santa Fe [S]treet [B]ridge leads feminine outbreak; rumor among servant girls that quarantine officers photograph bathers in the altogether responsible for wild scenes; streetcars seized and detained for hours; girls attack automobiles."[101] This polemic recognized yet belittled what often went unmarked in El Paso: the active presence of "Mexican" working women in the public spaces and private households in El Paso.

Open attacks by Mexican women on the southbound border-crossing privilege that came with automobiles and streetcars shocked the *El Paso Times* and *San Antonio Express* reporters. The rioters made the movement of streetcars and automobiles into Ciudad Juárez targets of their rage. The surprising challenge to the American privilege of automobiles probably pushed the *El Paso Times* reporter toward clichéd phrasing: "Those who witnessed the actions of the Mexican mob at the end of the bridge will never forget it."[102] He went on to state that the crowd, "composed largely of young girls, seemed bent on destroying anything that came from the American side. As soon as an automobile would cross the line the girls would absolutely cover it. The scene reminded one of bees swarming. The hands of the feminine mob would claw and tear the tops of cars. The ising-glass rear windows of the autos were torn out, the tops torn to pieces and parts of the fittings, such as lamps and horns, were torn away."[103]

The act of women collectively stripping the automobiles down to their basic essentials reversed the ways in which USPHS inspectors collectively stripped the clothes from Mexican women and men before certifying them for work across the border. The *Express* claimed that rioters wrecked and burned the streetcars, an eerie parallel with the firestorm six months earlier.[104] The perception that the mob would try "to injure and insult Americans as much as possible without actually committing murder" forced transportation businesses and the customs office to halt traffic into Ciudad Juárez.[105] By midday, the El Paso Electric Railway Company ended all attempts to move their streetcars into Ciudad Juárez. The *San Antonio Express* and the *El Paso Times* emphasized attacks on specific American men—streetcar operators, cameramen, racetrack regulars, and public health officials. A local businessman and member of El Paso's sporting life, David McChesney, caught in his automobile, was "beaten, scratched and his clothes torn from his body."[106] Again, the inversion of the USPHS's inspections is hard to avoid. Carmelita Torres personally attacked Nick McDonald, a motion picture operator for one of the movie weeklies, and forced him to stop filming the spectacle.[107] The crowd turned away motorists who attempted to enter Ciudad Juárez for the saloons and racetrack. Actions taken by working-class women on the bridge to defend their respectability threatened the privileges that El Paso's leisure class enjoyed in Juárez.

Coverage emphasized the sudden vulnerability of professional men (such as journalists, those involved in the leisure and sports community, or union workers) demonstrated the real threat that "young girls" posed to the privilege of border-crossing Americans. Young Mexican women were assaulting the experience of American men at the border, and this put the nation at risk. The humiliating experience of inspection was necessary to maintain the privilege of a nation's men on the move. The *Express* and *El Paso Times* coverage maintained the importance of this cross-border privilege by emphasizing the everyday presence and precariousness of propertied American men in Ciudad Juárez. For example, it was reported that women at the bridge trapped a party of midwestern "turf-men," men who owned horses and the land to train their animals. These Americans were potential investors in the Ciudad Juárez racetrack. Upon their return to El Paso, Colonel M. J. Winn, manager of the track, daringly requested that streetcars brave Ciudad Juárez and continue their movement between El Paso and the racetrack.

American reporters searched for ways to make the quarantine and the actions of this crowd of women familiar to their readers and touched on available stereotypes of Mexican political significance. In one of its head-lines the *Los Angeles Times* replaced the iconic Carmela Torres with a more familiar character in recent news coverage: "Viva Villa Shouted in Riots at Juarez."[108] Pancho Villa, of course, was the general and revolutionary being futilely chased across Chihuahua by General "Black Jack" Pershing and the Tenth Cavalry. The *Los Angeles Times* demonstrated that open resistance by notorious Mexican male political figures was easier to communicate than young women closing an international border. American press coverage also emphasized the weakness of male Mexican political authority in the face of "young girls." Andres Garcia, the consul general in El Paso for Carranza's government, drove across the bridge to Ciudad Juárez to inform the rioters that the USPHS was merely trying to disinfect all commuters from the Mexi-can city. A crowd surrounded his automobile, and "when he started back to the American side the crowd seized the wheels of his car," preventing his return to the United States.[109] When General Murguía's cavalry showed up, "women laughingly caught their bridles and turned the horses aside, holding the soldiers' sabers and whips."[110] This account, with its references to horses, sabers, and whips, connected the Mexican military presence to the defunct armor of the Spanish conquest and mocked the effectiveness of Mexican mili-tary authority.[111] To American male reporters wrapped in a rancorous debate over suffrage and preparedness, the female rioters also presented a disturbing vision of the authority wielded by women in societies at war.[112]

The Spanish-language edition of the *El Paso Times* challenged the vision of male Mexican weakness in the local English-language press. The writer rearticulated a patriarchal vision of Mexican gender culture by focusing on the more minor actions of men in the crowds and on the bridge. The paper reported, "Como es natural [as is natural]," Mexican male participants were so offended that their wives, sisters, or female relatives would be stripped naked, photographed, and then doused with kerosene and vinegar that they were forced to act violently.[113] This phrase placed the actions of these male participants in the realm of near biological common sense. Such an assertion pointedly ignored that women themselves acted against an attack on their place and respectability in El Paso's main thoroughfare.

Power and place shaped the lead editorial in the Spanish-language *El Paso Times*. The editor connected the push for quarantine to American privileges in Mexico: "While the ostensible purpose of the rigid quarantine rules is to prevent the spread of typhus fever, it is known that the real reason is based on the fear that Villa may capture Juarez any day and massacre the Americans."[114] Newspaper coverage treated typhus, epidemics, Pancho Villa, and the female Amazons nearly interchangeably. Assistant Surgeon Pierce pushed the symbolic fusion of disease and disorder, writing in a column that "United States soldiers have more to fear from disease than from Villa bullets."[115] The symbolic permeability of the U.S. Army and the USPHS led the *San Antonio Express* to claim that the El Paso typhus baths were meant to protect U.S. citizens who lived on the quarantined Mexican side of the international border as well, that somehow disinfecting women crossing into the United States would protect Americans living in Mexico from typhus.[116] The challenge at the border led the *Times* to confuse Americans in Mexico and the United States.

The local press rhetoric provided the narrative for the official story. Pierce underlined paragraphs of the Spanish edition of the *El Paso Morning Times* as evidence for the motivations of the crowd on the bridge: "The Mexican crowd was already very excited, as the leaders of the unruly mob had already harangued them telling them that Americans could do nothing to Mexico. As Pancho Villa had forced the exit of Pershing's Punitive Expedition was proof of this situation, they stood firm in their demands, insisting that the women pass without being fumigated or bathed."[117]

Pierce's highlights emphasized the impact of Mexican politics on the boundaries of medical authority in the United States. The voices in the crowd demanded that Mexican women be able to move freely into the United States. The political realities in El Paso after the death of Kluttz made this demand impossible. The *Times*'s editor also turned the demand to pass the bridge untouched and uninspected into a matter of Pancho Villa's politics, not commuting women in Ciudad Juárez. By underlining this demand, Pierce emphasized that Pancho Villa made the bridge into a revolutionary battleground and, perversely, turned public health into a political matter.

Pierce then highlighted the way the Spanish-language *El Paso Times* described his actions at the border. The press turned the confrontation at the bridge into a dramatic defense of American sovereignty. As the *El Paso Times* wrote and Pierce underlined: "In the face of these demands, American authorities declared that no one could pass without being examined, especially regarding their personal hygiene. The orders to enforce the quarantine were strict and the authorities could not disobey them simply because of threats communicated by foreigners."[118]

The emphasis on foreigners and passing explicitly excluded the legitimacy of any Mexican pressure on American policies. Pierce's defense of the line did not rest on the need for inspections to protect the people inspected from typhus. Instead, he emphasized that his orders to enforce a quarantine between El Paso and Ciudad Juárez came from the president of the United States himself. This was a vision of international law that drew sharp lines separating U.S. territory from the rest of the world. This vision implicitly ignored the widely recognized due-process rights of foreign subjects on American territory. More important, this crab-like rigid inside-outside view of American borders contradicted the original reason for disinfection.[119] The U.S. Public Health Service was in the business of certifying healthy Mexican workers for local American employers—not maintaining political agendas. Moreover, because typhus, lice, and rats ignored political borders, the USPHS had to track and contain potentially dangerous bodies after their entrance. The imperative to contain illness, which had led to the destruction of houses and more homelessness in El Paso, lay at odds with the demand to require submission to medical authority at the Santa Fe Bridge. In a more vivid contradiction, the political vision of sovereignty clashed with the practice of disease prevention: because typhus vectors did not recognize international borders, the best thing to do was to follow and control dangerous bodies.

The nationalized dynamics of this public health campaign pushed a vicious contrast between American modernity and Mexican resistance.[120] The American/Mexican duality obscured the daily movement of Mexican laundry women and domestic labor across American household boundaries to maintain what medical historian Nancy Tomes calls "the private side of public health," ignoring the everyday household labor needed to prevent the presence of germs within homes.[121] Pierce could have emphasized the city-wide importance of border-crossing Mexican working women who cleaned clothes and houses in El Paso; some of his medical counterparts took this angle in Atlanta when discussing black women.[122] But instead Pierce, trusting that Surgeon General Rupert Blue might give more authority to an explanation for Mexican actions written in Spanish, used the nationalist and patriarchal counterpoint in the Spanish edition of the *El Paso Times* to explain the insurgency on the bridge. Mexican men and Pancho Villa's partisans were the problem, not the relationship between USPHS officers and the people they served (and inspected) on a daily basis.

The U.S. military ignored Pierce's stark emphasis on political sovereignty.

General Bell withheld all military aid from Consul General Andres Garcia, Mayor Torres, and General Murguía until they cleaned up the threat of rioters and epidemic disease in Ciudad Juárez. General Murguía captured Carmela Torres and two men alleged to be ringleaders and turned them over to El Paso city authorities.[123] This action highlighted the way domestic demands in the United States forced political actions in Mexico. Much to Pierce's surprise, a city judge dismissed the charges against Carmela Torres and her peers, because El Paso had no legal jurisdiction over events in Ciudad Juárez.[124] The local judge endorsed a respectful but national division of political borders. This was yet another interpretation of the events on the bridge, in firm opposition to the army's informal exercise of influence and Pierce's unilateral declaration of sovereignty.

Drawing two separate medical and political spaces was much easier than connecting a shared responsibility for conditions on both sides of the border. As the riots on the transborder space of the Santa Fe Bridge receded from public memory, American cartoonists started using typhus as a larger metaphor for the situation in Mexico. In the Spanish edition of the El Paso Times, cartoonist Bill Blassingame drew a nearly unclothed Mexican peasant, almost a peon figure, in front of a national boundary as Uncle Sam looks anxiously in the background. The figure seems to be suffering from fevered delusions. At first glance, it seems as if Blassingame placed what looked like lice or red splotches (petechial bleeding) associated with the final throes of typhus all over this body. A closer look reveals that the splotches spell out "Istas." The cartoon has two titles. The longer caption is in Spanish: "La enfermedad mortal de Mexico, Mexico se debate en frente del Tio Samuel acosado por el personalismo político de todo ista [Mexico's mortal disease. Facing Uncle Sam, Mexico debates itself as it struggles with the "ista" scourge of personal political ambition].[125] The one in English simply states, "Mexico consumed by internal conflict."[126]

Blassingame represented Mexico in medical terms. He used a male body to represent the presence of disease, violence, disorder, and political change in Mexico. Unlike other cartoons, this one did not include a doctor with a ready medical solution. The cartoon highlighted the powerlessness American observers may have felt when their bridge was subject to Mexican authority. Perhaps it would have been difficult for Blassingame to represent this independent form of political power through a female body. The cartoon did not include the El Paso neighborhoods, the Santa Fe Bridge, and the streetcars as sites of medical intervention. By representing Mexico through a diseased male body as a space outside of the control but not the gaze of the United States, Blassingame demonstrated how people in El Paso were disavowing responsibility for the conditions that created typhus as well as the harm publicly inflicted on women by El Paso's typhus prevention policies. The spectacle of the riot effectively erased the connections women forged in their movement between El Paso and Ciudad Juárez.

Moving Divisions: Streetcars, Women, and Domestic Labor in El Paso and Ciudad Juárez

The bridge quarantine in the typhus campaign relied heavily on restricting streetcars. These vehicles were important to El Paso's self-image as a progressive metropolis. The transnational experience of a streetcar ride was transformed by the decision to stop movement. Before the campaign, Charles Armijo explained that his family just came over: "Everybody was allowed to go back and forth without any passport without anything else. Everybody was allowed to go back and forth whenever they wanted . . . and we came over on a streetcar."[127] Conrado Mendoza's statement reiterated the importance of the streetcar: "All one had to do was get on the electric trolley, or on the electric streetcar and cross over to the United States and no one told you anything."[128] The streetcar had been a place insulated from humiliating inspections. Now the vehicle had become a moving border zone where inspectors assigned bodies to national identities and then treated these persons based on their assessments. For Mexicans and Mexican Americans, the streetcar was no longer an escape from the humiliations of the border.

The vision of a streetcar peacefully making its way across a border must have been surprising to midwestern tourists, visitors, and recent settlers in El Paso. Many started to share postcards of a streetcar's movement on both sides of the border with their friends and family at home in the Midwest. Like Armijo and Mendoza, many tourists shared their pleasant memories by sending postcards highlighting the wholesomeness of their jaunt to El Paso.[129] This peaceful jaunt across the Santa Fe Bridge was symbolically crucial to El Paso's public identity.

Streetcar conductors had a different evaluation of these "easy" jaunts. The conductors responded to the violence they faced in Mexico and the United States by mounting their largest organizing drive between 1916 and 1917. Their

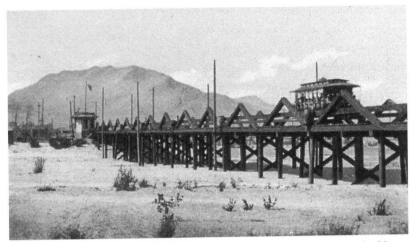

Figure 9. New International Bridge (El Paso, Tex.). Courtesy of the Victor A. Blenkle Postcard Collection, Archives Center, National Museum of American History, Smithsonian Institution.

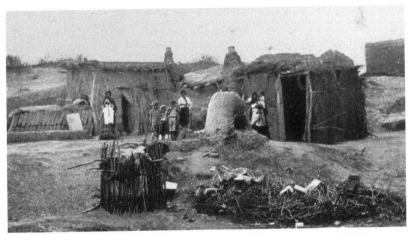

Figure 10. Suburban Residence (El Paso, Tex.). Courtesy of the Victor A. Blenkle Postcard Collection, Archives Center, National Museum of American History, Smithsonian Institution.

strike in May 1916 paralyzed downtown El Paso. Addressing an imagined Trades Union member reading the *El Paso Labor Advocate*, a writer asked streetcar-riding union members to "take a look at him up there in front of the car, with the responsibility of your life and the lives of many others in his care. Then turn around in your seat and take a look at some ugly vis-aged, peon Mexican laborer from the smelter or the cement plant. Compare the two. There is the American motorman or conductor, true Americans yet paid a slave's wage. Those Mexicans . . . are paid as much as those men upon whom the company places a burden of responsibility greater than wages."[130]

The editor of the *Labor Advocate* demanded that El Paso's union members embrace the American conductor over their fellow passenger, a Mexican smelter worker. The editorial asked members to endorse raising the average wage of streetcar drivers above that of Mexican smelter workers to protect the American standard of living. This implied that the editor found the idea of wage parity between Mexican and American workers troubling. The address rhetorically transformed his fellow union member, the smelter worker, into someone who is threateningly out of place: a man whose spending habits, presence, and wage are dangerous to the privileged free status of an "American" conductor. The writer asked his fellow union members to become unpaid volunteer immigration inspectors and exclude a large number of the employees of the ASARCO (American Smelting and Refining Corporation) plant from this streetcar/border zone. The striking conductors needed ethnic Mexican passengers as counterweights to their American identity. Thus the Mexican passengers were threatening and indispensable for the conductors' hold on a true American identity.

The conductors' union also used violence to maintain their hold on the streetcars and the picket lines. The El Paso Streetcar Company settled with the union after a number of pitched street battles around control of the streets and the streetcars. El Paso and Ciudad Juárez's dependence on open streets and on streetcars, complaints by local small business owners, and the supremacist demands of these "American" cross-border laborers forced the El Paso Streetcar company to negotiate with the union. The streetcar kept its role as a vehicle moving through contested borderlands terrain where local grievances carried international resonances. The Mexican Revolution, the typhus campaign, and General Pershing's Expeditionary Force transformed the streetcar into a vehicle for the creation of many competing imagined communities.

The USPHS's forced inspection removed some symbolic boundaries protecting people in the cars from the streets. For tourists, men in the sporting life, and many El Paso residents, streetcars provided an entry into a world of saloons, racetracks, gambling dens, and dance halls. For men and women like Carmelita Torres, the streetcar provided needed protection and mobility for middle- and working-class laborers in Ciudad Juárez making their way to El Paso. The firestorm and bath riots led to the eviction of riders, while pedestrians and onlookers recognized the streetcars as the vehicle for an (attempted) American domination of public space in El Paso and Ciudad Juárez. For some of these riders and their American peers, these acts of violence served as reminders of the precariousness of their settlement in Mexico and in El Paso. When General Bell placed armed guards on the streetcars to protect the passengers in the midst of a medical riot, he protected the passenger's slumming privileges in Mexico. The attacks on the streetcars and automobiles represented street-based challenges to the vehicles and mechanisms of U.S. expansion. The typhus campaign, the streetcar strike, the Columbus raid, and the American Expeditionary Force transformed the streets and streetcars into a transborder forum for volatile struggles over the meaning of gender, class, and national identity. In this case, public cleansing led to open reprisals.

On the East Coast, *Jacobson v. Massachusetts* set the boundaries of medical authority in public health campaigns.[131] In El Paso, street battles over the experience of bridge crossing pushed back against the American elimination of a sense of privacy among working-class Mexicans. The firestorm also put public authority over domestic cleanliness into crisis. Five people had died of typhus, but one of them was Morris Buttner, an immigration inspector. At the beginning of the campaign, eleven American men died during an exercise in typhus prevention.[132] The ensuing public health measures in El Paso rested on the links already made in the Southwest between lice, filth, and Mexican labor. In the circular published by the *El Paso Times* after Buttner's death, Pierce spelled out the general implications of a louse eradication project by stating, "The extermination of lice means the extermination of typhus."[133] This implied boiling, washing, and ironing clothes more frequently for every household. In addition to immediate cleansing, Pierce recommended more general measures: "Avoid all association with dirty people who may carry lice." Implicitly separating the readers from "dirty people," Pierce identified the places where contact with lice might occur, claiming that it was "unwise to visit moving picture shows, club rooms, and dance halls unless all the persons have been freed from lice."[134] Safety from typhus meant separation from accepted forms of sporting life and middle-class leisure that helped create a shared urban economy in El Paso and Ciudad Juárez. At the same time, the typhus campaign called for reinvigorated American household labor.[135] Healthy American households required the active elimination of filth, and the labor was put in by transborder female workers (who themselves were presented as "dirty people").

The active elimination of filth required more work from men and women in each household. Given the time and labor required to boil and iron clothes, this demand forced middle-class households to bring their clothes to the laundries that depended on Mexican women living in Ciudad Juárez and South El Paso.[136] This demand for additional labor created opportunities for domestic workers outside other people's houses.[137] Mexican women cleaned clothes as workers in the local laundry, independent contractors, and as domestic laborers across households in El Paso.[138] As Pierrette Hondagneu-Sotelo and Mary Romero repeatedly point out, higher standards of cleanliness have usually implied increased domestic labor employment and therefore increased dependence on hired Mexican labor.[139] Pierce noted the spatial aspects of this employment relationship when he advocated that local "citizens" adopt compulsory disinfection as a condition of household employment.[140] As Tera Hunter and Nancy Tomes have pointed out regarding Atlanta, higher standards of cleanliness also implied more employers and potentially higher wages.[141] The attempt to separate the "citizens" of El Paso through an emphasis on cleanliness grew volatile after 1917, particularly because more cleanliness depended heavily on the labor of Mexican women residing in South El Paso and Ciudad Juárez.

A more targeted struggle over the value of domestic labor in the United States engulfed the streetcar circuit, highlighting its material and symbolic importance to labor struggles in El Paso. In October 1919, in the midst of the typhus quarantine in El Paso, local laundry workers decided to organize the Acme Laundry. When Acme fired two veteran workers and union organizers during the drive, their coworkers closed down the plant. Within a few days, approximately five hundred Mexican female laundry workers joined the workers in Acme and walked out of five other laundries in El Paso. The workers staffed picket lines in front of the laundries as well as the Santa Fe Bridge.[142] Their public presence in front of their workplaces as well as the

Santa Fe Bridge contested the minimal recognition given to them as workers, family members, and U.S. residents and citizens.[143]

The workers went on strike for many reasons. The *El Paso Labor Advocate* reports emphasized reasons that highlighted connections between these workers and the readers of the *Advocate*. One worker conveyed her knowledge of Progressive era union strategies, emphasizing, "I find it hard to live on my wages, which I turn in to the family budget,"[144] and stressing the obligation she had to her family as well as the union effort. The *Advocate* was mindful of its nationalist past and illuminated an obvious dimension of ethnic Mexican working-class settlement in El Paso: "True it is, they are nearly all of Mexican origin, but they are by no means all of Mexican citizenship. The large majority are residents of El Paso and citizens of the nation."[145] The strikers moved to highlight their American status in the United States by picketing the Santa Fe Bridge to prevent workers living in Ciudad Juárez from taking their places. These women challenged the assumption that Mexicans could never be Americans or that all brown people are non-American Mexicans.

The laundry women who picketed the bridge actively rejected some of the propaganda deployed by their employers. For example, the owner of the Acme Laundry reiterated the dirtiness of Mexican labor and peoples to justify his employment of scabs: "Some of my Mexicans quit and I put Americans in their place. . . . The work was cleaner and whiter and better in every way."[146] Clearly silent on the way his earlier profits depended on minimal wages and dangerous workplace conditions, the owner used the logic of inspection, auto raids, and house fumigation to justify the expulsion of ethnic Mexican labor from his laundry. The El Paso Federation of Labor brought Eduardo Idar to work with the Central Federation of Labor in order to establish a contract with the five laundries, thus displacing the initial community-based organizers from this key dimension of labor leadership. Women had acted on their own behalf until the initial crisis dissipated.

Despite their exclusion from central organizing committees, women like Carmen Alonzo or even Carmelita Torres used the streetcar circuit to make their labor visible to a larger public by picketing at the border and the laundries. The ongoing contestations occurring on streetcars, streets, and the Santa Fe Bridge depended on recognizing the value of domestic labor. The American Federation of Labor forced the El Paso Federation of Labor to go against its earlier official anti-Asian and anti-Mexican policies to support a successful unionizing drive in El Paso's laundries in 1919.[147] The *Labor Advocate* temporarily included ethnic Mexican laundry workers within a nationalist demand that the United States treat workers as an equal part of the larger war effort because "a citizenship that has not been weakened by excessive toil and low working conditions can stand the test of war. Unions should be fostered."[148] This demand focused on the union status of workplaces and not the need to hire (Mexican) American workers.

When it came to the possible residences of many of the laundry workers, the *Advocate* followed rhetoric similar to the U.S. Public Health Service. In their articles "Erect No More Adobes" and "Jap Importation," the *Advocate* argued for the continued residential expulsion of Mexican and Asian neighbors. The *Labor Advocate* could envision sharing a union workplace. The same editor refused to consider the possibility of sharing neighborhoods and residential services. Because El Paso was "on the border of the United States and Mexico, . . . homeless thousands cross into the state and are offering their services at prices far below that which an American can live! [The Mexican presence in El Paso threatens] the sacrifice of manhood, of homes and all that go to build up and sustain a community. The Americans do not want or advocate the importation of any people who cannot be absorbed into full citizenship, who cannot eventually be raised to our highest social standard, and by co-operation sustain this standard."[149]

For the editor of the *Advocate*, the destruction of Mexican housing in South El Paso was necessary for the survival of a (white) American working class. The *Advocate* employed a normative version of American sanitary citizenship that used housing provided to Asian and Mexican laborers to justify why South El Paso residents should be expelled from "American" territory. The typhus campaign and the epidemic seized upon familiar Mexican stereotypes bandits (Pancho Villa), spitfires (Carmela Torres), workers (Nellie Oaxaca Quinn), and "bad" health practices. This disease-specific prevention campaign obscured the actual conditions that produced sickness.[150] The city of El Paso moved to "make the city beautiful" and raze much of South El Paso's housing stock in the name of public health. This left a number of people homeless.

Nellie Quinn remembered this part of the anti-Mexican disease campaign. "We barely had enough to eat. They could hardly expect us to pave the streets and put in the sewers and electricity. We were forced to drink that dirty water from the canal. Of course we had to boil it first, but the inspectors were right, many people were getting sick."[151] The USPHS and the city of El Paso decided to destroy the neighborhood in order to save it from its residents. The destruction and disinfection of poorer households in this frenzy of public health displaced more families and children into more precarious living conditions.

After the campaign one migrant remembered that the USPHS "disinfected us as if we were some kind of animals that were bringing germs."[152] Juarenses had to consider their coworkers, their friends in the neighborhood, their supervisors, their family members, and the inspector on the bridge when they chose their clothes for the day.[153] The typhus campaign brought medical perceptions into the daily urban life of people who risked being branded Mexican when they crossed the border.[154] The inspection and potential bathing became part of the modern border-crossing experience through 1942, when the USPHS ended the typhus quarantine.

The coverage of the two riots in the American press made the typhus campaign an extreme case of the split between individual consent and medical authority. Reporters delighted in the spectacular accounts of attacks on cameramen, news reporters, conductors, and track regulars, while the crux of the violence was buried. With the laundry strike, picketing women drew lines across the bridge and the entrances to El Paso laundries; they used the streets to mark the public dimensions of private cleanliness. The coverage of the riots and the strikes emphasized the apparent split between clean, restrained representatives of the law and dirty, disorderly, loose Mexican women. By presenting working women as resistant to routine cleaning by federal health officers, media coverage obscured the ethnic Mexican dimensions of the voice, power, and labor of those who cleaned and cared for households in El Paso. Such a media spectacle obscured the circuits that connected public space and private health in El Paso and Ciudad Juárez.

How do you tame a wild tongue, train it to be quiet,
how do you bridle it and saddle it?—Gloria Anzaldúa,
Borderlands / La Frontera: The New Mestiza

SIX

Bodies of Evidence

Vaccination and the Body Politics of Transnational Mexican Citizenship, 1910–1920

Surgeon John Hamilton of the USPHS left Laredo to inquire into a seemingly invisible smallpox outbreak around Rio Grande City. His superior, Surgeon General Rupert Blue, ordered him south to Starr County because Texas Representative John Garner demanded to know why the USPHS had not cooperated with local health authorities during that county's winter smallpox epidemic.[1] Hamilton found out there had been 150 cases of smallpox, and, to his pleasant surprise, he also discovered that Dr. Mary Headley, a Tejana and the Starr County physician, had isolated the smallpox cases and successfully vaccinated close to eight hundred of the remaining Starr County residents.[2] Hamilton asked Judge Monroe if it would be possible to end all skiff traffic across the Rio Grande and thus end smallpox in Starr County, but Judge Monroe said no. The judge believed "it would be almost impossible, that the same families lived and owned property on both sides of the border and it would work a hardship on them to prevent them from using their own skiffs, in visiting their close relatives."[3] Hamilton found this acceptance of informal cross-border traffic by a local political authority, who asked for federal assistance in a smallpox epidemic, deeply troubling. He asked permission from the surgeon general to have all acting assistant surgeons at key border towns "vaccinate all incoming aliens and immigrants, all year."[4] The surgeon general ignored his request.

Three years later, Hamilton found a means to coerce vaccination compliance from commuters moving between Laredo and Nuevo Laredo. He reported that "the bridge company was instructed not to allow persons without a vaccination certificate with USPHS stamp on to enter Mexico, so that all persons either going or coming from Mexico were vaccinated."[5] One year later, the USPHS inspectors in El Paso, Eagle Pass, Laredo, Rio Grande City, and Brownsville reported that they vaccinated every Mexican arriving from Mexico who could not prove their successful vaccination to the satisfaction of the immigration officer.[6] When people tried to demonstrate that they lived in the United States or that they had a previous vaccination or a previous experience with smallpox, the USPHS dismissed their oral testimony and the scars of the physical evidence. As Dr. Hunter stated, "Most Mexicans male or female will deceive me if they can, in any way they can."[7] Within the space of four years, the USPHS moved from ignoring to distrusting the words, the flesh, and the scars of Mexican bodies. This chapter explores the emergence of this invasive form of body politics, as well as a variety of Mexican responses.

The smallpox vaccination policy made the medical line between the United States and Mexico evident on Mexican bodies. Through it, the USPHS officers felt they exercised more control over the movement of people across the southern border of the United States. The same policies rendered individual Mexican control over the borders of their own bodies at the Texas-Mexico borders more tenuous and almost moot. The American decision to dismiss the evidence bodies provided was particularly troubling to northern Mexico's professional and aspiring classes. To many, vaccination was both a mark of civilization and a requirement for citizenship, not a badge of humiliation.[8] Communities in the lower Rio Grande Valley mobilized against this medicalized understanding of Mexican bodies and turned USPHS health officers into sites for Mexican state formation in the United States. Representatives of Mexican revolutionary factions used the mobilization against the vaccination policy to provide an avenue for their legitimacy in the United States and among Mexican communities in the United States.

The growing importance of coerced vaccination on the Mexican border during the Mexican Revolution emerged alongside a USPHS folklore about the untrustworthiness of Mexican words and bodies. The practice of forced vaccination itself arose from a complex set of pressures on USPHS officers stationed at the border. Local, state, congressional, and federal officials demanded an official practice that addressed the military dynamics and population movements during the Mexican Revolution. With each battle along the eastern railroad corridor connecting central Mexico to Laredo, the Mexican Central Railroad funneled a variety of people to the southern valley. Border county officials tired of the additional expenditures associated with the population growth in their counties and demanded assistance and reimbursements for medical expenses from the USPHS.[9] However, the pressure was not simply from Texas.

The movement of Mexican families into the greater United States paradoxically increased the visibility of border policies in Texas. Various investigations by USPHS officers into smallpox outbreaks in Arkansas, Tennessee, and California traced the initial outbreak to people who maintained contact with itinerant laborers from the Mexican border. These investigations fostered the impression that the border quarantine maintained inconsistent vaccination practices. In the aftermath of large costly vaccination campaigns and smallpox quarantines in California and Tennessee, local and state boards of health applied extraregional pressure on the USPHS to increase the extent and coverage of vaccination along the Texas-Mexican border. The state boards depended on the reliability of USPHS border vaccination practices to protect the citizens of their state from "the possible introduction of a more virulent strain of smallpox from Mexico."[10] The increased emphasis on reliable vaccination on the Mexican border derived from the failure to achieve full vaccination coverage within each state. For example, in California in 1915, "a considerable portion of the State [was] not vaccinated and the vaccination law does not make vaccination of school children absolutely compulsory."[11] Because of citizen apathy and constitutional and statutory limits on state-level action, the California State Board of Health requested "special steps to prevent the introduction into California of smallpox and other diseases prevalent throughout Mexico."[12] After the Banning smallpox crisis, California started suspecting the quality of vaccination at the Mexican border.[13] Dr. James S. Cumming used the presence of Mexican laborers to demand increased federal regulation of the Mexican border. He referred to the presence of smallpox among the laborers as a "fact that the disease had been introduced by Mexican peons who had recently entered the United States through El Paso. From Dr. Geiger's report it will be seen that the children responsible for introducing the disease had been vaccinated at the border but that the vaccination was not successful. We have no evidence as to whether the Mexicans had not interfered with the vaccines in hope of preventing a take."[14]

Dr. Cumming demanded a federal investigation of Mexican attitudes toward federal vaccination procedures: Did Mexicans crossing the border interfere with the lesions where the vaccination material was placed within each incision? Did this mean the lesions that might otherwise be the visual guarantee of a successful USPHS vaccination were suspect on all Mexicans? Smallpox among Mexicans in California was proof that vaccinations were unreliable at the Mexican border. Employers across the United States wanted consistently reliable Mexican labor, and each smallpox case undermined their sense of reliability.

For USPHS officers, the concept of "untrustworthy" Mexican bodies provided a solution to rising challenges to the legitimacy of their practice on the border. These national demands encouraged USPHS officers to frame ethnic Mexican actions and attitudes toward communicable diseases as unreliable, separate, and irreducibly different. This near biological difference that inhered in Mexican immune systems required a rougher and more uniform policy. As USPHS officers reacted to various smallpox crises in the United States, they used the conditions particular to specific parts of the Mexican border during the Mexican Revolution to justify a blanket approach to vaccination policy on the Mexican border. First, the military and economic dynamics of the Mexican Revolution in northern Mexico meant that the political factions conscripted doctors—USPHS's political contacts—to treat soldiers at a variety of battlefields. After three years of revolution, USPHS officers considered political authority in northern Mexico transitory, unreliable, and probably temporary. Hard experience forced towns and cities across northern Mexico to recognize a variety of inoculation and vaccination scars as proof of smallpox immunity. This meant ethnic Mexicans, Mexican Americans, Mexican medical officers, and USPHS officers had different approaches regarding the most appropriate means of smallpox prevention. The USPHS officers understood these physiological and medical differences as proof of Mexican unreliability, not Mexican participation in a wider debate of the practices of inoculation and vaccination. As the USPHS officers narrowed the spectrum of acceptable public health practices, the methods that Mexican nationals and Mexican public health authorities adopted to defend their body's medical history started to pose an unacceptable challenge to the appearance of professionalism coveted by the USPHS.

This chapter also provides a window into the short-lived period when Carrancista representatives actively sought the consent and recognition of

Mexicans and Mexican Americans living in the United States. The local representatives of Venustiano Carranza's revolutionary factions searched for issues that could make them relevant to Mexican communities along the border. Carranza, the revolutionary leader based in Nuevo León, competed against Pancho Villa and the Constitutional Convention for American recognition of their authority. Their pressure on the federal USPHS policies on behalf of Mexican border communities in the United States provided another way to prove their importance to the local communities and the American federal government. This chapter argues for the importance of Carrancista legal mobilization against the USPHS smallpox vaccination policies to the medical history of due process rights in the United States. It will also show how the local representatives and consuls along the lower Rio Grande Valley became forums for a particular grievance: the refusal by USPHS officials to recognize Mexican participation in a shared medical modernity.[15] The subsequent USPHS and Texas State Health Office reactions shaped the boundaries of force and the limits of Mexican consular authority along the Rio Grande border. The legal challenges by middle-class Mexicans confirmed the deep untrustworthiness of Mexican bodies, a perception required by the "vaccinate all Mexicans" ideology.[16]

This USPHS ideology emerged in response to the *sedicioso* uprising, the multiple coups in Mexico, and the ongoing rumors of battles and attacks. The seemingly constant change in authority wearied the USPHS. Although many Mexicans and Mexican Americans had been vaccinated, USPHS officers at the border grew increasingly wary of the evidence provided by vaccination scars on Mexican bodies. By 1915, some public health officials thought the deeply untrustworthy nature of Mexican laborers would contaminate the previously reliable evidence provided by vaccine lesions. Vaccination scars, certificates, and plentiful oral testimony could not overcome an American fear that Mexicans would do something contrary to American expectations. In Arizona and California, public health authorities initiated various smallpox-inspired "Mexican roundups." These states pushed for increasingly tight universal vaccination policies in Eagle Pass, El Paso, Laredo, and Brownsville. After 1915, incoming immigrants were restrained for an additional ten minutes and placed under observation to guarantee that they did not attempt to remove vaccine material from their scars.

The USPHS also observed that Mexicans on both sides of the river relied on the border's urban economies. Assistant Surgeon Hamilton recommended the establishment of vaccination stations in the main transportation hubs between Mexico and the United States. He noted that laborers, farmers, and peddlers had to come through these hubs to participate in the cash economy. Instead of reaching out to recalcitrant Mexican smallholders through chaparral and private ranch properties, Laredo-based Assistant Surgeon Hamilton recommended that vaccination become a condition of legal entry into the United States at the main transportation hubs along the Mexican border, a requirement for anyone entering the legal marketplace in the United States.[17] While this policy was in place, inspectors could vaccinate any Mexicans, regardless of class, occupation, or past vaccinations, on their whim. No Mexicans or their scars were trustworthy enough to pass freely. Moreover, by centralizing medical inspections in the transportation hubs of South Texas, the USPHS could weather the transitions in political authority that accompanied military dynamics in Mexico. The burden of proof now lay on arriving Mexicans, not the inquiring doctors. Legal and respectable entry into the United States potentially turned vaccination, the mark of civilization, into another badge of humiliation.

Revolutionary Politics and the USPHS, 1912–1916

American public health officers worked at the margins of the Mexican Revolution. Officials witnessed the consequences of the conflicts in northern Mexico after General Victoriano Huerta's coup d'état against Francisco I. Madero. The battles between Carranza, Villa, and Huerta affected the border towns on the Texas border in very different ways. Venustiano Carranza's sphere of influence included the greater portion of lower Rio Grande Valley towns: Del Rio, Eagle Pass, Laredo, Rio Grande City, and Brownsville. Because Pancho Villa controlled Chihuahua, the towns of Presidio and El Paso were most directly affected by developments in Chihuahua. Villa and Carranza's relationship to U.S. military policy shaped the timing of refugee flows and troop movements along these two corridors.

Popular uprisings in Chihuahua and Nuevo León followed news of Ambassador Henry Lane Wilson's involvement in the coup. In Chihuahua, the assassination of Abraham González, Francisco I. Madero's popular appointed governor, announced Huerta's new rule.[18] The local military divisions rose up in protest. The conflicts in Chihuahua that accompanied the assassination of González by federal forces occurred mostly in the states of Chihuahua, southwestern Coahuila, and Durango. In Coahuila and Nuevo León, Carranza refused to recognize Huerta's position as president of Mexico. The Laredo and Brownsville borders were relatively free of military disturbances, because Carranza directed the largest military contingent in the region between Monterrey and Laredo, and he never allowed federal troops into his region. Battles between Huerta's federal troops and Carranza's local conscripts took place between Monterrey and central Mexico. The supply lines and the rail connections between Mexico and the United States determined the battles, defeats, and refugee movements in Mexico.

The USPHS, whose job was to prevent disease in the United States, did not formally track or seek to explain the dynamics of the revolution. If this list of names and battlefronts is confusing, the situation must have looked far more complex to American health officials in 1913. Woodrow Wilson's election and Huerta's coup occurred within two months of each other. By the time full military conflicts were occurring along the rail corridors that joined Chihuahua and Monterrey to Mexico City, Wilson had refused to recognize any faction as legitimate representatives. Customs officers, however, looked the other way and did not enforce embargo on arms shipments on the requests made either by Carranza or by Villa's Division del Norte.

The revolutionary conflicts in northern Mexico after President Madero's execution radically changed the landscape of smallpox prevention on the border. Under Madero's short-lived regime, duly elected and/or appointed *presidentes municipales* and state governors appointed local health authorities. After Huerta's coup and Ambassador Henry Lane Wilson's push for American recognition of this new regime, a patchwork of local resistance, accommodation, and outright civil war emerged across Mexico. However, the reaction of the majority of Mexico to Huerta's execution of President Madero showed that even informal U.S. foreign policies could be met with rampant disapproval and open, violent opposition. The civil wars that emerged in the wake of this coup and execution undercut any consistent cooperation between USPHS and Mexican state health officers. Any cooperation between USPHS officers and local Mexican authorities implied a political investment in Mexican affairs with risky long-term consequences.

The illegal coup in Mexico City had consequences for the USPHS. The increased operating costs of the USPHS after 1912 bore traces of the response to the illegal intervention of Ambassador Henry Lane Wilson (and the Department of State) into Mexican electoral affairs. Even though President Taft's economic embargo of Mexico fell within the boundaries of international law, the

promises of recognition and financial support—sanctioned by Taft and secretary of state Philander Knox and given to Huerta by Ambassador Wilson—
were clearly illegal under international law. The tacit American support of the
overthrow and execution of a president voted in by 98 percent of the Mexican
electorate stretched the boundaries of international law. Still, no USPHS officer
officially approved of Huerta's overthrow of Madero.[19]

After his inauguration in 1913, Woodrow Wilson refused to recognize
Huerta, established an arms embargo around Mexico against Germany, England, and Japan, and, in mid-1914, occupied Vera Cruz. Wilson cited Huerta's actions as necessitating these foreign policies. President Wilson's opposition to Huerta's presidency was also apparent in the lax policing of military
weapons and supplies into northern Mexico.[20] The movement of arms into
Mexico's civil wars also implied the continued movement of Mexican residents away from the battles and, perhaps, toward the United States. The USPHS
border stations were starting to face some of the costs of contradictory American foreign policy initiatives in Mexico. Informal American investment and
Mexican refugees rode the same rails, but in opposite directions. USPHS vaccination policy took place in the middle of this two-way movement created
by wars in Mexico.

In the process of reacting to the movement of people (soldiers, refugees, exiles, laborers) across the border, USPHS health officials tried to create mechanisms to compensate for the unpredictability of war and hunger in northern
Mexico. The USPHS heard news of a variety of smallpox situations in Mexico,
and its officers were interested in preventing and containing smallpox from
a place awash with unreliable rumors. The USPHS decided to treat the border
bridges and ferries as places to inspect Mexicans, whether they were entering
or exiting the United States.[21] This USPHS action forced individual Mexican
men and women who crossed over bridges to answer to difficult situations in
Mexico. The USPHS ended up projecting the indeterminate and unpredictability of revolutionary politics onto Mexican bodies. An unpredictable nation
fostered unreliable bodies.

The USPHS, Mexican Complaints, and the Unreliable Mexican Body

Unreliability worked in both directions. On September 4, 1916, Juana Garza
took the ferry from Camargo, Tamaulipas, to Rio Grande City, Texas, to meet
up with her sister Juliana Solis. As she expected, she submitted to the inquiries

made to her by the inspector and a doctor. She was bathed and she and her two daughters, Epimenia and Ofelia, were all vaccinated. At the end of the process, the female attendant brought her to a room where the doctor, the inspector, and a clerk asked her to take an oath and answer a set of questions thoroughly. The inspector translated the questions the doctor asked into Spanish and then communicated her response back to the doctor. She told the inspector that she was from Los Aldamas, Nuevo León, and that Amado Garza, the father of her daughter Epimenia, paid for her passage to Rio Grande City. She reported that she was going to stay with her sister Juliana Solis. They pointedly asked if she was the sole means of support of her two children. Although the passage had been paid by Amado, Juana claimed responsibility for her two children.[22] At this point, Dr. Hunter read the statement that Juana Garza, as the sole support of Epimenia Solis and Ofelia Solis, was to be excluded because both children suffered from afflicted conjunctivitis, a "loathsome and contagious disease."[23] Edward Flannery told her that she had to return to Mexico because her children were sick.

On the ferry back to Camargo, Garza broke down, exclaiming that she and her children had gone through the bath and undergone the vaccination but the doctor still prevented her from meeting her sister in Rio Grande City. An older Mexican gentleman consoled her, telling her that in Roma, there were no inspectors, no doctors, and no border stations. She gathered her two kids, made her way to Roma, crossed the river, and, within five days, made her way to Rio Grande City.[24] That gentleman turned out to be Leoncio Revelas, the Mexican consul in Rio Grande City. This small exchange between the Mexican representative and Juana Garza points to the ways the dynamics of the Mexican Revolution disrupted established class and race hierarchies and temporarily forced solidarities among different classes of Mexican nationals and Mexican Americans. That Revelas and Garza were on the same ferry was the result of a USPHS policy requiring that only one ferry run between Camargo and Rio Grande City. Revelas, as someone who crossed the border regularly, was very aware of how Mexican nationals were treated by Inspector Edward Flannery and Dr. Hunter at the ferry landing. Flannery and Hunter enjoyed great authority over the legitimate border-crossers. Revelas may have enjoyed undercutting their authority by having Juana Garza take another ferry.[25]

Within two weeks, Revelas filed or coauthored the first of three diplomatic complaints against the practices adopted by Flannery and Hunter in Rio Grande City.[26] The first complaint involved Garza's vaccination and subsequent deportation. The second complaint involved Miguel Barrera, a Mexican businessman based in Sam Fordyce, Texas, who was outraged by the process through which he was vaccinated against his will. In the third complaint Efraim Domínguez, the director of a teacher's academy in Saltillo, challenged the full disrobing, inspection, and vaccination process. The act of filing the complaint with the State Department introduced Revelas as the new consul and community advocate to the USPHS. His presence added an international relations wrinkle to the exercise of federal medical authority in the lower Rio Grande Valley. For Revelas, Hunter and Flannery's insistence on inspection and vaccination regardless of vaccine or immigration status demonstrated their immense disdain for Mexico and Mexicans. Revelas used the complaint to defend the interests of a large number of border-crossing residents.

In the ensuing investigation, Inspector Reynolds told Consul Revelas he informed Juana Garza that her children had "a loathsome and contagious disease [conjunctivitis]" and that the absence of her husband made Juana Garza likely to become a public charge. In accordance with well-worn USPHS policy, either of these situations was grounds for deportation in any version of American immigration law.[27] Her exclusion because of her status as an unaccompanied mother of two children made her a very representative candidate for the most common exclusion in all ports: "likely to become a public charge" (LPC). The LPC exclusion highlighted the gender inequity implicit in using immigration control to shape the kind of labor admitted to the United States. Inspectors assumed men would be able to contribute to the American economy through their labor; a single mother would be unlikely to find the kind of jobs inspectors considered work. Inspectors actively privileged some forms of manual labor over the skills and domestic labor markets available to working-class Mexican women.[28]

Juana Garza was just one of five thousand people excluded upon arrival by the USPHS at the Mexican border in 1916.[29] Her exclusion fit the larger ways the USPHS sought to shape the contours of a healthy, adult, male immigrant industrial labor force in the United States. Amy Fairchild argues that USPHS medical inspection emphasized inclusion over exclusion, even in the face of anti-immigration pressure by labor unions, anti-immigrant leagues, and even Progressive reformers.[30] In 1916, after all, the USPHS cleared close to 150,000 people for entry into the United States. These 150,000 arrivals shared the process of inspection, a disciplinary spectacle that introduced arrivals to their secondary position in the United States.[31] For the large numbers of Mexican,

Chinese, and Syrian nationals working far beyond the Rio Grande border, the border inspection was a key humiliating passage in their journey or settlement deeper within the United States.[32] In contrast, Garza's deportation in Rio Grande City symbolized the risks and consequences of the ongoing medical humiliation for men and women who regularly crossed into the United States.

The struggle for authority between revolutionary factions led the relatively visible consul in Rio Grande City to use Juana Garza's case as a vehicle for Mexican state formation in the United States. Although factions could assert their military control of a given territory in Mexico, most found it difficult to achieve a stable commercial relationship with other parts of Mexico and the United States. By advocating on behalf of Mexican communities in the United States, Carranza's representatives made an argument that they had the approval of large portions of Mexicans in the United States and—by extension—Mexico. Filing a case with the State Department meant the Carrancista consul was now the legal representative of his aggrieved client. The inspection stations formed an important part of the daily lives of border residents; challenging the humiliations of inspection spoke to border Mexicans as a class. Leoncio Revelas's public challenge to this form of American medical authority aimed to resonate across border communities.

Diplomatic challenges to medical authorities might seem to be a less risky way to challenge authority at the border. Mexicans and Mexican Americans in Laredo, Rio Grande City, and Brownsville were still recovering from an earlier more military declaration of solidarity by the Sediciosos who published the *Plan de San Diego*. This manifesto declared that their killings and theft inside the Texas border were the first steps to a violent Mexican overthrow of Texas. Anglo ranchers and farmers in the farther reaches of South Texas responded to news of this declaration by violently attacking the Mexican presence in their midst. General Frederick Funston estimated that the Rangers and associated ranchers killed approximately three thousand Mexicans in South Texas in 1915. Mexican sheepherding and cattle-ranching families fled from their residences to the relative safety of Laredo, Rio Grande City, and Brownsville. This legal challenge to federal medical authority would probably not inspire the same anger and revulsion among Anglo border residents.[33]

The translation of Juana Garza's story into a State Department deposition in 1917 demonstrates that a legally based diplomatic strategy for the defense of Mexican communities in the United States coexisted with more dramatic and violent efforts to transform the conditions of Mexicans along the border.[34] Still, civil rights and due process claims complicated the easy exercise of public medical authority, as in Mary Mallon's initially successful legal case against the New York Board of Health.[35] As it turned out, the legal window to match Mexican to American rights of passage was small. The Mexican consular office never filed official claims against USPHS vaccination practices after 1920.[36]

Venustiano Carranza used his consuls to counter the hostile political space Porfirian exiles maintained in the United States. With the State Department's recognition of Eliseo Arredondo as the confidential agent of the de facto Mexican government in Atlantic City in October 1915, Carranza became the de facto president of Mexico in American eyes.[37] In November 1916, Mexican foreign ministry circulars ordered consuls to work with local American officials to help "immigrants with justice problems."[38] This demand meant consuls had to appear to be representative of Mexican interests in local situations. Local conditions and local Mexican grievances therefore shaped the structure of consular authority in the United States.

Consular authorities became one of the few public and peaceful forums available to concerned and affected Mexican residents in South Texas.[39] Official and unofficial representatives of the de facto Mexican government filed complaints with the State Department against the practices implemented under the border quarantine. In the process of challenging these vaccination practices, the claimants described the ways they considered forced vaccination part of the structure of domination on the Texas-Mexico border. When the consuls registered these complaints, they were part of the reestablishment of consular authority in Mexican communities in the United States.

Once all the immigration stations incorporated the 1915 demand that medical officers vaccinate all incoming Mexican arrivals, the political field shifted. Mexican health officers and consuls adopted a variety of informal, official, and legal strategies to challenge the perceived exclusions of the USPHS immigration policy. Although Mexican officials named and challenged the indiscriminate vaccination policies adopted by the USPHS, the complaints took place within a challenge to the untrammeled authority medical inspectors claimed over all incoming Mexican bodies. In the process, consular authorities came to adopt the increasingly narrow rules of evidence demanded by the

Department of the Treasury. By 1920 local Carranza representatives' reliance on legal channels forced them to transform public Mexican demands against vaccination policies into individual complaints.

This highlights a potentially exclusionary paradox of Mexican consular politics for ethnic Mexicans in the United States.[40] In the case of antivaccination claims along the Texas-Mexican border after 1915, Mexican consuls advocated the unfettered traffic of most Mexican residents across the Rio Grande. When consuls used specific cases to challenge public health policies on the Mexican border, they chose cases where the need for redress, in light of the relative injustice and the respectability and status of each client, would be immediately recognized. The unspoken emphasis on respectable claimants in the demands for federal redress led to an emphasis on property-owning, literate, and powerful men, even though the cases were supposed to represent the full community. The vehicle of consular redress emphasized the private and individual loss of autonomy of each case, not the greater Mexican community at the border. The cases filed by Mexican nationals against the vaccination and inspection process underscores the difficulty in achieving legal redress when officials need to balance respectability with the need to represent community rights, especially when individuals stand in for larger social processes.[41]

The new consular forum opened up the possibility of change in American immigration stations. Once Woodrow Wilson recognized the Carranza revolutionary faction as the de facto government in Mexico, Carranza's representatives filed a complaint against the USPHS and Texas Board of Health quarantine policies. On January 28, 1916, Arredondo asked that the quarantine between Camargo and Rio Grande be lifted because of the financial hardships it imposed on Camargo and Tamaulipas.[42] Three months later Arredondo included the question of indiscriminate vaccination. Unlike the situation in Nuevo León and Chihuahua, which affected the cities of Piedras Negras, Nuevo Laredo, and Chihuahua, the Mexican consul in Rio Grande City claimed there were no reported incidents of smallpox in Camargo, Tamaulipas.

The USPHS insisted on the vaccination of all incoming Mexicans, despite the absence of smallpox around Rio Grande City. According to Arredondo, this policy served no practical purpose, and the medical inspectors at the station did not differentiate between incoming Mexican arrivals because "vaccination [was] indiscriminately practiced."[43] Even though the confidential agent of the Carranza regime in Atlantic City filed the two complaints, the

State Department did not devote time to address either of these complaints. The State Department did not share the concerns Arredondo, Revelas, and the Camargo residents had about indiscriminate vaccination.

Official Mexican differences with indiscriminate and forced American vaccination policies also took place within informal arenas. The U.S. consul stationed in Piedras Negras, Nuevo León, reported a clear official challenge to the strict vaccination policies in Eagle Pass. Responding to rumors of two smallpox deaths reported by the U.S. consul in Piedras Negras, the USPHS ordered the vaccination of all persons (meaning Mexicans) entering Eagle Pass from Piedras Negras on January 16, 1916.[44] After two months of this practice, military authorities on the Mexico side in Piedras Negras decided to mimic the American inspection policy. The military authorities in Mexico informed the State Department that if the USPHS maintained its vaccination and inspection requirements, local Mexican military authorities would impose their own understanding of identical inspection requirements in Piedras Negras on March 6, 1916.[45] The following day, local Mexican military authorities established quarantine regulations, kicking off a racial status crisis in Eagle Pass.[46] The Mexican quarantine regulations implied that "respectable [white] American ladies" would be forced to expose themselves to, and be touched by, Mexican soldiers.[47]

The U.S. Army decided that military policies required military responses. An army colonel reminded the authorities in Piedras Negras that the quarantine would threaten their access to necessary military and financial resources for Carranza's forces in Mexico. Within a couple of hours, the U.S. consul sent a follow-up telegram reporting that the "quarantine on Mexican side [was] raised and differences amicably settled."[48] Border-based U.S. military authorities used Carranza's tenuous diplomatic situation during the recognition process between 1916 and 1917 to exert administrative pressure on federal policies in Mexico.[49] Informal military intervention quelled the possibility of conflict between local Eagle Pass authorities, Texas state authority, and Carranza's military forces after just one day of Mexican border inspection.

Eliseo Arredondo adopted a more indirect strategy in his third complaint regarding vaccination and inspection practices in Rio Grande City. He did not directly challenge the quarantine; instead, he requested "a more liberal application of sanitary restrictions."[50] The State Department forwarded this request to the Department of the Treasury, where Ambassador

Creel bluntly restated the Treasury's position: "Quarantine restrictions will fall once national authorities in Mexico cooperate more closely with United States authorities."[51] Surgeon General Rupert Blue informed Arredondo that the restrictions were already liberal and loosely applied. Furthermore, local USPHS authorities had to defend the modified quarantine against the demands for an even stricter quarantine by elected officials and public citizens in the state of Texas. In either case, the amount of cooperation between Mexican and U.S. authorities was sorely lacking. Until the Treasury perceived a drastic change in the official climate in northern Mexico, the USPHS would maintain its practices in Rio Grande City and elsewhere. At the time, Arredondo and the State Department were negotiating the conditions for peace and recognition between the United States and Carranza in Atlantic City. These border grievances against the USPHS became pieces in the larger chess game in Atlantic City between Mexican and American diplomats.

Deaths at the border could have audiences all the way to Atlantic City. The death by drowning of Jose Montelongo in the Rio Grande in Laredo was a key case where local grievances tested the limits of Mexican consular authority on the U.S. side of the border in this period. There were persistent rumors in Greater Laredo that all Mexicans who attempted to elude the rigors and financial expense of the bridge crossing and were detained would be "forced to return to Mexico by water."[52] Jose Montelongo's case appeared to confirm the rumor. Two medical officers escorted Montelongo's wife and two children across the bridge. Texas State Health Officer H. C. Hall and three quarantine guards brought Jose and his brother-in-law Francisco Urrutia back to the riverbank. After a short scuffle, Urrutia and Montelongo were forced into the river. Ten minutes later, people on the bridge observed Montelongo's body floating past the bridge, coming to a halt on the Nuevo Laredo riverbank two hundred yards downriver. Nuevo Laredo City authorities immediately organized an investigation around Montelongo's death and this new quarantine policy in Laredo.[53] On August 25, 1916, Arredondo demanded that the State Department prosecute Officer Hall for his role in Montelongo's death.[54]

The city authorities in Nuevo Laredo initiated an investigation into the causes of Jose Montelongo's death. Francisco Urrutia, Dominga Urrutia, and Petra Sanchez identified the body as Jose Montelongo, brother-in-law to Francisco, husband of Dominga, and son of Petra. Francisco Urrutia swore that he and Montelongo were, "at two thirty in the afternoon, beaten by an

American official on the American side."[55] The judge identified two wounds, one on the side of Montelongo's head, and the other on the right side of the eye.[56] The police authorities then brought Montelongo's body to the Maclovio Serrena hospital. Dr. Adolpho Salinas Puga and Dr. Francisco Serrans completed an autopsy. In their deposition they stated that the body gave clear evidence that Jose Montelongo died by drowning and that "the body showed two more wounds to the head, having been made with violence, as both cut the scalp and discovered the skull."[57] The doctors claimed that an animal caused the wound above the eye but that the two other blows must have come from another person. The doctors submitted their witness to the Mexican foreign office on August 22, 1916, in Nuevo Laredo.

The Foreign Office asked the consul in Laredo, Melquiades Garcés, to follow up on this public and international incident. He deposed the public health office in Laredo and asked Dr. Hall if he remembered the incident. In the deposition Hall "admitted that he had given the order and seen when the men were forced to jump into the river."[58] Hall recalled, "Quarantine Guard George Hill, on duty at the footbridge noticed three Mexicans crossing the Rio Grande above the footbridge, in plain view and contrary to quarantine regulations. Guard Hill went after them, and one of the Mexicans tried to get away, and was hit and knocked down. The Mexican hit was not hurt very much, but was able to walk and did not know that he felt the effects of the blow, a few moments after."[59] Having found that both Hill and Hall acknowledged that Hill had delivered force to "one of the Mexicans," Garcés pursued additional avenues to address Montelongo's death. Consul Garcés moved responsibility for the Montelongo case to Arredondo, the de facto representative of the Mexican foreign office and key negotiator in Atlantic City. Mexicans in both Laredos wanted a response to the public beating they had seen earlier that week.

The matter of Jose Montelongo moved from the murky river water into a murkier political realm. American diplomatic recognition of any Mexican revolutionary faction was a near military intervention in Mexico's civil war. Arredondo, arguing that the evidence "above implies a deliberate crime on the part of Dr. Hall," demanded that the State Department initiate specific procedures so that the "offender be brought to justice and punished accordingly."[60] This public death occurred during the delicate dance of negotiation over mutual damages that occurred during the Revolution before the Joint Mexican-American Commission in Atlantic City. Given that the State

Department wanted Carranza's government to assume liability for damages that had occurred during the previous decade to American citizens in Mexico, the State Department felt obliged to pursue the investigation. On September 5, 1916, Secretary of State Robert Lansing requested that the governor of Texas initiate an investigation. The Montelongo case could establish a strong precedent for wrongful deaths and property claims by Americans in Mexico.

The governor's office in Texas decided to cooperate with this effort. By September 11, 1916, Texas State Health Officer Al Lincecom had completed initial inquiries and concurred with the account presented by Arredondo. Lincecom confirmed that Hall and his quarantine guard used force to place Francisco Urrutia and Jose Montelongo into the river; Lincecom deferred on the question of responsibility, claiming that Hall was not responsible for the river's condition. That same day Chief State Health Officer Collins wrote Robert Lansing in defense of Hall's actions, charging that "the Montelongo complaint [was] registered with the department for the purpose of injuring Dr. Hall and of encouraging the law breakers along the border."[61] The legal authority embedded in the quarantine laws of the state of Texas, Article 4333, authorized the use of force in enforcing compliance.[62] Both Dr. Collins and Dr. Lincecom claimed that the State Department could, under the Texas Criminal Code, prosecute "excusable homicide" at best. In response, on October 11, 1916, the solicitor general of the United States requested that the state of Texas prosecute Hall for excusable homicide, because "the Department is called upon not infrequently to insist that the Mexican authorities shall take legal measures against persons charged with crimes committed against American citizens."[63] The State Department felt publicly compelled to pursue this legal precedent. Governor Ferguson complied with this request.

The Mexican pursuit of a precedent against medical officers at the border circled back to Laredo. On October 31, 1916, Governor Ferguson transferred responsibility for inquiry into the death of Jose Montelongo to the Webb County district attorney's office. District Attorney John Valls convened a grand jury for November 20, 1916, to establish a bill of indictment to guide the possible prosecution of Hall; however, "after so very thorough investigation of all the witnesses and all the circumstances the grand jury did not find any bill of indictment in the case."[64] Despite Montelongo's public death, the mutually acknowledged blows, and the medically documented strikes to Montelongo's head, the "representative" Webb County jury did not think the evidence merited charging Dr. Hall with excusable homicide.[65] Despite fairly strong pressure by the State Department, the governor's office, and Mexico's consular corps, all three agencies were unable to bring the matter of Jose Montelongo's death to trial. Despite the very visible evidence provided by Jose Montelongo's body and the depositions provided by his family, the Mexican foreign office's commitment to diplomatic pressure failed to overcome the reluctance on the part of Webb County residents to prosecute a long-term member of their professional circle. The State Department could not move heaven and earth to make common cause with the indictment in Nuevo Laredo for murder or "excusable homicide."

Vaccination complaints followed this pattern of public Mexican outrage, consular complaints, federal investigations, and local Anglo refusal to cooperate with executive branch orders.[66] Two of the cases dealt directly with the revaccination of ethnic Mexicans along the bridges. For others, inspection and the presence of a vaccination needle prompted the possibility of intimate Anglo scrutiny of their bodies. The Montelongo decision was a clear defeat of direct Mexican diplomatic challenges to state-certified Texas medical authority. State and federal health officers now had a public precedent to defend their impunity in the face of Mexican border-crossers.

In the aftermath of their legal victory, Dr. Hall and his employees gave themselves a wider latitude in the use of force as they enforced the vaccination and inspection regime between Laredo and Nuevo Laredo. The Texas State Board of Health, the USPHS, and the Mexican consul in Laredo never documented the extent of this informal application of force. However, when Mexican immigration inspectors on the southern side of the footbridge over the Rio Grande filed a complaint against specific quarantine guards, they included allusions to extensive and illegitimate violence by these guards. Recently appointed Mexican authorities considered the quarantine guard's use of force authorized by the grand jury's decision in the Montelongo case to be abusive.[67] The consul utilized the quarantine authority's use of violence against specific Mexican bodies in the next consular challenge to Hall's authority.

Rather than pursue depositions carried out in Mexico, officials in Nuevo Laredo asked specifically abused Mexican individuals to give their physical evidence in person in the United States. Immigration Inspector I. Juarez asked one injured man, Severiano Valle, to present himself with a letter of introduction to Melquiades Garcés's consular office in Laredo. This way there would be an actual body of evidence alongside sworn depositions. The letter of introduction made reference to the clear evidence of abuse that Valle had recently suffered. The translated body of the letter follows:

> Yesterday several persons came to me to complain that an employee of the sanitary department of that republic, Charles Ramsay, treats Mexicans with the utmost brutality. As proof of facts and that the consulate in your charge may take up the matter energetically to avoid such ruthlessness, I am sending you with bearer of this note, Mr. Severiano Valle, one of the five victims yesterday afternoon of said sanitation employee. At the customs house of this port is to be found another of the persons who has suffered at the hands of said employee. I regret to personally have to add that the conduct of some of the quarantine department employees of this state has really become intolerable, and they are going to the length of frequently physically beating our fellow-citizens, and of these, we ourselves can cite very many cases.[68]

Inspector Juarez assumed that Garcés (and anyone else) could see the traces of violence on Valle. The physical presence of Valle as a body of evidence was very different from the body of evidence available in Hall's trial. In court, there was no body, only the textualized medical interpretation of official violence that Drs. Puga and Serrans put to paper after their autopsy of Jose Montelongo. The witness provided by the Urrutia family and the shared memory of the public spectacle of Jose Montelongo's body floating down the Rio Grande through downtown Laredo supplemented the autopsy report. Here, Valle's body could actually provide witness to the violence that was done to him and four other people a day earlier. The letter, witnessed by a notary public in Mexico, placed Valle on the bridge and named Charles Ramsay as the perpetrator of this violence. Garcés placed the key evidence that upheld the Valle incident off the written page. Valle's body and presence certified the physical violence exercised in all five incidents. These five stories would then provide representative evidence of the extent to which quarantine guards were "frequently beating our fellow citizens."[69] If more evidence were necessary to prove the extent to which Ramsay and other sanitary employees exerted physical violence on ethnic Mexican border-crossers, Inspector Juarez would be happy to "cite very many cases."[70] Garcés sought to use Valle's body as a forum through which Ramsay and the practices of the Texas State Board of Health could be placed under federal scrutiny.

The possibility of a forum to address Mexican grievances against federal personnel addressed was, potentially, the most novel result of this legal encounter. Inspector Juarez and Consul Garcés hoped that diplomatic negotiation could compel restraint on the part of the Texas State Board of Health employees. Garcés's faith in power of the recently appointed ambassador in Washington, D.C., Ugnacio Bonillas, was tenuous but present in this plea: "Earnestly beseeching that you may enter complaint with the corresponding authorities, I renew the assurance of my consideration."[71] The creation of a forum for these five cases would rest on Bonillas's ability to negotiate with the State Department and the appropriate federal agency.

The State Department was not willing to negotiate with Bonillas on this matter. The State Department forwarded the complaint to the Texas Board of Health. Secretary of State Robert Lansing demanded an official response from the Texas State Board of Health regarding the alleged abuses by the quarantine guard in Laredo. Despite Hall's recent conflicts with Mexican authority over Montelongo's death, Texas State Health Officer Collins demanded that Hall investigate and report on the conduct of the quarantine guards under his authority in Laredo, Texas. In other words, Dr. Hall was ordered to investigate Dr. Hall.

The results of this investigation provide a privileged insight into Hall's understanding of his work at the Laredo bridge. Hall addressed the "mistreatment of Mexican passengers" accusation in three ways. First, he emphasized that quarantine practices were already under an informal legal scrutiny. In the case of illegalities in the practice of the quarantine, Hall informed the guards that the Mexican consul had encouraged the use of local courts to address grievances against the quarantine guard. The local courts would then judge "the merits of these difficulties."[72] As a result, "any transgression of theirs will in due course reach this jurisdiction."[73] Dr. Hall's supervisory measures placed responsibility on "Mexican passengers" themselves and assumed that Mexican nationals had free recourse to the courts. Hall probably knew how the courts would respond, based on the Montelongo decision. He banked on local indifference.

The second argument emphasized that special conditions at the border required special policies. Hall claimed that the conditions in Laredo under which quarantine guards worked were uniquely stressful. The guards were busy because they surveyed the movement of five hundred people across an eighteen-foot bridge entrance. Furthermore, the work interests of a number of these bridge-crossers were in conflict with quarantine procedures. Hall associated any interpersonal difficulties with quarantine guards with membership in this class: "99 percent of the difficulties have been caused by a class of passengers, from the hack-men, hotel runners, and persons passing the night in Nuevo Laredo, Mexico, on account of our 9:30 closing against saloons."[74] In other words, Mexicans who worked in the transportation industry, from railroads to the horse-driven equivalent to taxicab drivers, were naturally predisposed against the routines of quarantine. Second, there was always potential conflict between the State Health Office's work schedules and the unsavory workplace environments of this class of Laredo residents. Any quarantine guard who pursued his job "with efficient service" created a hostile audience for himself.[75] In this case, this "element of interurban traffic" singled out the exemplary and dutiful actions of Charles Ramsay.[76] According to Hall, this claim by five different people was yet another example of the wide spectrum of Mexican indifference and hostility to the work of the employees of the Texas State Board of Health. The complaints had nothing to do with Ramsay's willingness to use violence against a wide range of Laredo residents to compel consent.

Finally, the challenges to the practice of the quarantine challenged the ability of both the Texas State Board of Health and the USPHS to police the public in Laredo and Nuevo Laredo. Given the commitment to trade and the close connections between both cities, Hall stated, "these two communities must be considered as one, from a health viewpoint, so long as traffic is kept open as we have been doing for the past two years."[77] Hall claimed that the quarantine was the reason there had been no outbreak of smallpox in Laredo since 1915. Unlike El Paso, all 125 typhus cases had been peacefully isolated in the Maclovio Serrena hospital in Nuevo Laredo. He claimed that the friendly cooperation between Mexican and American bridge authorities enabled this success. Ironically, the friendly Mexican immigration inspector, Juarez, was the person who assembled and initiated the complaint that Ramsay allegedly assaulted five people. In order to make this claim, Hall ignored the immediate history of the complaint against Ramsay. In any case, Hall did not regard as legitimate this State Department pressure to change the tone of the quarantine. As Hall succinctly stated, "We do not consider it within our province to change Texas State Laws in parley or conference."[78] Federally mandated cooperation with Mexican officials was acceptable only if the cooperation did not challenge local custom or Texas state laws and procedures. The absence of smallpox and typhus in Laredo demonstrated the necessity for this unquestioned authority. Dialogue was too much of a challenge to the established inspection procedures in Laredo.

Ultimately, the possibility that any Mexican authority could question Texas state authority troubled Hall. Dr. Hall's argument proceeded in the following manner. Ambassador Bonillas filed a specific complaint with the State Department. The State Department investigated the complaint. In response to this investigation, Hall claimed that he would recognize only county courts as a legitimate vehicle for complaints against Board of Health employees. In the case of a complaint, Hall would only recognize specific complaints against his employees by legitimate and respectable residents of Laredo. Because Hall continued in charge of the state quarantine in Laredo, any consular complaint, regardless of the evidence presented, would not be able to achieve the minimum conditions for a hearing or an investigation. Hall's suggestion— that "future difference should be taken up at once, while witness could be obtained, and the local courts settle same"—undermined the authority of both the State Department and the Mexican foreign office to settle grievances in Laredo.[79] This move to the county jurisdiction for diplomatic complaints afforded test cases that lived up to this new standard of evidence. Questions of everyday harassment were too routine. The Mexican consuls stationed in Laredo did not file another complaint against a USPHS or a Texas State Board of Health employee. Instead, the consuls started relying on the administrative authority of the federal government.

Passport to Modernity: Banking on the Vaccination Scars of Porfirian Modernity

For a century before the USPHS required all arrivals to submit to an inspection, Spanish and then Mexican state authorities used vaccination scars as a mark of distinction. When lymph from the Balmis Expedition arrived in San Antonio in 1808, Coronel Antonio Cordero y Bustamante brought men and women in surrounding towns to San Antonio to witness the first successful vaccination in Texas.[80] The frequent smallpox epidemics that appeared after Mexico's independence created new opportunities for the paternal exercise of spatial power. Gobernación—the Mexican equivalent of the executive branch—frequently authorized the transfer of lymph from vaccine farms in Jalisco and the valley of Mexico to gubernatorial allies in Nuevo León, Baja California, Sonora, and Tampico during various epidemics.[81] Vaccination was part of a larger movement to make Mexico modern. During the decade of armed conflict known as the Mexican Revolution, the legibility of vaccination scars on Mexican bodies became the site of conflict and authority between two different state authorities, the USPHS and an emerging Mexican foreign office. Officers of the USPHS decided to ignore any evidence provided by Mexican bodies. Mexicans, on the other hand, wanted the evidence of the body to be recognized as evidence of a modern medical act.

In 1916, the USPHS required inspections of all uncertified Mexican bodies at the border. This demand outraged Mexicans because they had to disrobe and display their bodies and, after this humiliation, their vaccination scars were not considered worthy of American medical recognition. After having undergone vaccination in Rio Grande City's immigration station, Miguel Barrera filed the only case that directly addressed receiving a vaccination against his will and against the evidence supplied by his vaccination scars. In the letter Miguel Barrera filed with Leoncio Revelas, the "Consul de Mexico City," Barrera stated the following:

> I call your attention, for the purpose or for whatever use you may want to make of this letter that today on arriving at the immigration office at this side of the river, and coming from Camargo, Tamaulipas, notwithstanding my old age of seventy-four (74) years. And in spite of having my residence in Sam Fordyce, the doctor refused to hear my arguments and vaccinated me.
>
> When a boy I was vaccinated at the age usually done in Mexico, said vaccination having taken; but to be vaccinated at the age when the danger of infection may be said to have passed is in my opinion altogether unnecessary and above all, what calls my attention and which I want you to understand is that the doctor appears insensible to the just reasons that may be exposed to him by persons like myself are used to deal with the TRUTH.
>
> Without other subject than to let you know that I am ready to uphold what I have said, whenever it may be necessary, I beg to remain,
>
> > Yours respectfully,
> > Miguel Barrera.[82]

Part of the outrage felt by the people Leticia Garza-Falcón calls *gente decente* (literally "decent people," but more accurately the aspiring classes) lay in the USPHS's refusal to recognize their early investment in modernity. Barrera's vaccination "at the age when it was usually done in Mexico" revealed a substantial commitment in his original district to modern hygiene practices during the tumultuous era before the Porfiriato in Mexico.[83] Parish boards, local business owners, landowners, and municipal bosses committed to the expense, supervision, and energy necessary to maintain arm-to-arm vaccination across a given region. This regional commitment to medical guarantees of human capital of the district went national in the age of "order and progress" in the Porfiriato.[84] In 1874, Don Porfirio committed himself to guarantee the peace necessary to move Mexico into the modern world and away from the perceived disorder associated with civil wars, mestizos, and foreign invasions.

The Porfiriato justified itself to the world through a new political stability, publicly visible and expert administration, visible efforts to improve the hygiene and public health of Mexico, and increased levels of foreign investment. The metaphor of modernity even transferred to the ways the Porfiriato smothered dissent. Observers knew federal authority would frequently use "the sanitary rifle" against rebellious bandits, unruly campesinos, difficult workers, and other ills that stained the appearance of productivity in Mexico.[85] Bureaucrats in Mexico City were concerned with the image of cleanliness, order, and progress they exported to the rest of the world. For Don Porfirio Díaz and his advisers (the *científicos*), the appearance of cleanliness and hygiene were essential to the cultural transformation of Mexico's residents into citizens of the modern world. These words also implied anxieties around the depth of the change—around the possibility that it was illusory.

Modernity was also a local project. A number of municipalities provided public schooling and industrial education to make sure that modernity would not melt into air. The literacy of workers and middling classes was proof of one commitment to change in Mexico. In order to receive some services in Monterrey, urban residents had to have vaccination scars and proof of certified vaccination.[86] Increasing numbers of self-styled modern work sites required vaccination as a condition of employment. The Mexican Central Railroad required vaccination among all its employees.[87] The American Smelting and Refining Corporation required vaccination as a condition of employment.[88] Vaccination demonstrated, perhaps, a deeper commitment to the new rhythms of industrial Mexico. These requirements followed a parallel commitment on the part of northern Mexican middle classes to vaccination. American public health officer John Hamilton remarked on the wide extent of vaccination among middle-class Mexicans in Matamoros, Laredo, and Monterrey in his 1910 report on smallpox in the lower Rio Grande Valley. After twenty years of compulsory vaccination in Nuevo León, vaccination scars had become both a badge of distinction and a necessary passport into the modern workforce. When someone displayed these scars to a public official in northern Mexico, they asserted their sense of citizenship and belonging against an attempted exclusion. The lines that separated modern from disorderly Mexico were forcefully drawn in individual bodies across public spaces; these exclusionary lines shaped the public significance of vaccination scars.[89]

This modernizing Mexican context sparked Miguel Barrera's outrage toward the USPHS medical officer at the Rio Grande City office. His vaccination scars failed to prevent him from being vaccinated at the border. His complaint called the recently arrived Mexican consul's attention to the framework through which Dr. Hunter understood Barrera's presence in the inspection station. Barrera respectfully dissented from federal policies that Hunter sought to enforce. Barrera assumed that a class of men like himself, who argued with "just reasons," who were willing to stand by their statements "wherever it may be necessary," and who used the bridge to move between Camargo, Tamaulipas, and Sam Fordyce, Texas, should be able to argue with their peers and equals on the other side of the USPHS scarification process. The rhetorical weight of Barrera's outrage fell not on Hunter's forced revaccination but on his attitude toward the arguments that Barrera and other men like him probably deployed as they made their legal way into the United States. Hunter appeared "insensible" to arguments that were based on "truth."[90] The USPHS framework was a direct affront to the investment Miguel Barrera and his family had made in Porfirian medical technologies.

In the process of delivering his complaint to the recent consular appointee, Barrera demonstrated the distance between the county court and the adjudication of Mexican claims. Even though Consul Revelas was new to Rio Grande City, Barrera considered the consular office a better vehicle for grievances than the recently elected "Good Government" county court.[91] This vehicle was important to Starr County residents. Evan Anders has documented the ways that Jacobo Guerra, the Starr County sheriff, was unable to protect the Mexican residents of Starr County from abuses by Texas Rangers, vigilante parties, and lynch mobs between 1915 and 1916.[92] The consulate provided another forum for Mexicans of all nationalities to air their grievances against public authority.

Commitment to the forum began to grow. Jorge Olivares followed Miguel Barrera's tracks when he filed his tentative case with Leoncio Revelas. In his complaint about the USPHS, Olivares made reference to the extent to which the consul might be a better vehicle for legal redress. Olivares made reference to an unspoken claim that Carranza's recent recognition by Woodrow Wilson's government might have an effect on American federal policies on the Mexican border: "I understand that if the Mexican government would take an active part, this situation may have changed in a radical way, it would render a valuable service to us who have to cross the river on business and would avoid the continuing for a longer time for the mocking of our race. In these hopes I call your attention to all the preceding events."[93] This plea emphasized that USPHS policies endangered the binational status and practices of a specific class "who have to cross the river on business."[94] Respectability forced them to comply with these new USPHS regulations. This is one reason the regulations fell much more heavily on the *gente decente* of the Texas-Mexican border. Residents of the border could take a ferry in towns with no USPHS service, cross the river illegally by foot or boat, or try to evade the USPHS service as they crossed the bridge. However, if someone working on the northern bank of the Rio Grande had to show papers that the business they were negotiating complied with all regulations, they would have to share the USPHS certificate of vaccination, disinfection, and inspection. Revelas's authority among the varied sectors of Rio Grande's Mexican community as the "Consul de Mexico City" depended on his advocacy of this particular sector.[95]

Jorge Olivares considered his experiences at the hands of Dr. Hunter to be representative of most ethnic Mexicans who legally crossed the border. Buttressing this contention, Olivares incorporated himself into this deposition as a claimant and a witness to the abuses committed in the Rio Grande quarantine station:

> Owing to my trip to Camargo to-day, I had an opportunity to witness on my return, in the immigration office on the American side, the abuses daily committed with our people by those two persons who are in charge of the service and who ostensibly show their anti-Mexicanism daily. I am aware that the doctor has here an employee devoted to inspect the head of everybody coming across the river, to search for lice not taking into account that the person may be some times tidy. Having the absolute necessity to come to this country, or rather to return, since I reside here, I was compelled, not without first having to smother my wrath, to pass through all the vexations

to which all Mexicans must invariably submit themselves, if unfortunately they need to cross this river at this crossing, the only one, of which may be said the daily abuses have reached a high degree.

I understand that if the Mexican government would take an active part, this situation may have changed in a radical way, it would render a valuable service to us who have to cross the river on business and would avoid continuing the mocking of our race.[96]

The Olivares testimony made it clear that universal vaccination entailed "the mocking of our race." Surgeon General Rupert Blue's demand that every incoming Mexican arrival be inspected and vaccinated had an immediate impact on the aspiring sort in Mexican communities. The USPHS treated Olivares, on his return home from Mexico, like any other incoming Mexican on arrival. Despite his respectable status, the USPHS inspectors forced him to submit to the vexations of the quarantine. The inspection for lice and vaccination scars placed the practice beyond the boundaries of legitimacy. Olivares used phrases like "the mocking of our race," "vexations to which all [and only?] Mexicans must submit themselves," and "daily abuses" that "ostensibly show[ed] their anti-Mexicanism" to describe the intimate experience respectable Mexicans underwent when they crossed back into the United States.[97]

Since Rio Grande City was a local transportation hub, the northernmost link to Brownsville in the southern part of the valley, the presence of a town between Rio Grande City and Laredo where no quarantine officers were stationed offered a clear contrast between unrestricted and humiliating traffic across the Rio Grande. Olivares knew that there was a potential crossing twenty miles north of Rio Grande City with no quarantine station, so the practices that were "continuing the mocking of our race" must have seemed arbitrary to this man whose business ties forced him to cross at Rio Grande City. The location of the crossing and the continued humiliation associated with the vaccine scar inspection made quarantine practices an ideal target for visible reforms advocated by Leoncio Revelas, the local Carranza consular appointee.

Revelas filed his next complaint a day after he received the deposition of Efraím Domínguez, a professor in the Escuela Normal de Profesoras in Saltillo, who came to the United States to purchase supplies for the school. Revelas used Domínguez's situation to illustrate the USPHS officials' abuse of respectable Mexican professionals. Domínguez's position as a professor made him an ideal person to challenge the indignities of vaccination and inspection practices. Consul Revelas began his narration with the recounting of the shame associated with inspection practices. Professor Domínguez had "suffer[ed] the shame of submission to the (denigrating to us) practices that, instead of necessary, are capriciously enforced by the two American officials of whom I made reference earlier, even though he gave evidence that he clearly was a respectable person."[98] Efraím Domínguez had stepped off the ferry into Rio Grande City after a train ride from Saltillo, dressed in some of his best clothing. Upon his arrival, the two officers stripped him to inspect the quality of his underwear, even though his commitment to cleanliness should have been clear "from any distance."[99] They then publicly inspected his naked person, "with a harshness that revealed their hate [*con una aspereza reveladora de odio*]," for evidence of smallpox and lice.[100] Given the financial constraints on his time, Professor Domínguez submitted to the inspection process without complaint or obvious resistance even though he would have preferred to return to Mexico and cross at another port.[101] Consul Revelas argued that, if any Mexican citizen could avoid the indignity of the inspection practices, Efraím Domínguez would be the most likely candidate.

For Revelas, this proved that the inspection practices had gone too far, tying the respectable northern Mexican middle class to the condition of common laborers in Mexico and Texas. In Revelas's hands, Domínguez's case was an example of a widespread pattern of federal harassment and humiliation. As he commented to Ambassador Bonillas, "Because similar and more appalling abuses had been frequently committed by the employees of the sanitary agency and not just with men but with the gentler sex, judging from communications in Camargo, I have found it an urgent necessity to inform you of all these abuses, with the hope that through this gesture you may be able to obtain some remedy for this aberrant situation."[102]

If the newly won recognition by the U.S. government was to mean anything to the residents of the border, the Mexican foreign office of Ygnacio Bonillas should force the federal government to change these practices. The complaints moved directly into the sphere of administrative law, away from civil and criminal court. Revelas further claimed that the indignity of the quarantine station was accompanied by a lack of respect for the time spent by people forced to cross legally between Rio Grande City, Texas, and Camargo, Tamaulipas. Both Dr. Hunter and Inspector Flannery opened the ferry at seemingly random intervals, their lunch breaks went over the scheduled time,

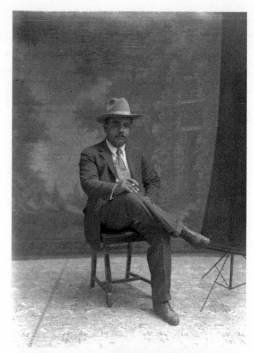

Figure 11. Robert Runyon, "Pablo Ramirez." Courtesy of the Robert Runyon Collection, "run05086," Center for American History, The University of Texas at Austin.

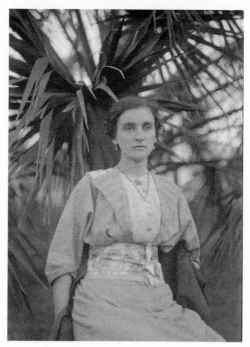

Figure 12. Robert Runyon, "Felipa Medrano." Courtesy of the Robert Runyon Collection, "run09263," Center for American History, The University of Texas at Austin.

and they frequently closed the ferry early. If passengers arrived at the ferry late, the ferry demanded more payment for passage back to Camargo. This meant additional overnight costs. And once they crossed, they were forced to confront, submit to, and suffer at the hands of the local inspectors. In Revelas's opinion, Hunter and Flannery were "two employees zealously pursuing their obligations who never bothered to conceal the heights of their anti-Mexican sentiment. Even submission to their demands was no guarantee of safe passage, as there were a number of people who, after they were vaccinated and bathed in gasoline, were not allowed to pass into the United States."[103]

Beginning with Miguel Barrera, Jorge Olivares, and Efraím Domínguez, Consul Revelas argued that the quarantine at Rio Grande City was both arbitrary and indiscriminate. Revelas used Ambassador Bonillas's office as a means to challenge American federal administrative practices along the Rio Grande City–Camargo corridor. Bonillas outlined the arguments that Consul Revelas laid out in his report for Secretary of State Lansing. Given the racial and diplomatic tensions that accompanied Pershing's exit from Chihuahua, and the earlier tensions around the *Plan de San Diego* in South Texas, Ambassador Bonillas implied that the arbitrary and indiscriminate application of the quarantine by American sanitary authorities served "no practical purpose whatsoever."[104] Bonillas enclosed Leoncio Revelas's three depositions in his letter to Lansing to bear witness to the treatment to which Mexican citizens were subjected.[105] Bonillas urged Secretary of State Lansing to use his office to force these practices to cease, as they seemed to serve no practical purpose.[106]

The translators in the Department of State provided a very different letter to Secretary of State Robert Lansing. In the translation, Ambassador Bonillas did not send the incendiary report filed by the consul at Rio Grande. Rather, Secretary Lansing received the report of "a concrete case of lack of consideration on the part of sanitary authorities toward Mexican citizens."[107] In the translation, Bonillas argued that these practices "caused misunderstandings between the authorities and the communities on the border, to the detriment of the cordial relations that should prevail."[108] Secretary of State Lansing read a letter requesting that the State Department investigate this specific case regarding two employees because of these "misunderstandings." In the original text in Spanish, Bonillas demanded that Secretary of State Lansing use his authority to stop these USPHS practices. The English translation Secretary Lansing read was much narrower than the original complaint written by Bonillas. In the process of translation, the status of the claims filed in Rio

Grande City went from a report with depositions to a request for an additional investigation.

The emphasis of the complaint changed drastically in the State Department translation. The translator changed the pattern of abuses to just one case that demonstrated "a concrete lack of consideration."[109] Secretary of State Lansing complied with the language of the English translation and demanded an investigation of this one event from the Department of the Treasury, the Department of Labor, and the office of the governor of Texas. The governor's office merely requested a response in writing from the federal employees in Rio Grande City to the charges laid by Consul Revelas against Inspector Flannery and Dr. Hunter. The Department of Labor commissioned Inspector Reynolds, posted in Brownsville, to investigate whether the quarantine stationed operated at regular hours, whether Inspector Flannery of the Immigration Service or Assistant Surgeon John Hunter harbored racial prejudice toward Mexican nationals, and whether Hunter's vaccination policies conformed to federal directives. In their initial responses, Flannery and Hunter both challenged Consul Revelas's authority and emphasized their perception of Mexican unreliability. Reynolds focused on the inspector's intent, not the medical officers' treatment of the patients within their inspection station.

Following the language in the translation, Flannery addressed the problem of courtesy and lack of consideration. He wrote that he always treated applicants "with the courtesy due them from an American standpoint."[110] Flannery maintained his commitment to American courtesy, "even in the face of insolence, abuse, insults and other provocations from Mexican applicants totally lacking in the instincts of refinement."[111] Perhaps Consul Revelas and his peers disapproved of his direct mode of address, but he would "never follow and never intend to follow the silly Mexican customs of effusive embrace and the use of obsequious phrases of address."[112] Even in the matter of the courtesy due to what he perceived to be the Mexican upper classes, Flannery drew on Spanish fantasy stereotypes to separate himself from upper-class Mexican refinement. That is, if the matter was general discourtesy, in Inspector Flannery's view the real problem was the insolence and disrespect Flannery received from Consul Revelas and the long-term Mexican residents of Rio Grande City. Starr County did not feel like an American place to Flannery.

Flannery assumed that Texas State Health Officer Spivey and Governor Ferguson understood the code behind the phrase "American standpoint," which probably accrued its meaning from recent international and state-level politics. Judging by Revelas's commentary, Flannery was a relatively recent arrival to Rio Grande City and Starr County.[113] He may have been another farmer, Good Government advocate, and Republican who worked out of the customs house.[114] He may have also advocated the sole enfranchisement of men who conformed to the image of literate, propertied, white, American, and publicly motivated male citizens that powered many Good Government disenfranchisement drives.[115] If he participated in Texas electoral politics, he took part in electoral campaigns where both candidates were openly white supremacist and advocated the disenfranchisement of unqualified voters. His descriptions of Starr County and Rio Grande City depict an urban region *dominated* by a Mexican population. This rhetoric belied the large number of Anglo immigrants arriving in Rio Grande City at the time.[116] The wave of migration from the Midwest was changing the politics in Starr County.

Flannery swore under oath that his attitude toward the majority of ferry passengers was neither racist nor disrespectful.[117] He explained the challenge of his job to Inspector Reynolds in blunt terms: "Rio Grande City is strictly a Mexican town, with Mexican ways and Mexican customs, and the local officers here are Mexicans, including the sheriff and all the deputies. . . . The people in this section, as well as aliens, have been used to crossing the Rio Grande River for years without any immigration or public health restrictions whatever, and they do not take kindly to the immigration and public health laws and regulations."[118] Flannery drew a national distinction between himself and the majority of residents of Rio Grande City when he claimed that because of the un-American status of Starr County, federal immigration requirements would be unpopular: "The population of Rio Grande City consists of four or five thousand Mexicans and about 18 Americans, and when an American officer [like Edward Flannery] comes to a place like this and tries to do his duty without fear or favor, and without partiality, he at once becomes unpopular."[119] The disjuncture between "American" legislation and "Mexican" practices in Starr County led to situations where "numerous aliens prevaricate to us when the truth would serve them better. Also, aliens have perjured themselves under oath a number of times. They attempt to come over here at times in a drunken condition, and act unseemly, and very impudent, and refuse to answer simple questions, and tell us to go to H—, or said, 'what the h—do you care where I am going?' or 'what I am going for?'"[120] Inspector Flannery considered the investigation itself—because it was initiated by Consul Revelas, who refused to ask Flannery and Hunter about the reason behind their practices—further proof of the illegitimacy of any Mexican testimony.[121]

Dr. John Hunter expanded the unreliability of Mexican evidence to include the physical evidence provided by vaccination scars. Hunter twice addressed the charge that, against their expressed consent, he had vaccinated Mexicans in his Rio Grande City quarantine station who had already been vaccinated. The first time he addressed the charge was during his deposition by Inspector Reynolds on June 6, 1917. Hunter claimed the legal complaints arose from the relationship between Mexican ideals (on both sides of the border) and American legal practices: "The Mexican is inimical to restraint and our immigration and health laws and if he can't have things just his own way, he resents it."[122] Even in the best of relationships—as in Efraím Domínguez's case, where he "was treated courteously and made no objection to anything which was done," in the eyes of the health officers—Efraím and other ethnic Mexicans still resented USPHS authority and filed complaints.[123]

Inspector Reynolds considered Dr. Hunter's explanation of Mexican complaints in his station to be adequate. Dr. E. W. Spivey, the state health officer charged with clearing Arthur Bates, the Texas State Health Office quarantine officer in Rio Grande City, of the same charges required more detailed answers from Hunter. In Spivey's subsequent inquiry, he demanded that Hunter directly address the question of whether he had vaccinated people who had already suffered a bout of smallpox. Dr. Hunter described this vaccination practice as he sidestepped the question of consent.[124] Hunter considered the hue and cry around this vaccination procedure ongoing evidence of Mexican unreliability. As Hunter stated in response to Spivey,

> The additional charge that I vaccinate persons who have had smallpox, I am not prepared to deny, I may have done so, so it is not improbable. My instructions are to vaccinate all who do not clearly show recent vaccination scars or clearly evident marks of smallpox. I follow my instructions. Most Mexicans male or female will deceive me if they can, in any way they can, so great is their prejudice to vaccination and submission to our laws. Each one is given the option of being vaccinated or returning to Mexico. They claim every little scar to be smallpox and if one has had chickenpox his whole family will swear he has had smallpox.[125]

This is a succinct statement of the double bind the USPHS created for every ethnic Mexican who took the ferry from Camargo to Rio Grande City. Because they took the ferry, this fleeting embrace of American legality placed them in temporary USPHS custody on landing at the Rio Grande City landing site. Once in custody, they placed themselves under the inspector's gaze. If their bodies displayed no evidence of vaccination or smallpox in the inspector's eyes, Hunter claimed he would offer them the choice of vaccination or a return to Mexico.[126]

If the incoming Mexican ferry passengers had submitted themselves to vaccination in Monterrey or Saltillo, the scars that accompanied their vaccination experience proved their commitment to the medical practices of state citizenship in northern Mexico. By the same token, the display of smallpox scars from their inoculation and vaccination experiences in northern Mexico should have been similar to the displays mandated by state-level and national-level decrees in the United States. As Hunter made clear in his written response to Spivey, the official framework through which this display of scar tissue was understood by the USPHS was drastically different. Dr. Hunter offered all incoming Mexican ferry passengers the same choice, regardless of their smallpox vaccination status in Mexico. They could either submit to the vaccination process or return to the ferry and cross the river back to Camargo. Any attempt to demonstrate to Dr. Hunter that the vaccination, inoculation, and/or smallpox scars on their bodies were medically legitimate was further proof that the incoming Mexican arrivals suffered from a great "prejudice to vaccination and submission to [U.S.-based] laws," therefore their bodies and words were unreliable witnesses to their own experiences.[127]

For Inspector Reynolds, these complaints were proof that both Dr. Hunter and Inspector Flannery were efficient in their work as inspectors. As he proudly reported to Secretary of State Lansing, "[Hunter and Flannery] have excluded quite a number of aliens there for good and sufficient reasons under the immigration laws and these cases are all recorded in their board records, and it seems that these excluded aliens and their relatives are offended."[128] The inspectors conformed to the broad guidelines of the definition of undesirable immigrant bodies. Besides exclusion based on loathsome and communicable diseases, Flannery and Hunter excluded people they considered "likely to become public charges, also professional beggars, feeble minded, idiots, totally blind, public prostitutes, aliens who attempt to import prostitutes, contract laborers, etc."[129] For Reynolds, these were "the kinds of people who are offended at not being permitted to enter the United States."[130] Efraím Domínguez, Miguel Barrera, and Juana Garza would have been shocked that their refusal to submit to a humiliating medical treatment placed them on the same level as sex workers, beggars, and human traffickers.

This was the heart of the conflict in Rio Grande City. There was a clear contrast in the attitude toward complaints about medical procedures. Revelas advocated legal redress for citizens whose commitment to modernity, hygiene, and respectability was difficult to impugn. Reynolds's attitude toward their act of legitimate protest tied the Mexican claimants even more closely in the mind of USPHS officers with the sectors of Mexican society they probably disdained. Reynolds stressed three matters to Revelas in his final interview. First, the vaccination and inspections were not meant to be burdens. Rather, the vaccination was a service that the federal government was providing free to all incoming Mexican ferry passengers. "[Any incoming alien] is also required to submit to vaccination and a thorough medical examination and if they are not overly sensitive it does not seem that any person should be offended by answering these questions and by submitting to vaccination which is given gratis."[131] Second, the passage by ferry was also a journey into another national sovereignty. By immigration statute and congressional mandate, the medical and the immigration inspector were meant to select the best classes of immigrants and residents. "The purpose of immigration laws is to admit healthy and desirable aliens and to keep out diseased and undesirable aliens, and, if in the performance of that duty we should offend certain inadmissible aliens, that cannot be helped."[132] The inspectors offended ferry passengers through the inspection, but this was an unavoidable result of the admissions process. Because insult was embedded in the ritual of inspection, Reynolds thought Revelas should not entertain the notions of some of these "inadmissible immigrants" that they deserved to be treated any better than they had been. Finally, by tying the U.S. secretary of state and the Mexican ambassador to vaccination complaints in Rio Grande City, Reynolds thought Revelas involved too many levels of diplomatic bureaucracy, when matters could be addressed locally. The consul should bring local matters to federal authorities stationed at the border. The Mexican complaint process unnecessarily stigmatized the efforts of the USPHS in Rio Grande City and other stations with their supervisors at other levels of the Department of the Treasury. Reynolds's instructions paralleled USPHS surgeon John Hamilton's response: let local federal institutions address these local border matters.

The consul was the local federal Mexican institution. Here, Leoncio Revelas understood something very different from this diplomatic intervention. According to Revelas, both Dr. Hunter and Inspector Flannery adopted a less intrusive and authoritarian mode of medical inspection after the investigation. Even though many local Mexican residents of Camargo and Rio Grande maintained their hostility to the ritual of inspection, the mode of address in the inspection process became less "anti-Mexican."[133] Revelas took the opportunity to lay a case for further intervention by the layers of the Treasury bureaucracy that might yield to Mexican diplomatic pressure. As Revelas informed Spivey, "After Inspector Reynolds' visit last month, their [Flannery & Hunter's] way to attend to their duties has changed considerably according to reports given to me, and this shows that these two employees needed some reproach from their higher officers to show all persons due respect."[134] Revelas understood that their alleged change in behavior resulted from the increased administrative pressure on the part of State Department authorities in Washington, D.C. If complaints yielded these minimal changes in attitude, diplomatic pressure accompanied by the careful testimony of respectable Mexican nationals on the border provided a potential bargaining tool.

The first cases highlighted a shared experience to challenge the physical violence and public humiliation that accompanied their passage across the river. Mexican consular officers maintained similar themes in their complaints regarding the smallpox inspection: the process was disrespectful of their autonomy and their immediate history; there was an implicit exchange between vaccination and legal entry; inspectors were unable to differentiate between Mexican nationals and Mexican residents; finally, the attempt to challenge vaccination practices through the rules of evidence was considered further proof of the unreliability of Mexican oral and physical testimony. The class basis for Mexican consular complaints regarding the conduct of vaccination turned elite Mexicans into potential political trouble for border inspectors. A short case demonstrates the way American medical officers feared the wrath of Mexican consular defense of elite privilege.

Mexican consul Teodoro Frezieres made arrangements with the immigration inspectors at Eagle Pass to allow the Peraldi sisters, the sisters of the commanding general of the Piedras Negras military district and the nieces of General Carranza, a medical-inspection-free passage into the United States. The inspectors agreed to expedite the paperwork. Three days later, when the two sisters presented themselves at the immigration station, the immigration inspectors allowed them into the United States and forwarded them to the quarantine office in the same building.[135] The two sisters were inspected for lice, and their arms were examined by a "medical inspectress" to ascertain whether they were vaccinated and whether those vaccination scars were sufficient evidence of immunity to smallpox.[136] The medical inspectress determined that the Peraldi sisters were already clean and that they seemed to have been recently vaccinated; she gave them free passage into the United States. Consul Frezieres witnessed their exit from the medical inspection room. As this was clear evidence that Inspector Ostrom had broken his informal promise, Frezieres created a "totally unnecessary and unjustifiable scene." According to Inspector Parker, Frezieres used so many words to inform Ostrom that he "was no gentleman" that Parker did "not have sufficient command of the English language to state how insulting Consul Frezieres had been."[137] In the subsequent investigation, all three inspectors maintained that Mexican consul Frezieres threatened to force any "Immigration man, going to Mexico" to a bath, "even if he had to do it himself."[138] In this case, the Mexican foreign office exerted informal diplomatic pressure. This time the immigration office initiated an investigation into Consul Frezieres's misconduct. These cases highlight the unequal modernity that the USPHS imposed on the Rio Grande border.

The claimants asked for recognition of a shared medical modernity. In response, the USPHS and immigration service officers emphasized the opportunities local Texas governance offered Mexican claimants. Given that between 1910 and 1920 the majority of upper and lower Rio Grande Valley border counties had a majority ethnic Mexican electoral base, Democratic machine politicians were able to fend off a number of insurgent Good Government League attempts to disenfranchise their electoral base. In the process of defending their American status during the violent phases of the Mexican Revolution, there was little electoral gain for machine politicians in challenging the increased federal presence of the USPHS. This agency was, after all, a presence they themselves had requested to address their position at the railroad hubs between Mexico and the United States.

County courts offered Mexican claimants little solace. The use of consular redress to challenge indiscriminate vaccination and its associated practices tied local Mexican challenges to the vagaries of international diplomacy. Despite the clear evidence they provided of their commitment to medical modernity, the USPHS systematically deported ethnic Mexicans from their position within the larger community of citizens committed to medical progress. In these protests, ethnic Mexicans challenged the indignity of indiscriminate vaccination. They, like the officers that vaccinated them against their will, shared a commitment to disease prevention through vaccination.

The field of border inspection shifted with the ratification of the 1917 Constitution in Queretaro. Both the Mexican-American Commission and the Constitution included universal vaccination coverage for all Mexican nationals as a demand.[139] Beginning in 1918, the new Secretaría de Salubridad began the industrial production of higher-quality calf-lymph vaccine serum. The Secretaría required vaccination certificates from citizens who initiated transactions that required federal and municipal certification. In the same vein, the Mexican immigration service required adequate vaccination certificates as a condition of entry into Mexico.

For some U.S. nationals, this new requirement was a shock. In 1921, the U.S. Shipping Board filed an official complaint about Mexican vaccination certificates with the American embassy. The shipping board charged that the Mexican Bureau of Public Health did not allow select members of various crews on American ships to disembark because they did not present adequate proof of recent vaccination and they refused to get vaccinated.[140] Ambassador George Summerlin responded to the complaint within two months. The policy was legal; the Mexican Bureau of Public Health required adequate vaccination certificates to establish who needed revaccination.[141] If crewmembers wanted to disembark in Mexican ports, the decision to allow crew members in without adequate certification lay under the Mexican health officer's authority. The health officer also exercised the power to require revaccination as a condition of entry into a Mexican port. Both Carranza and Obregon adopted compulsory vaccination and increased medical discretion as part of their nation's imagined border rituals.[142] Vaccination moved from being the scar of a shared modernity to becoming another burden in the increasingly fraught passage across this American medical border.

We fought against poverty, high infant death rates,
disease, and hunger and misery. I would do the same
thing again.— Emma Tenayuca, in Zaragosa Vargas,
Labor Rights Are Civil Rights

SEVEN

Between Border Quarantine and the Texas-Mexico Border

Race, Citizenship, and National Identities, 1920–1942

Margarito Pomposo and Juan Morales earned their place on the 1932 Mexican Olympic team. Pomposo won the right to run the marathon, Morales the right to represent Mexico in the 10,000 meter event. For observers in Mexico, Pomposo's and Morales's visibly Indian looks and their position in these two premier long-distance events demonstrated how Mexico was turning Indian labor into an asset for the modern world. According to Don Gaspar, the sports editor for *Excelsior*, Mexico City's premier daily, Pomposo and Morales represented "our famous Indians, who run like the wind and are notorious for their ability to withstand long workdays."[1] For physical education advocate Colonel Lamberto Alvarez Gayou, Mexico had a comparative advantage in long-distance events, because "Mexico's prevalently indigenous background [made it] one of the most physically enduring countries in the world."[2] Their success in the Los Angeles Olympics would be a symbol of Mexico's Indian present and modern future.

The Mexican long-distance running team faced one hurdle before the final leg of their journey to Los Angeles: the El Paso border and the U.S. Public Health Service. When their train arrived there, Dr. Richard Allen, the USPHS medical inspector, refused to allow the team off the train into the United States without an inspection and demanded that the whole team undergo medical inspections like other Mexican workers coming into the United

States.[3] The team representative probably responded that the U.S. Congress had already extended "the privilege of free entry and usual customs courtesies and facilities accorded distinguished foreign visitors" to all Olympic teams, including the Mexican team.[4] Because the team needed to get to Los Angeles in time for the Olympics, the consul asked the trainer to encourage team members to accept the inspection and the potential revaccination.[5] Compelled to accept by Dr. Allen's refusal to allow a congressional edict to affect his sense of medical authority, the Olympic team consented to the heightened inspection and possible vaccination procedures at the bridge inspection station. Allen then decided to vaccinate Pomposo and Morales, the members of the team whom he thought did not have satisfactory evidence of vaccination.[6] The USPHS treated a group of the healthiest people in Mexico like any other group of laborers coming to the United States, like possible medical threats. The decision to vaccinate members of the Olympic team demonstrated the way USPHS authority at the border had come to mean the authority to decide which Mexican bodies to inspect, detain, vaccinate, certify, and deport. The public health service office had already wielded impressive authority over Mexican Americans and Mexican nationals in the United States. One year earlier, the USPHS turned its holding pen into "a large *corral* by the Customs House, where early in January more than two thousand *Repatriados* camped and starved, huddled together, waiting for a kind government to help provide them with transportation so they could move on."[7] Allen's decision to ignore American diplomatic and congressional edicts simply confirmed the central place of the USPHS in maintaining racial hierarchies at the Texas-Mexico border.

Events at the Olympics ended up bringing a critical focus on Dr. Allen's decision to take American laws into his own hands. Pomposo and Morales performed well, but not spectacularly. Juan Morales started the 10,000 meters slowly, but once he realized that the winning pace was faster than he expected, he applied a "superhuman effort" to pass a number of competitors, and arrived in eighth place. This disappointing performance put more pressure on Pomposo. The day before the marathon, the *Excelsior* claimed that "the well-known strength and endurance of the Mexican race would be put to the test."[8] This prediction seemed to bear out in the early half of the marathon. Pomposo kept at the head of the pack, even leading Argentinian Juan Zavala, the eventual winner, at the twenty-mile mark.[9] The combination of his training, the heat, and his early push robbed him of his position. Pomposo was the last finisher, ahead of all others unable to finish but still last among twelve.[10] After the marathon, the *Excelsior*'s lead editorial announced "Olympic disasters" and claimed that "even our famous Indians ... performed dismally."[11]

Despite the alleged Indian affinity for arduous labor, the *Excelsior* argued that Pomposo and Morales could not overcome athletes who had trained from their childhood, accumulated years of coaching experience, and endured special athletic diets.[12] Lamberto Alvarez Gayou, the official observer from the *Secretaria de Educación Publica*, found the coaching for Juan Morales and Margarito Pomposo to be near incompetent. Morales ran barefoot and therefore had no traction on the slick track surface.[13] He also had no sense of the caliber of the competition. Gayou reported that Pomposo ran the marathon almost as if he were trying to avoid the amateurish mistake Morales made in the middle-distance event; Gayou mentioned that Pomposo also had the second best time in the world for the twenty-six-mile race, just behind Juan Zavala. In fact, Pomposo led Zavala at mile 20. The decision to chase Zavala in the marathon, rather than focusing on placing, led to Pomposo's collapse. Gayou held the runner's limited experience competing at the highest international level responsible for their disappointing results.[14] The athlete's burden of representation—the national allegory for their Indian distance running skills—ultimately changed the meaning of Allen's vaccinations in El Paso.

Their athletic performance in the Olympics turned the medical inspection at the border into a national Mexican spectacle. Angry reporters in Mexico started claiming the American medical rite of passage was a direct attack on the physical integrity of the Olympic team. The *Universal Grafico* reported four weeks after the border crossing that "the protest made by the Mexicans on account of this procedure became actual mutiny, due to the unusually rigorous measures used against the athletes, as though it were intentionally sought to disable them by breaking down their physical powers."[15] However, physical violence was only one among many outrages that people like Pomposo and Morales faced in El Paso. Vaccination was the reason the Indian runners did not prevail. The editorial writer felt that "the abovementioned procedure caused much feeling among the treatment—considered almost barbarous by the interested parties—employed by American health authorities, for they inoculated the majority of [the Mexican athletes] against smallpox, tuberculosis, malaria, etc., the reactions to which brought on sickness and not a few ran high fevers for several days."[16] Moreover, the newspaper claimed that the vaccinations against smallpox, malaria, tuberculosis, and cholera, caused weakness and dehydration in Los Angeles, a problem given the heat and the long-distance events.[17] The Olympic vaccinations were a graphic example of the American fear of Mexicans.[18] In the subsequent State Department investigation, Allen confirmed that he inspected and vaccinated members of the Olympic team.[19] The Olympics brought the USPHS practice of unchallenged (Mexican) vaccination at the Texas-Mexico border back into public contention. The diplomatic identity of the Mexican Olympic athletes challenged the "Mexican narrative" Dr. Allen used in his everyday border quarantine practice. The political and social changes underfoot among the Mexican and American communities around the medical border hubs in El Paso, Eagle Pass, and Laredo began to catch USPHS personnel by surprise.

Typhus and the Border Quarantine, 1920–1945

The Olympic incident in the border quarantine highlights a historical paradox: USPHS quarantine routines were central to the experience of crossing the border during the interwar years, but the quarantine procedures grew increasingly irrelevant to national USPHS concerns after the First World War. One reason that USPHS procedures were not changing was that USPHS personnel was not changing. In 1938, Dr. Allen noted that, with the exception of the recently hired Dr. Para in Brownsville, all of the head USPHS doctors in the border towns were born in the decade after the American Civil War.[20] Their service started during the Mexican Revolution. The USPHS brought personnel in other American locations on clinical research, venereal disease intervention, TB containment, and sanitary engineering. After all the innovations leading up to the Mexican Revolution, the USPHS did not adopt any Texas border counties for new forms of medical outreach until the advent of the Second World War. Chicago, New York, and Tuskegee, Alabama, seemed more relevant to the leading edges of public health efforts through the New Deal.[21]

The relative lack of interest by USPHS personnel in the professional status of their colleagues at the border may have followed from the relative improvement of social, political, and thus health conditions in Mexico after the Revolution. There were no significant epidemics of typhus or smallpox at the border between the First and Second World Wars. Typhus cases in Revolutionary Mexico fell with the end of famine and open military conflict in northern Mexico. The last large outbreak of typhus in the United States was on the San Juan Indian Reservation in 1921, where the USPHS reported sixty-three cases and twenty-seven deaths. Dr. Charles Armstrong implicitly blamed the outbreak on the porous racial boundaries in the working-class Arizona borderlands when he linked typhus to "itinerant laborers [who] carried the infection from across the international border where typhus is endemic. Or some Indians, as occasionally happens, may have traveled beyond the reservation boundary, where the Indians are known to mingle with the lower elements of society."[22] Armstrong considered the presence of typhus a clear medical consequence of the ongoing transgression of American racial boundaries by Indians, Mexicans, and others in the American-Mexican borderlands. The absence of typhus in other places confirmed the righteousness of American public health efforts in other parts of the United States.

The reports of small outbreaks of typhus in Mexico after the Revolution distracted public health officers from the relatively short-lived presence of epidemic typhus in the United States. As Wilbur Sawyer pointed out in 1944, there were 229 cases of epidemic typhus in the United States over the previous twenty-five years.[23] According to Margaret Humphreys, there is still no adequate medical explanation for the absence of large typhus epidemics in the United States, given the strong commercial connections with Ireland, Germany, Poland, Mexico, and Russia, all countries with a history of typhus epidemics.[24] Despite general fears during the Gilded Age and the First World War, epidemic typhus never became endemic to the United States. The fears, not the (absent) epidemics, led to typhus disinfection at the Texas-Mexico border. The USPHS committed itself to inspection and disinfection routines to address the powerlessness of American medical treatments in the face of an actual case of typhus.

There were alternative typhus narratives. The USPHS reported on the domestic presence of typhus. Poor black and white communities across the southern United States suffered from murine typhus, and shepherds suffered from Marfa fever along the Rio Grande.[25] There were rickettsial diseases across the United States, not just central Mexico. Moreover, typhus inspection and disinfection commanded the lion's share of resources at the Rio Grande border stations. Norberto de la Garza, the inspector at the International Footbridge in Laredo, focused on "searching for live nits on all male persons; vaccination of those showing insufficient evidence of successful vaccination against smallpox; making primary inspection of those suspected with disease and taking temperatures when deemed necessary."[26] His coworker, attendant fumigator Jose I. Gutierrez, was also the mechanic and the bath inspector.

His duties included "supervising the bathing of male unclean persons, [and making] primary inspections for venereal and skin diseases in the bathrooms while the men [were] undressed."[27] Anna G'Sell was charged with inspecting women at the footbridge and supervising their bathing at the bathhouse, vaccinating whenever necessary. The Laredo office had two mounted guards (Anglos) to prevent illegal entries along the thirty-six miles separating Laredo and Palafox.[28] Assistant Surgeon Joe Sanders completed "line inspection: examination, bathing, delousing, vaccinating aliens, and fumigating their bedding and baggage" at the Del Rio crossing.[29] He inspected 10,692 people, he gave twenty-three of these people an intense examination, and he barred three people from entering the United States. As Del Rio's tiny medical rejection rate in 1940 demonstrated, typhus prevention seemed to serve a ritual purpose across the different USPHS border stations.

Each station inspector took a different approach to the importance of delousing Mexicans. Dr. Lumsden, the surgeon in charge of the New Orleans district, completed an inspection of the Rio Grande border stations and found drastic differences across El Paso, Eagle Pass, and Laredo, the three main railroad hubs into the United States. Between July and September 1934, the El Paso station estimated that inspectors reviewed 1,259,758 people crossing into the United States, of which they inspected 7,707 people (see table 7.1). The station gave 5,006 delousings to these people, approximately 65 percent of people inspected. In Eagle Pass, the station estimated there were 139,793 people subject to the USPHS medical gaze. The Eagle Pass inspectors chose 977 of these border-crossers for a more intensive inspection and gave 1,276 delousings to the people they inspected, approximately 150 percent of the people they inspected. Both efforts lay in a stunning contrast with the Laredo station, who counted 501,073 people crossing into downtown Laredo, who inspected 9,589 people, and who provided 441 delousings. The Laredo and Eagle Pass stations performed roughly the same percentage of vaccinations (29 percent and 36 percent), while the El Paso station vaccinated nearly 58 percent of all people they brought in for a more thorough medical inspection.[30] All three stations followed the surgeon general's USPHS border vaccination directive that "it is considered that one of the most important quarantine functions performed along the Mexican border is keeping a high degree of immunity against smallpox among the local population through the medium of vaccinating arriving persons as indicated."[31] Lumsden, the director of the New Orleans office, noted in his 1934 inspection of Eagle Pass, El Paso, and

Table 7.1. People inspected at El Paso, Eagle Pass, and Laredo stations, July–September 1934

	El Paso	Eagle Pass	Laredo
Medical Inspections			
Quarantine inspections. Total number of people tallied walking through USPHS station.	1,259,758	139,793	501,073
Aliens Inspected. People given a medical inspection by USPHS health officer.	7,707	977	9,589
Permanent Entry	92	33	222
Temporary Entry	1,623	944	5,833
Local-crossers	5,727	944	3,481
Warrant cases inspected before final deportation	265	0	55
Immigrants certified for permanent medical exclusion	715	10	91
Arriving Railroad Passengers			
Passengers from interior Mexico	22,585	3,225	26,406
Passengers deloused, bathed, and fumigated	5,006 (22.1%)	1,276 (39.5%)	441 (1.6%)
Passengers vaccinated	4,512 (19.9%)	289 (8.9%)	3,486 (13.2%)
Baggage disinfected	142	1,379	558

Source: L. Lumsden, "Recent Inspections of El Paso, Eagle Pass, and Laredo, TX," November 7, 1934, RG 59, USPHS, Decimal File 711.129, NACP.

Laredo that "so far as quarantinable diseases are concerned, health conditions on the Mexican side seem as good as those on the United States side of the river region."[32] Dr. Crawford at the Laredo station reflected this understanding, as he had his inspectors delouse barely 5 percent of bridge-users. On the other hand, Dr. Lea Hume at Eagle Pass station committed the administrative impossibility of delousing more people than they inspected. Local inspection station cultures overrode any general agreement regarding the threat of typhus at the Texas-Mexico border.

Local USPHS culture shaped the definition of "border-crosser" and the threat of disease. There were vast differences in the ways Dr. Allen in El Paso and Dr. Gorman in Laredo implemented their inspection standards (see table 7.2). The Laredo office recognized approximately 85,000 local border-crossers in 1937 and 1938.[33] The El Paso office only gave 8,873 to 13,271 local-crosser

Table 7.2. Medical inspection outcomes at El Paso, Eagle Pass, and Laredo stations, 1936, 1937, and 1938

	El Paso		Eagle Pass		Laredo	
	1936	1938	1936	1938	1937	1938
Permanent Entry Applicants	330	766	0	0	1,311	1,544
Inspected		766			1,311	1,544
Intensely Examined		766			1,311	1,544
Passed		766			1,241	1,486
					(94.6%)	(94.6)
Excluded		0			70 (5.3%)	70 (5.3)
Temporary Entry Applicants	12,624	667	11,806	7,472	2,304	1,593
Inspected		667	11,806	7,472	2,304	1,593
Intensely Examined			47	44	16	20
Passed		516	31	44	2,301	1,587
		(77.3%)			(99.8%)	(99.6%)
Excluded		151	16		3	6 (0.4%)
		(22.7%)			(0.2%)	
Local Crossers	13,271	8,873	5,987	6,121	85,554	85,529
Inspected	13,271	8,873	5,987	6,121	85,554	85,528
Intensely Examined				28	179	150
Passed		8,166	0	28	85,457	85,400
		(92%)			(99.8)	(99.8)
Excluded		707	1		97	129
		(8%)				
Border Patrol Detainees	2,230	3,060	0	0	138	254
Inspected	22,230	3,060			136	254
Intensely Examined					136	254
Passed	1,952	2,833			118	232
	(87.5%)	(92.5%)			(86.7%)	(91.3)
Excluded	278	227			18	22
	(12.5%)	(7.5%)			(13.2%)	(9.3%)
Total Medical Inspections	*28,125*	*13,366*	*17,793*	*13,593*	*89,540*	*88,687*

Source: Richard Allen, "Of Quarantine Operations at El Paso, Texas during Fiscal Year June 30, 1936," RG 59, USPHS General Classified Records, Subject Files 1850–95, El Paso Quarantine, NACP; Richard Allen, "Of Quarantine Operations at El Paso, Texas during Fiscal Year June 30, 1938," RG 59, USPHS Decimal Files, Subject File 1850–95, El Paso Quarantine, NACP; P. J. Gorman, "Narrative Report Covering Transactions at the U.S. Quarantine Station, Laredo, Texas, July 8, 1937," RG 90 USPHS General Classified Records, Subject File: 1850–15–Laredo Quarantine, NACP; P. J. Gorman, "Narrative Report Covering Transactions at the U.S. Quarantine Station, Laredo, Texas, July 7, 1937," RG 90 USPHS General Classified Records, Subject File: 1850–15–Laredo Quarantine, NACP; Lea Hume, "Annual Report Eagle Pass Quarantine Station," July 7, 1936, RG 90, USPHS, General Classified Records, 1936–1944, Subject File: 1850–1915, Eagle Pass Quarantine, NACP. Lea Hume, "Annual Report Eagle Pass Quarantine Station," July 7, 1938, RG 90, USPHS, General Classified Records, 1936–1944, Subject File: 1850–1915, Eagle Pass Quarantine, NACP, USPHS.

certificates, only around one-tenth as many as Laredo.[34] Maybe the demand for harvest labor was more obvious in the lower Rio Grande Valley; maybe Dr. King defined local more generously than Dr. Allen. This generosity extended to the intense medical examination. In Laredo, the officials seemed willing to allow applicants for temporary legal entry more medical leeway than El Paso officials, for Laredo allowed more than 99 percent of applicants to come into the United States. In El Paso, the officials found 22 percent of applicants to be medically ineligible for entry into the United States. The Department of Labor demanded the medical certification of Border Patrol detainees and both Laredo and El Paso inspectors were willing to certify that deportees face medical exclusion if they chose to return to the United States legally. The variety in numbers is even more astonishing, given that both surgeons in charge estimated somewhere between 12,000 and 20,000 bridge passengers a day. Moreover, the difference in medical inspection routines across the three stations made it very difficult to compare them directly. Perhaps the difference in political standing for Mexican communities in Laredo and El Paso may help explain why USPHS officers took different approaches to Mexican medical inspection in their stations.

The relatively weak political power of Mexican communities in El Paso shaped the prominence of the typhus baths and delousings in the USPHS stations. The availability of the baths emerged from the cordial relations each USPHS office established with city and county authorities in each city. In El Paso, USPHS officer Dr. McNeil reported that in March 1936, he deloused 47 to 78 city prisoners a week, and he counted the prisoners as local-crossers.[35] In 1936, El Paso also used the USPHS baths to disinfect people and goods in the city transient camp.[36] Two years later, Dr. Allen reported that it was still "customary, during the winter months, to bathe and delouse the city jail prisoners every Saturday morning."[37] El Paso medical inspectors told themselves that "all aliens presenting an unclean appearance were bathed and also deloused if indicated." Inspectors in El Paso openly acknowledged the random basis of delousing and inspection. As Dr. Allen told the USPHS, "With the number crossing the bridge daily probably exceeding an average of twelve-thousand persons, it is not possible for each individual to be inspected, but by assigning inspectors at what seems to be the best advantage, the crowds are observed as closely as possible and suspicious cases are held for further examination by a medical officer."[38] In 1940, Allen shared the news that, "as a routine, immigration prisoners are given a blood test for syphilis."[39] He reported that 98 of

343 detainees tested positive on the Wasserman test, a test result that barred people from legal entry into the United States for life.[40] The cordial relationships USPHS officers established with city authorities in racially segregated El Paso forced people crossing a bridge to ponder the risks of being treated like unclean, criminal, homeless, and potentially sexually diseased people. Although the risk was very small, given the large numbers of crossers, the inspectors were always there, looking for the unclean among the crowds of people coming into El Paso.

The USPHS baths in Eagle Pass provided an even closer reflection of the local racial order. P. J. Gorman, the senior USPHS surgeon in charge of the service's border quarantine, reported his shock at ways the baths became ingrained into everyday life in Eagle Pass. He disagreed with USPHS officer Dr. Miller that the station should continue to "bathe local people living in Piedras Negras coming to Eagle Pass to work in the onion and spinach fields." Gorman thought it perfectly appropriate that Inspector Cecilio Rodriguez run the baths, even though Dr. Miller thought "a white man should be in charge of fumigation," and Dr. Hume believed his Mexican American employee had "too many amigos to be trusted."[41] Gorman saw no need to waste federal resources bathing public school children in Eagle Pass, especially given that local Eagle Pass inspectors told him that during the school session "50 to 75 percent of fumigation efforts are dedicated to people living in Eagle Pass."[42] Dr. Gorman's criticism of the hierarchical racial mores in Eagle Pass and New Orleans reflected the structure of peace among Mexican, American, and Mexican American professional communities in Laredo. Moreover, the racial mores in the Eagle Pass USPHS station explained why they disinfected more people than the Laredo station, and bathed more locals than people crossing into Eagle Pass. The baths were a vivid reminder that the established political community in Eagle Pass believed that the emerging Mexican American community was still unclean and foreign and needed disinfection before participating in basic American institutions. The threat of typhus provided the ideological space, and the typhus baths provided the material space, that turned Mexican American children into alien citizens of the United States.

The daily presence of kerosene and vinegar baths, louse inspections, the fumigation of clothing, and the near-ritualized disinfection of working-class border-crossers were the most visible dimensions of the American medical border in the interwar years. Because of this visibility, USPHS surgeons complained about the general neglect the fumigation equipment faced across the different border stations. In 1936, Lea Hume reported that the Eagle Pass Station inspected 453,331 people, deloused 1,480 people, and vaccinated 1,468 people. He complained that, "as has been brought to the attention for several years, the fumigation plant is in a worn-out condition, and is terribly hot in the summer and cold in the winter."[43] Some USPHS officials almost ventured to argue that the routines were nearly pointless. Quarantine hours were limited, although traffic across the river never ceased. Lumsden found that "such quarantine operations are obviously inconsistent and might be designated by some health inspectors as actually quite absurd."[44] Richard Allen, the El Paso–based medical director in charge of border inspections reported that in Laredo in 1937, "the fumigation equipment at the old bridge station is in need of repair . . . but the installation of fumigation equipment should be held in abeyance."[45] Allen had already put some of the typhus equipment into abeyance in El Paso. The army requisitioned the USPHS women's bathhouse and turned it into an Army Prophylactic Station, where they provided three thousand treatments a month to soldiers and seventy-five treatments a month to civilians.[46] The typhus quarantine was crucial, but syphilis among soldiers in El Paso trumped the threat of Mexican typhus in the Second World War border.

The advent of war in Europe and East Asia revived fears of typhus in the United States. The State Department circulated a public health pamphlet to all its consulates and embassies in February 1941. Breckinridge Long, the head of the Visa Division, warned the embassy staff that refugees and asylum-seekers were a medical threat. He warned his staff, "Typhus is an ever present threat in time of war, or emergency mass movements of people, because some of the customary health measures are usually obtainable with difficulty to great numbers of people. Immunization is in the experimental stage so no inoculation can be recommended at present. It is thus important to avoid contact with persons or personal effects likely to be sources of contamination and observe other measures."[47] His general fear of typhus fit nicely within his well-documented disdain for Jewish asylum seekers.[48] The handbill reminded embassy staff of the same routines that the USPHS established at the Mexican border twenty-five years earlier. Wilbur Sawyer, the one-time director of the California Board of Health, reflected a little less dramatically on typhus. He told his audience that the current risk of typhus was "quite different from 1916. Mexico is free from civil war and there are no extensive typhus epidemics, though typhus is present . . . [but] there are labor shortages on account of the war, much movement of people, an acute housing shortage and overcrowding around war plants."[49] The USPHS was aware of the sporadic presence of typhus among rural villages in central Mexico. When the Bracero program got started in 1942, the USPHS decided to reimplement the practices it implemented twenty-five years earlier in El Paso and Laredo. They simply reestablished the "detention and delousing of laborers entering the state in temporary observation camps . . . [and] the systematic delousing of infested laborers at the Mexican border by the U.S. Public Health Service."[50] The USPHS mandated border disinfection even though its own inspectors reported that their efforts in "the stadium in Mexico City rendered . . . splendid examples of Mexican hardihood."[51] Both the American surgeon general and Mexican doctors feared what they considered the "disposition of the men to go home and pick up lice or to contact a venereal disease after their acceptance."[52] The USPHS acknowledged the relatively small presence of typhus in Mexico, and even supported the control of typhus fever through DDT field trials in Mexican villages and rural populations.[53] Still, the need to portray control, even to allay some American medical fears of rural Mexican men, led to the reimplementation of typhus quarantine inspection and disinfection procedures in the Bracero program.

The translation of typhus quarantine routines into the various Bracero quarantine stations produced a familiar resentment among people working with the program. As Pedro del Real Pérez remembered, "After you were contracted, things changed, but there was still an element of discrimination. The doctors who inspected you at the border gave you this feeling . . . they undressed you, to examine you, they messed with your hair, they put white powder on you, all that was discrimination, and it was not right."[54] Elías Espino remembered that, when he entered the Santa Fe Bridge Station, "the doctors started to put white powder on us. And we protested. And complained. And then they stopped putting the powder on those of us from Chihuahua."[55] Faye Terrazas recalled that "they were sprayed with some type of disinfectant . . . and that was not a good thing. They had the white powder in ears, their face, their clothes."[56] Alberto Magallón Jiménez found the experience difficult to narrate to Anaís Acosta, his interviewer. As he said, "You couldn't imagine what they did when they touched you; they were giving you a cleaning, forgive me, but they undressed you. Completely. And they sprayed you. With the same thing you use on your plants."[57] Retelling these stories allowed the enrollees in the Bracero program to recount the humiliating dimensions of the disinfections. The disinfection process staged their humiliation; retelling the inspection process allowed Braceros and others in the Bracero program to mark their differences from the perceived callousness and indifference of American, Mexican American, and Mexican medical authorities. The possibility of delousing marked an enduring memory of legal entry into the United States.

Smallpox, Citizenship, and the Border Quarantine, 1920–1945

The possibility of smallpox vaccination was also embedded in the image of legal passage across the Rio Grande. Both the United States and Mexico moved to make vaccination a requirement for entry into their countries. City and state governments across the United States moved to make vaccination a requirement for access to public benefits. These decisions were part of a longer medicalization of public institutions and social reforms in the United States and Mexico. As legislatures and city councils moved to pass mandatory school attendance laws for children, these mandatory requirements turned children into a readily available site to implement progressive medical reforms. Progressive activists pushed for compulsory vaccination laws as well as the active presence of school nurses as schools had a wider reach and provided a more enduring passage into citizenship than border inspection stations.[58]

Partly because of this wider reach, more parents objected to the ways schools usurped parental authority. Some reformers embraced the possibility of expanding established medical benefits through the schools to better the general public health of the nation, to transform the social body, or to temper the threat of immigrant children in the American public arena. Other reformers saw this as an unfortunate incursion of an authoritarian medical establishment, a form of technological rationality that boded ill for workers' autonomy. Texas came late to the establishment of vaccination and other compulsory public health measures in the schools, compared to states on the East Coast and West Coast.[59] The Texas-Mexico border provided a prominent example of compulsory vaccination, and border vaccination had a quiet—if weighty—place in the debate in El Paso and Texas over the expansion of public health to public schools.

United States citizenship emerged more prominently in the vaccination question in the aftermath of the Mexican Revolution. Once open military maneuvers were over in Mexico, El Paso County medical authorities began to focus on vaccination coverage in El Paso. Immigration authorities in Mexico had begun to require certificates of vaccination of U.S. citizens crossing into Mexico.[60] Public Health Service officers stationed in Naco, Ajo, and Nogales, Arizona, claimed that there was substantial vaccination coverage in their particular sections of Sonora and that any case of smallpox among ethnic Mexicans could be traced to contacts in northern Arizona and Colorado.[61] As Dr. Quinn wrote the USPHS from his vantage point in the coal-mining town of Monclova, Coahuila, "Keep your eye on the smallpox situation and if possible get the Texas people to see that those who were born and raised there are vaccinated against smallpox and you will avoid for your department a whole lot of annoyance and useless expense."[62] Medical authorities at the border were confident that places in the United States outside of immediate USPHS border jurisdiction were more likely to have smallpox outbreaks than the more industrialized mining and trading towns of northern Mexico.

State medical authorities in Arizona, Colorado, and Texas committed to new compulsory vaccination statutes to change this situation. In March 1923, El Paso health officer John Brown, in conjunction with USPHS officer Major Tarbett and the El Paso County Medical Association, proposed that "persons conducting an educational institution" file a list of the place and date of vaccination for all students, teachers, and employees with the El Paso Board of Health.[63] Physicians on contract with the Board of Education were required to provide certification that they had been vaccinated in the last seven years.[64] The city gave the Board of Health the power to require vaccination of students, teachers, and employees and the authority to fine people who refused to comply with the ordinance between $10 and $100 for each day they refused to comply.[65] This ordinance lay well within the growing state interest in children's welfare in public schools.[66] The key exception was the clause covering adult teachers, employees, and contractors with the El Paso school system.

El Paso was slowly becoming aware of the Mexican presence in its public schools, and debates over public health measures in public schools began to have a quiet Mexican underpinning. As A. Hughley, chief superintendent of the El Paso school system, reminded readers of the El Paso Times readers before the beginning of the 1923 school year: "El Paso's education and Americanization work must be paid for. This is why some people consider the school tax rate too high. The burden of educating the poor families of Mexican descent falls upon the more fortunate Americans. The school tax rate may be high but it is lower than in most Texas cities."[67] The city council entwined the fear of smallpox with the burden of Americanizing Mexican children in El Paso's (Mexican) public schools.

The question of compulsory vaccination and general medical scrutiny of city employees opened a public debate over the privileges of U.S. citizenship.[68] City health officer Brown, Dr. Hugh Crouse, and the El Paso County Medical Association mounted a campaign advocating the public benefits of compulsory vaccination. Antivaccination activists in El Paso responded with procedural questions, alternative medical claims, and a libertarian challenge to compulsory vaccination. The antivaccination partisans emphasized that American citizens exercised sole authority over their own and their dependents' bodies and that state-mandated vaccination threatened this American freedom. The USPHS station lay at the edges of this debate over the legal expansion of medical authority over American bodies.

The symbolic importance of children to the nation protected some Progressive era reforms from the national backlash against public policy interventions after the First World War. The USPHS opened and maintained syphilis treatment clinics across larger cities across the United States.[69] Congress passed the Sheppard-Towner Act, opening maternal and child health care centers across the United States.[70] After a number of small outbreaks of smallpox in Texas in 1922 and 1923, the Texas State Board of Health initiated a statewide push to establish uniform compulsory vaccination statutes across different municipalities. In Dallas, the City Health Department and the Texas State Board of Health faced widespread noncompliance among large numbers of parents and children in public schools.[71] The Texas State Board of Health requested that the USPHS help persuade Dallas residents of the importance of this statute. Here, federal medical authorities impressed on the Dallas municipal electorate that a compulsory vaccination campaign was commonsensical, medically practical, and constitutionally legitimate.[72] To accrue this form of cultural authority, compulsory vaccination had to be made "comprehensible and persuasive to socially powerful groups and the lay public."[73] Here lies the importance of El Paso and border vaccination policies to the larger vaccination question in Texas.

Many native-born American citizens did not share the Public Health Service's well-established faith in vaccination. A cursory review of USPHS smallpox files between 1918 and 1923 reveals public challenges and widespread noncompliance among public school supervisors with compulsory vaccination mandates in Arizona and Colorado.[74] In Denver, Dr. Leo Spears, a local chiropractor, placed advertisements in the *Denver Post* that he and potentially thousands of other Denver residents would "absolutely refuse vaccination" and risk jail for their beliefs.[75] In St. Louis police authorities arrested Dr. Edgar Anderson in Union Station for urging detraining passengers, likely African Americans leaving the South, to refuse the vaccination requirement for all people seeking residence in St. Louis.[76] Scholarship on antivaccination movements suggests that the combination of antimaterialist religious communities, alternative medical practitioners, a working-class distrust of elite politics, and libertarian challenges to government policies coalesced to mount legal challenges to compulsory vaccination. Legislative antivaccination challenges in Colorado, Oregon, and Arizona in the post–First World War American West fell within this framework.[77]

In El Paso, a coalition of Christian Scientists, libertarians, and labor advocates stood against the national regulatory trend and actively organized against USPHS surgeon Major Tarbett's proposed compulsory vaccination ordinance.[78] The coalition saw compulsory vaccination as a threat to their civil liberties, and they used the city council to limit the scope of compulsory vaccination.[79] When rumors "that all and sundry, and not merely the children who entered the public schools would be forthwith and immediately be vaccinated" became news, coalition members organized against this infringement of their autonomy and sense of liberty.[80] The Carpenters' Union joined members of the Liberty League, Christian Scientists, and local chiropractors to petition against the compulsory vaccination ordinance.[81] They demanded a stay of the ordinance in the council, claiming that no governmental body could pass a law to force adults and their minors to get vaccinated.[82] This argument followed both a libertarian and a Christian Science understanding of the Fourteenth Amendment. In the legal struggles between Christian Science practitioners and public health advocates, Mary Baker Eddy encouraged her followers to argue that "the Constitution of the United States does not provide that the *materia medica* shall make laws to regulate man's religion."[83] No state power, she argued, "can quench the vital heritage of freedom—man's right to adopt a religion, to employ a physician, to live or to die by the dictates of his own rational conscience and enlightened understanding."[84] This constitutional argument fell in line with a libertarian common sense that city laws should not intervene in the medical decisions made by family members and, therefore, the city should not apply the compulsory dimension of vaccination ordinance. R. W. Still summarized this argument when he told Dr. Crouse,

"Vaccination is undoubtedly a medical, or rather a surgical, procedure, but compulsory vaccination assuredly is an ethical, a fundamental American, even a political issue."[85] Vaccination was identical to other medical procedures: a private matter between patient and doctor, outside the regulatory purview of the state. Chiropractors required this distinction to defend their craft in Texas. Antilicensing medical activists and religious dissenters agreed with this argument. Both Rogers and Still also invoked a libertarian ideal: no state power should be able to intervene in the private domain of a citizen or a corporation.

The presence of the Carpenters' Union in the public opposition exposed the instability of this antivaccination coalition. The libertarian arguments mirrored the defense of individual contracts used by employers and the judicial system to overthrow the legality of labor unions. After 1919, unions in the American Federation of Labor (AFL) labored in an informal legal arena, where companies used court injunctions to challenge union restriction on the right of all laborers to enter into contracts with local employers.[86] In *Adkins v. Children's Hospital of New York*, the U.S. Supreme Court overturned the labor protections enshrined by *Muller v. Oregon* because, with the vote, women were entitled to the same workplace freedom as men.[87] Any attempt to legitimize the liberty of contract in public debate also threatened the legitimacy of local labor unions. Moreover, the Carpenters' Union was already suspect, because it had a large minority of Mexican American and Mexican members. The Carpenters' Union was one of at least eight AFL unions in El Paso that admitted Mexican Americans.[88] The El Paso AFL supported unions in crafts—like hod carriers, cigar workers, and laundry workers—dominated by Mexican immigrants. The *El Paso Herald* published a weekly bulletin detailing tasks, city contracts, and associated union members. This list made the ties between the Carpenters' Union and city hall maintenance, the construction and maintenance of public works, and patronage agreements a matter of near-public record.[89] There were at least ten Spanish surnames among the sixty members of this union.[90] During the relative labor shortage in the First World War, Samuel Gompers called on AFL locals in the Southwest to organize Mexican immigrant labor because "the internationalization of capital has made necessary the internationalization of the labor movement."[91] The presence of Mexican workers in this patronage-based trade union implied a close attention to the privileges of formal citizenship on the part of its members. This link was clearest for sanitation workers, whose employment depended on Ike Alderete as city sanitary commissioner.[92] Mexican American mobilization mattered intensely to both the Davis administration and the mayoral campaigns of Richard Dudley. The public challenge to the anti-Klan city council majority on the vaccination question complicated the Carpenters' Union's political situation. Even though participation in this debate might limit the negotiating position of local AFL craft unions, the Carpenters' Union opposed the compulsory vaccination ordinance.

The opposition to compulsory vaccination threatened the El Paso County Medical Association's monopoly over medical licensing. Dr. Crouse, the president of the El Paso County Medical Association, understood this public movement to be a threat to certified and licensed medical authority.[93] If policies written by a "panel of experts" and the USPHS could not find the approval of the El Paso City Council, there might be a difficult future for the advisory role for the El Paso County Medical Association. Both city and county medical authorities invoked the cultural authority of the USPHS to gain support for these ordinances among El Paso residents who considered Ciudad Juárez an open threat to the health of El Paso's white citizens.[94] The El Paso County Medical Association invited Tarbett to cooperate in the overhaul of the public health codes for El Paso.[95] Once they finished the code requiring vaccination for school attendance, Dr. John Brown mailed written samples of potentially controversial legislation to city health officers and nationally recognized medical authorities. The El Paso Herald published the responses to his questionnaire and pointed out the wide support among health officers across the United States for this progressive legislation.[96] The article banked on established medical authority, mentioning that even Victor Vaughan, "recognized as one of the greatest health authorities in the United States," supported compulsory vaccination.[97] City health officer Brown and Dr. Crouse presented the proposed code to the city council after a highly contentious mayoral and council election campaign.[98] Mayor Dudley built on this base of support and asked that the city council consider ratifying the uniform health code. Passage of this code would show his supporters that, in contrast with the furor over Klan influence in the school board, there was increased cooperation between local and federal authorities.[99]

The city council scheduled open meetings to discuss compulsory vaccination.[100] Seeking to shed some light on this discussion, the El Paso Herald arranged to meet with A. O. Scott, the president of the Texas State Medical Association, as he made his way to the summer resort in Cloudcroft, New Mexico. In this interview Scott reminded the journalist,

> The fact that there were few deaths of smallpox in the greatest assemblage of armed forces during the recent world war is the best proof of the value of vaccination. . . . Some years ago we vaccinated all the employees of the Gulf Coast and Santa Fe Railroad, about eight thousand in all, and there was not a single case in which a complication occurred. In Michigan University a few years ago a student who had never been vaccinated returning from his vacation developed smallpox and exposed several hundred students. There were 17 cases in all and in no instance did the disease appear in one who had been vaccinated.[101]

Scott and the reporter emphasized the benefits and the clear risks of indifference to vaccination in schools. This discursive field of statements linked vaccination to the national male experience of soldiering, elite public higher education, and corporate rail labor. Although people, courts, and voters in the United States moved to repudiate many of the public reforms of pre–First World War America, reformers and corporations still considered publicly mandated vaccination a rational use of public goods. The activists who objected to vaccination as a condition of employment had to challenge the power of this common sense.

Crouse requested that the city council debate the merits of compulsory vaccination inside the William Beaumont Army Medical Hospital in Fort Bliss. In this locale, the defenders of compulsory vaccination could find a specialist for every argument advanced by the different sectors of the opposition.[102] The city council adopted a debate format to understand the vaccination question, turning political differences into political entertainment.[103] Those who opposed compulsory vaccination emphasized that forcing parents to vaccinate their children or remove them from school challenged patriarchal privileges: "The liberty granted by a democratic form of government guaranteed to every individual the right to accept or reject anything that the individual might decide upon, either for himself or his minor child."[104] Moreover, "there had never been a law passed by Congress ordering vaccination."[105] On both points, the opponents of compulsory vaccination celebrated the authority (male) citizens had over their bodies and their children's bodies. They called the legal authority over vaccination claimed by the USPHS, the El Paso County Medical Association, and the city of El Paso potentially tyrannical.[106]

The debate collapsed distinctions between all people and all citizens. For citizens, the Supreme Court recognized the constitutionally granted requirement of consent for all surgical operations by sanctioning punishment for willful resistance to compulsory vaccination ordinances; *Jacobson v. Massachusetts* sanctioned fines and detention. Adult Mexican nationals—who were people but were not U.S. citizens—had not been able to legally challenge the practice of vaccinating every incoming Mexican arrival that could not provide acceptable proof of vaccination. Dr. John Tappan used the spectacle of inspection and vaccination in the USPHS station to demonstrate to the El Paso City Council that compulsory vaccination was, in Evelynn Hammonds's formulation, "comprehensible and persuasive to socially powerful groups and the lay public."[107] By challenging the assertion that Congress never passed a law that mandated vaccination, Tappan bypassed the question of immigrant medical consent. He claimed that no "emigrants" were exempt from having to demonstrate a successful vaccination or undergo a USPHS vaccination as a condition of entry into the United States.[108] Furthermore, dissident medical beliefs about vaccination, like conscientious objection and Christian Science, "counted for naught in securing entrance to this country."[109] Congress passed a law mandating vaccinations for aliens. This federal testimony refuted the opposition's statement that Congress had never passed an act compelling vaccination.[110] Tappan demonstrated his clear knowledge of the limits and powers available to the USPHS under *Jacobson v. Massachusetts* and *Schloendorff v. Society of New York Hospital*.[111] Ironically, despite the association of El Paso public schools with ethnic Mexican families, the debate revolved around medical regulation and the rights of American citizens. The legal status of vaccination and noncitizens was never at issue. The vaccination of Mexicans, whether they were Mexican or U.S. nationals, was part of the urban routine in El Paso and Ciudad Juárez. These vaccination events were so commonplace that when proposals to make vaccination compulsory for Anglo-American adults charged with the care and education of public school children were based on a law that Congress had never passed, antivaccination partisans did not call for a legal distinction between public school employees and Mexicans subjected to inspection and forcible vaccination.[112]

Courts started citing *Jacobson v. Massachusetts* to support public medical authority in the 1920s in courts hostile to the expansion of public authority. The decision in *Buck v. Bell* in 1927 sanctioned Virginia legislative acts that placed accredited doctors in a position of authority over wards of the state. As Justice Holmes stated in *Buck v. Bell*, "The principle that sustains compulsory vaccination is broad enough to cover cutting the fallopian tubes."[113] In the debates over compulsory vaccination in El Paso, the focus on border medical authority obscured the libertarian principle that a compulsory vaccination law could be "unreasonable, arbitrary, and oppressive, and, therefore, hostile to the inherent right of every freeman to care for his own body and health in such way as to him seems best."[114] In 1923, medical policies in the El Paso bridge station helped exclude these procedural protections—like the importance of actual and robust consent to medical authority—from public debate on the Texas-Mexico border. El Paso's medical and legal protections against (Mexican) smallpox sawed away at the due process that helped define American citizenship in the United States.

Questions regarding vaccination and the privileges of American citizenship kept emerging at the border. Like El Paso's antivaccination activists, American tourists and businesspeople wondered why vaccination at the Mexican border applied to them. In 1920, the United States Shipping Board complained about the required five-year certificate of vaccination for all ship employees disembarking in Tampico.[115] In 1921, Ambassador Summerlin reported that the Mexican Department of Public Health ordered revaccination among entries only when it was expedient.[116] In 1930, George Lucas wanted to know whether revaccination would apply to him upon his return to the United States after a business trip to Mexico.[117] In 1932, Consul Farnsworth reported that the Mexican Department of Public Health was requiring vaccination certificates because of a smallpox epidemic in El Paso.[118] In 1935, Burris Jackson, the president of the Lions Club, requested that the State Department ask the Mexican government to waive the vaccination requirement for Lions Club conventioneers on the way to Mexico City.[119] In 1939, Gordon Reid warned U.S. consuls that, because of smallpox outbreaks in Dallas and Houston, the Mexican Department of Public Health had started vaccinating tourists once they entered Mexico.[120] The 1949 smallpox epidemic in New York City led to the vaccination of American tourists coming back into El Paso, Laredo, and Eagle Pass.[121] As *La Prensa* reported,

Dr. Crawford of the USPHS stated that this requirement is not in place because of new smallpox cases in Mexico. Rather, he says that this is the fault of an individual who came back from Mexico through Laredo nearly fifteen months ago and once he got to New York city he came down with smallpox and died in that city, which began the vaccination of nearly three million people including President Truman, and this started vicious recriminations against Laredo for not vaccinating everyone who crossed the International bridge. Dr. Crawford added that the people who object most strongly to the vaccination are the very same American tourists, that Mexicans put up very little resistance. He explained that they are vaccinating everyone from the interior of Mexico and all of Laredo's residents and that everyone will receive a new vaccination certificate.[122]

Crawford resentfully emphasized the way national USPHS authorities forced the Mexican border to address national failures on the East Coast. Border authorities reported eight cases of smallpox in Edinburg, Texas. Hidalgo County embarked on a countywide vaccination campaign, but the USPHS did not institute emergency measures anywhere else on the border or the United States.[123] The USPHS assumed little overlap between Mexican and American communities in Texas border counties. The vaccination queries after 1923 began with the presence of business interests at the border and began to include individual businesspeople, humanitarian organizations, and, finally, the reappearance of the tourist trade on the eve of the Second World War. The few revaccination requirements came from Mexican and American fears that smallpox epidemics might follow tourists and businesspeople to their homes far away from the Rio Grande border. Smallpox inspection, vaccination, and certification made the political border real to visitors, immigrants, and investors.

The 1923 debate was the last open political challenge to vaccination policies at the Texas-Mexico border. As Mexican families settled in El Paso, in Laredo, and across South Texas, cities and counties started building schools to address the need to separate Mexican families from the children of the recently arrived midwestern and southern immigrants to South and West Texas. Sheriff Emilio Forto surmised, "Everything relative to the Mexican becomes repulsive to the American who has been fed on anti-germ theories for a lifetime."[124] The language of typhus disinfection and smallpox threat suffused Paul Taylor's Anglo informants in the 1920s and 1930s. A Nueces County farmer told Paul Taylor, "I don't believe in mixing. They are filthy and *lousy* [my emphasis], not all, but most of them."[125] In Dimmit, a school official stated, "There would be a revolution if Mexicans wanted to come to white schools. Sentiment is bitterly against it.... We have an exaggerated idea of their inferiority. Mexicans have head and body lice and do not want to bathe."[126] In the 1923 University of Texas–authored report on illiteracy in Texas, the authors claimed that "the American children and those of the Mexican children who are clean and high-minded do not like to go to school with the 'dirty greaser' type of children. It is not right that they should have to do so. There is but one choice in the matter of educating these poor children and that is to put the 'dirty' ones in separate schools till they learn how to clean up and become eligible to better society."[127] In Eagle Pass, school administrators physically brought schoolchildren to the baths in the immigration office. David Montejano has argued that the "dirtiness" reflected the class order that came with the establishment of capital-intensive commercial agriculture in South Texas, that Mexican families were stained by their association with manual labor, and that the germ theory provided a language to rationalize this class structure.

The language of dirtiness, lousiness, and germs helped shape class order in South Texas, border towns, and West Texas. Moreover, these medical encounters shaped the relationships connecting Mexicans and American public institutions. County officials and families implemented the medical language and the medical practices to establish ostensibly temporary separate educational facilities in the 1920s and 1930s. These "temporary" schools lasted through the 1960s. Hector Garcia noted that he was able to have some of these schools condemned as health hazards in the 1940s in Nueces County.[128] For George Isidore Sanchez, the conditions of the schools were a material example of the simultaneous anti-Mexican open hostility and eager exploitation of Mexican farmworkers in border counties. Still, for twenty-five years, the daily inspection for lice by medical inspectors at the border gave a federal imprimatur to the term "lousy Mexican." The border quarantine and the separate bathhouses and fumigation stations provided a concrete example of allegedly temporary but practically permanent segregated medical facilities used to protect "clean American" residents. The institutional dimension of the border health encounter provided a powerful and flexible frame for the relationship between Texas, the United States, and emerging Mexican communities.

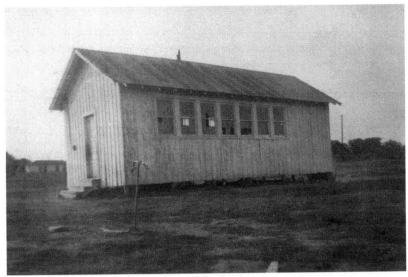

Figure 13. George Isidore Sánchez, "Sandia Elementary School Mexicans Only" (1946). Courtesy of the Nettie Lee Benson Latin American Collection, University of Texas Libraries, The University of Texas at Austin.

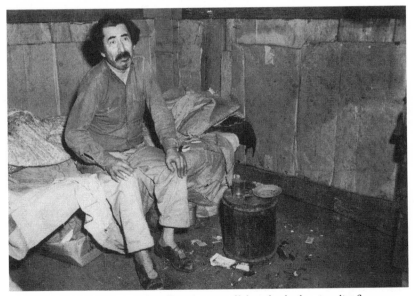

Figure 14. George Isidore Sánchez, "Inside view of labor shack, showing dirt floor, no washing facilities, and no cooking facilities whatsoever" (1934). Courtesy of the Nettie Lee Benson Latin American Collection, University of Texas Libraries, The University of Texas at Austin.

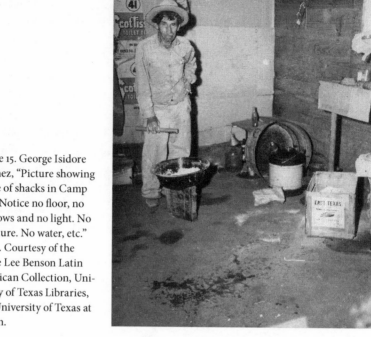

Figure 15. George Isidore Sánchez, "Picture showing inside of shacks in Camp No 1. Notice no floor, no windows and no light. No furniture. No water, etc." (1934). Courtesy of the Nettie Lee Benson Latin American Collection, University of Texas Libraries, The University of Texas at Austin.

Deaths, Citizenship, and the Border Health Paradigm, 1920–1940

The growth of Mexican communities in Texas after the Mexican Revolution overlapped with a federal emphasis in the United States on the registration of birth and death records. The federal push started in 1880, when the Census Bureau sought to get boards of health to store, record, and tally the information that came with local death certificates. John Shaw Billings, the director of the census, established a uniform survey and tabulation procedure and encouraged county health officials and census enumerators to follow the same format. In 1902, the Census Bureau became a permanent agency in the federal government. Wilbur Cressy, the chief statistician, used this authority to encourage national registration areas—places where states, counties, or cities registered more than 90 percent of deaths in the area—across the United States. Cressy argued that vital statistics registration was "an index to the degree and civilization and refinement possessed by each community," partly because the statistics would allow for more precise and more necessary plans for public health interventions. By 1915, every state had some version of vital statistics (birth and death registration) on the books, but only twenty-seven states met the 90 percent standard for the national registration area. With the cooperation of the twenty-seven states, the USPHS initiated its list of the top ten causes of death in the United States.[129] The growing numbers of states joining the national registration put pressure on other states to enter "the pale of civilization" and encouraged doctors and midwives to cooperate with the birth and death certificate recording efforts in each state. The vital statistics movement in the United States provided a national standard through which each state and registration area could evaluate its progress.

Vital statistics also exposed the hypervisibility of epidemic disease in a given registration area. In 1917, the USPHS inaugurated the typhus and small-pox quarantines along the Rio Grande border to prevent epidemics in urban areas across the United States. Two years later, the service published the top ten causes of death in the United States, and the top three were heart disease, pneumonia, and tuberculosis. Diarrhea was the most important cause of death for children under the age of two, though overall it ranked sixth, behind kidney failure and apoplexy.[130] Typhus, smallpox, and yellow fever did not make the top ten causes of death for the year. Moreover, the national survey was incomplete, as only twenty-seven states met the federal standard of a 90 percent registration rate for deaths within the state.[131] The illnesses that people in Texas suffered were invisible in these national surveys because Texas vital statistics did not conform to national registration area standards.

Conforming to the national standards was not simply a matter of enumerating deaths and births. Billings created a machine to eliminate variation and speed up the tabulation of each death certificate. Moreover, registrars had to ensure consistency across regions; for example, they had to ensure that doctors and registrars in New York and El Paso distinguished between typhus and typhoid in the same manner. This consistency in recording allowed for consistent statistical enumeration across the United States. The Census Bureau initiated ongoing registration workshops to ensure this consistency across the United States. Birth and death statistics also had to be consistent over time, to allow analysts to determine change over time in the prevalence of a given disease. These two analytical demands—consistency over time and uniformity across regions—meant a near-institutional hostility to regional variations and emerging differences in local demographics. Predictable and reliable analysis of national vital statistics required strict adherence to national vital statistics standards.

Texas had numerous problems conforming to these national standards. Not least among them was the long-term medical encounter with the growing presence of Mexican communities in Texas. The national tabulation for color and race gave two choices: "white" and "colored."[132] Most communities in Texas had three working racial categories: "white," "black," and "Mexican."[133] The San Antonio registrar included "Mexican" as a racial category in addition to national origin. The need for this separate inquiry became alarmingly evident to the Latino communities in San Antonio in 1926, when the registrar reported the deaths of seven Anglo infants and seventy-seven Mexican infants.[134] La Prensa told its readers that "on its own the number is nearly meaningless, but in context compared to the mortality rate for other nationalities, is enormously shocking."[135] Registrars across Texas knew that life conditions for Anglos, Mexicans, and African Americans were enormously different; others used racial language to explain or justify inequalities across diverse workplaces, social statuses, and living conditions.[136] Nationally, however, "Mexican" was an anomalous racial category, despite its temporary visibility as a racial category in the 1930 census.[137] In 1930 the El Paso County registrar, Alex Powell, started marking Mexican births in a separate racial category. After presenting information that there were seven thousand Mexican births and only two thousand (white) American, he joked to the La Prensa reporter that "if the Anglo Saxons do not hurry up, El Paso will be a completely Mexican Town."[138] County registrars across Texas must have had difficulties explaining this regional racial variation to the Census Bureau, let alone their local communities.

Registrars also faced the issue of community cooperation. The national registration area required that birth attendants certify each birth with the registrar. In Texas, parteras and midwives attended the majority of births in the poorer and more ethnic sections of the state. Each birth registration gave the attending partera a de facto official status. After the state of Texas required the registration of 90 percent of the births in 1933, the registrar suddenly became responsible for recognizing the legal status of each birth attendant. This hidden drama behind each number came to a head in El Paso in 1935. Felicitas Provencio went into the county courthouse to report the birth of her neighbor's child. Powell, the registrar, recognized Felicitas—a blue-eyed, healthy, energetic hundred-year-old midwife—and charged her with practicing midwifery without a license. Provencio defended her position with pride. She stated to a *Prensa* reporter who interviewed her while she was in jail "that she had never had anyone die on her, and that her track record and references speak more eloquently than a useless piece of paper."[139] Powell claimed that he and T. J. McCamant, El Paso's public health director, warned her not to deliver any more babies without a license. Provencio defiantly claimed that she "had been committing that crime for the past 60 years." She reflected that she had been doing this work when "this city was not even a miserable ranch. It was a river that crossed deserts and prairies, dotted with little adobe houses and even then I was a *partera* who helped my neighbors in their time of need."[140] Powell's desire to certify each birth in El Paso County by his standards brought him into hostile contact with local Mexican mores. The registrar's decision to arrest Felicitas Provencio clearly did not encourage cooperation among El Paso's long-standing Mexican communities.

The next city decision regarding vital statistics gave Mexican and Mexican American communities in El Paso a national stage. In 1935, the Census Bureau asked registrars across the nation to classify Mexicans as colored.[141] McCamant and Powell, after reviewing the registered death certificates in Mexican neighborhoods in El Paso, decided that the "colored" category was more appropriate than "white" to describe the life chances of Mexicans in El Paso. The high infant mortality and TB death rates made El Paso look like a very unhealthy city, although the majority of these deaths lay in the city's Mexican community.[142] McCamant and Powell told protesters that this decision would allow them to make two accurate lists, one white and one colored, and allow them to follow the patterns established in Dallas, Houston, Fort Worth, Austin, San Antonio, and Webb County.[143] McCamant and Powell must have been tone-deaf to Mexican community concerns, as all of these cities openly segregated and disenfranchised African Americans and, in the case of Dallas, Houston, Austin, and Fort Worth, openly discriminated against Mexican Americans.

Ten years earlier, the El Paso political community witnessed Dr. Lawrence Nixon's legally successful but politically fruitless campaign against the exclusion of African Americans from the white (Democratic) primary.[144] In 1934, Mexican Americans and the people who depended on the Mexican American vote successfully parried an attempt by some Democratic partisans to define Mexican Americans as nonwhite and therefore unable to vote in the "white primary."[145] Cleofas Calleros inelegantly stated the political dimensions of the decision by Powell, McCamant, and the Census Bureau: "Classifying Spanish-speaking people as colored is against Texas law. Mexicans as a race are red if they are Indians and white if they are not Indians."[146] This statement did little to clarify the status of Mexicans who were black. For Calleros and other Mexican Americans involved in Texas legal and political matters, the decision in the small Office of Vital Statistics seemed the beginning of the end of their career in Texas politics.

Participants in the debate used the terms to proclaim their disdain for African American communities in Texas. *El Continental* was shocked that Powell "was unaware of the insult he has given to every Mexican living inside or outside El Paso."[147] Gomez stated that "they would raise all necessary funds to bring the campaign to Washington to avoid being placed in the colored category."[148] Calleros called on everybody to donate and pay their poll tax, to defend the political privileges of official whiteness. Pablo Delgado pointed out, in a letter to the *Herald-Post*, that Senator Chavez's children would now be Negroes, and that the Mexicans should not be classified with African Americans because "the Negroes that are here are the offspring of the Negroes brought for slavery in this country."[149] The sense of difference and the tone of outrage was part of the campaign started in San Antonio, El Paso, and Los Angeles. In Los Angeles, La Union Latina demanded that Franklin Delano Roosevelt "recognize our equality under the law, and reject the odious agreement that classifies Mexicans as a colored race [*raza de color*, my translation]."[150] *La Prensa*, on the other hand, stated that "we Mexicans should not be offended when people refer to us as people of color. We know ethnic categories mean nothing to the spirit and the capacity of a people . . . and neither science nor religion can point out any markers that determine the superiority of one race over the other."[151] The terms of the debate over the applicability of the "colored" census category made it difficult not to express disdain for African Americans along with anger and dismay at this racial reclassification. The *La Prensa* editorial was a deft response to this awkward question.

The racial reclassification turned into a political opportunity. The Committee to Defend Mexicans and the Veterans of the Great War, or LULAC, came into being in El Paso through this challenge. In Mario Garcia's analysis, Powell and McCamant gave Mexican American public employees, lawyers, and minor political officials the opportunity to wage a national battle against American racial categories. The communities were engaged in a politics of citizenship. Their sheer presence must have shocked Powell and McCamant, as Calleros thanked "the hundreds of Mexicans who protested against the registrar's decision and who supported our suit against the Department of Public Health. There were people of Mexican citizenship, American citizenship and all walks of life. Splendid!"[152] He reminded people that the state of Texas determined that there were nearly fifty thousand American citizens of Mexican descent, but far less than ten thousand paid their poll tax to take advantage of their political rights. The discussion of the insult and the defense of Mexican access to the white (Democratic) primary exposed the racial underpinnings of electoral politics in Texas. The registrar's decision also brought the racially segmented life outcomes for Mexican Americans into clear view.

The legal battle overwhelmed the public health dimensions of the conflict with the Census Bureau and the Office of Vital Statistics. In El Paso, people challenged the indifference toward Mexican lives. Salvador Franco Urias, the editor of *El Continental*, emphasized that a broader public health mandate would make a bigger difference to mortality rates than reclassification:

Shuffling vital statistics is not the response we want to see for the infant mortality crisis in El Paso. The solution is a broader public health department, more able to take on the problem. El Paso has to lower this infant mortality rate by using a clearer and more intelligent analysis of the dangers threatening thousands of Mexican residents—dangers whose source is far outside the Mexican community. The solution is to eliminate filth in the neighborhoods and the dangerous sources of germs. El Paso has refused to do so for a long time. It is embarrassing that there should be clean and paved streets in south El Paso, because the mud and the floods are a disgrace for any self-styled progressive city.[153]

This argument did more than just challenge the El Paso Public Health Department's decision to place births and deaths for people of Mexican descent in the colored category. Franco Urias emphasized that the city of El Paso was responsible for the floods and the lack of clean water, sanitation, and paved streets that plagued South El Paso. The solution to the problem lay not with the Mexican community but with the racial hierarchy that allocated city funds for basic needs. The editorials objected to the way the new statistics might affect a claim on federal resources. Urias conceded that the changed statistics would allow two points: El Paso would look better to people outside El Paso, and the county health department would be responsible to the federal government only for the deaths in the white category. As he sarcastically put it: "Beautify these statistics and send them to Washington . . . a white list saying 'look at how well our public health department is doing.' And he would probably add, 'here is a list of people of color but this data has little importance. Don't really bother, since the list is pure Mexican and not worth taking into account.'"[154] Franco Urias and *El Continental*'s mocking humor revealed a public bitterness over the way Powell and McCamant papered over the health consequences of spatial segregation and political exclusion.

The previous year, Franco Urias wrote and *El Continental* published a short series of articles that linked infant mortality in El Paso to the economic consequences of the Great Depression.[155] They covered the news that El Paso had more deaths than any other city in the nation in the previous week, and announced that city health officer McCamant thought the children "died of hunger, and a lack of access to milk."[156] In a follow-up article, *El Continental* found it "terrifying that the majority of children dying in El Paso were Mexican."[157] The report in 1935 pointed out that 90 percent of the deaths were located in South El Paso. Franco Urias argued that, because infant mortality rates were so high in South El Paso, "the remedy should be given to sick, not the healthy; that prenatal clinics and dispensaries should be established . . . that they are tired of witnessing money being raised for those in need going to those with no need."[158] Material issues were paramount in their analysis. Franco Urias emphasized that the infant wing of the county hospital only had twelve beds, but that thirty families had already sought to have their children placed in the maternity ward.[159] In 1937, *El Continental* demanded a TB clinic in South El Paso, because that was where most of the cases occurred.[160] Deeply aware of the differential treatment accorded Mexicans and African Americans in El Paso and Texas, *El Continental* emphasized the absence of relevant health services in Mexican neighborhoods. Franco Urias did not want a public health practice that promised to create racial grounds for disenfranchisement in Texas. He was part of a border generation that demanded "sanitation, not discrimination."[161]

The Texas Office of Vital Statistics offered sanitation and discrimination. The director asked registrars in South Texas counties to tabulate Mexican (and then Latin American) deaths alongside white and black deaths. In his privately distributed report, *The Latin American Health Problem in Texas*, George Cox, the state's director of maternal and child health, argued that the segregated and unequal conditions facing *Latin Americans* meant higher death rates for them than for Anglos and African Americans. In 1938, the TB death rate for Latin Americans was 212.8 per 100,000; for African Americans, it was 98.2 per 100,000 and for whites it was 34.3 per 100,000 (see table 7.3). The Latin American rate was comparable to rates in segregated northern cities. In Baltimore, the average TB mortality rate was 66.5, the white TB mortality rate was 40.6, and the black TB rate was 175.5. The TB rate for Latin Americans in Texas was 25 percent higher than the national black TB rate, and almost double the rate than for African Americans in Texas.[162] The mean infant mortality rate for counties where more than 20 percent of the population was Latin American averaged between 114 and 118 deaths per 100,000 (see table 7.4). For counties where Latin Americans were a minority, the death rate hovered around 54 per 100,000, 50 percent lower than in counties with a higher percentage of Mexicans. Cox used these sharp differentials to ask that South Texas counties be excised from the general count to make for a more accurate (and positive) portrayal of health in Texas. He explained that the death rates rose in counties where the percentage of Latin Americans approximated 25 percent, because "in the counties where Anglo-Americans predominate, zoning and high land values have produced aggregation and unhygienic surroundings which can be described by no other term than slum. These small-town slums, familiar throughout South Texas, are ideal soil for TB and all other contagious diseases."[163] Cox clearly connected the health outcomes to the class structure in South Texas, but instead of demanding higher wages or housing conditions, Cox requested Spanish-speaking health workers to help Mexicans in rural Texas seal their milk and build fly-proof cribs. He concluded, "Results in selected areas have shown that striking improvements in infant mortalities can be achieved without elevating the general level of environmental sanitation up to the present Anglo American standards. Milk and water can be kept sterile without refrigeration and at negligible cost. If open privies cannot be eliminated and houses cannot be screened, at least the baby can be kept in a fly-proof crib."[164] Cox acknowledged the financial expense and political burden necessary to bring paved streets, running water, city sewage, and electricity to Mexican communities across the state. He simply hoped health education in Spanish would be enough to address the problem.

The root of "the Latin American health problem in Texas," according to Cox, was the presence of Latin Americans.[165] He granted that social and economic factors might explain why "the more Latin Americans, the more infant deaths per one thousand live births." Despite the open political campaigning

Table 7.3. Tuberculosis deaths per 100,000 population, organized by the percentage of Latin American population in Texas counties, and then by population grouping [Latin American, African American, Anglo American], 1938.

Counties by Percentage of Latin American Population	Number of Latin American Deaths	Latin American Death Rates (per 100,000 Population)	Number of Negro Deaths	Negro Death Rates (per 100,000 Population)	Number of Anglo-American Deaths	Anglo-American Death Rates (per 100,000 Population)
Urban	720	228	35	120	252	74
70%	49	148	0	0	4	37
60–70%	44	158	0	0	3	21
50–60%	161	175	4	181	22	28
40–50%	139	210	4	96	9	12
30–40%	140	229	12	88	21	21
20–30%	58	234	15	105	5	8
Total	1,311	212.8	70	109.1	296	42.6
Less than 20%	275	212.8	843	97.3	1,334	33.1
All of Texas	1,586	212.8	913	98.2	1,630	34.3

Source: George Cox, *The Latin American Health Problem in Texas* (Austin: Texas State Department of Health, Division of Maternal and Child Health, 1940), 6–7. Nettie Lee Benson Rare Books and Manuscripts, University of Texas at Austin.

by the Spanish-language press and various political organizations against the decisions made in his own office, Cox believed that Latin Americans did not participate in modern culture in Texas. As he reminded the policy makers who read his report, "Most of this group have not had the advantage of the schools, the press, and the radio in dispelling ignorance. They have almost no concept of medicine and they prize the bottle of medicine which results from a medical visit far above the advice given."[166] For Cox, the health problem lay in the combination of an unequal class and public health structure with a pill-centered population. The solution was public health education, not sanitation.

Public health authorities in Texas placed the public health issues in the border counties squarely within the Mexican community. They also knew the USPHS was devoting resources to preventing illnesses that were nearly absent in northern Mexico, West Texas, and South Texas. Texas health officer John Brown encouraged an American Public Health Association (APHA) commission to focus on the Texas borderlands. In 1934, the Public Health Engineering caucus consulted with Brown; Dr. K. E. Miller of the USPHS; and

Table 7.4. Death rates for infants and from diarrhea and tuberculosis in Texas counties, by concentration of Latin Americans in county population. Select mortality rates for counties with percentage of Latin American population higher than 10 percent. Infant deaths per 1,000 live births, diarrhea deaths under 2 per 100,000 population, and tuberculosis deaths per 100,000 population. The counties are organized by the resident percentage of Latin Americans, per 1930 census.

Concentration of Latin Americans by Percentage in County	Mean Population	Infant Death Rates	Diarrhea Death Rates	Tuberculosis Death Rates
Urban Group	701,054	113.1	92.5	150.1
70–80%	44,251	118.7	100.1	126.6
60–70%	42,495	134.9	85.4	107.3
50–60%	173,318	132.1	129.4	102.1
40–50%	137,221	102.9	74.5	94.7
30–40%	175,720	102.4	50.0	96.0
20–30%	99,256	82.6	85.8	72.4
Totals for Counties with Percentages above 20%	1,373,555	112.7	85.1	124.0
Totals for Counties with Percentages below 20%	4,976,335	54.9	10.8	51.4
Totals	6,349,630	70.0	26.9	67.1

Source: George Cox, *The Latin American Health Problem in Texas* (Austin: Texas State Department of Health, Division of Maternal and Child Health, 1940), 3–4. Nettie Lee Benson Rare Books and Manuscripts, University of Texas at Austin.

Dr. Miguel Bustamante, a specialist in communicable diseases and the head of public health in Mexico. Dr. Victor Ehlers, the head of the Public Health Engineering caucus, reported,

> The Federal Quarantine Service is only a fragmentary safeguard of health between the two countries. Federal quarantine is concerned only with plague, cholera, old world typhus, yellow fever, leprosy, trachoma and smallpox. The only disease among these that is of any great practical importance at this time is smallpox. The federal quarantine is not charged with, and therefore, can have no control over most of the present day health and sanitary problems common to the border. . . . Neither the river nor the imaginary line crossing from El Paso to the Pacific Coast offers any bar to the passage of typhus rats back and forth across the boundary line. The same applies to mosquitoes infected with malaria and yellow fever, and typhoid carrying flies. In similar manner, though carriers and active

cases, diphtheria, scarlet fever, and other diseases under the present circumstances enjoy an unobstructed passage between the citizens of both
countries.[167]

Ehlers equated flies to people, emphasizing that the full spectrum of
disease-carriers enjoyed relatively free movement across "the imaginary line."
Ehlers seemingly implied that free passage of mice and mosquitoes was as
problematic as the presence of disease on both sides of the border. His discussion of mosquitoes, malaria, and yellow fever acknowledged that both sides
of the river were part of the same environment. Because the political border
made this public health landscape unique, Ehlers recommended a political
solution to an environmental and sanitary problem: he advocated the creation of an international boundary health commission. The commission itself
would consist of representatives from the USPHS, the Federal Department of
Health, and the border states and territories in both nations. The commission
would establish basic public health guidelines for the region and establish a
way to address disputes in public health matters. The APHA recommended a
policy shift away from borders and quarantines toward a more amorphous
and flexible borderlands approach to public health issues.

The Texas legislature enthusiastically endorsed the idea of an international border health commission. Their recommendations transformed the
commission into an "International Public Health District along the international boundary between the two countries for a width of not more than
one county's depth." Using the rhetoric that "communicable and infectious
diseases do not recognize any man-made boundary," the legislators sought
to include malaria, tuberculosis, and the full spectrum of childhood communicable diseases in the mandate for the International Public Health District.[168] United States Senator Morris Sheppard and Representative Thomas
Connally demanded a response from the State Department and the USPHS.[169]
The Texas Commission report recommended federal-level funding and a
treaty-level agreement between the governing bodies of the countries. Texas,
the USPHS, and the surgeon general of Mexico would have permanent seats
on the international district board, while New Mexico, Arizona, and California would rotate one representative, and Tamaulipas, Nuevo León, Coahuila,
Chihuahua, Sonora, and Baja California would rotate two board members.
The district would set general policies for the political units adjoining the

international border, and El Paso would be the headquarters for this massive public health district.[170] The Texas recommendations shifted responsibility for TB and childhood illness to a board funded by money outside Texas. If Congress and the Mexican government had approved this International Public Health District, Texas could have shifted responsibility for the growing political scandal over the obvious racial inequality in infant mortality and tuberculosis mortality rates to an international authority, effectively "Latin Americanizing" the medical impact of Texas racial politics.

Cordell Hull, FDR's secretary of state, informed Senator Sheppard that the proposal was "neither desirable or practicable."[171] He did not recommend ceding or sharing political authority over difficult public health matters in Texas to an international agency. Rather, he argued that the agreements that created the Pan American Sanitary Bureau already provided tools that willing state governments could use to cooperate with their political authorities on the other side of the border. The State Department emphatically refused the possibility of federalizing or internationalizing TB or childhood illness. The international border (and the Fourteenth Amendment) meant that local authorities were still responsible for public policies that shaped public health outcomes for people living in their jurisdiction.

The Second World War brought this loose cooperative Pan American approach to fruition. As thousands of troops made their way to the bases in Fort Huachuca and El Paso, health authorities in these cities called for the creation of a forum where they could work together to address the challenge of soldiers and sailors seeking a break from their military routines. Allen openly worried about this contact. He reported that the troops in Fort Huachuca, a segregated black training base, "frequently visit the towns opposite Naco and Nogales. They cross the border in their army uniforms." He guessed that the uniforms were the reason why "there has been an increase in venereal cases at the Fort."[172] In El Paso, he worried about white troops from Fort Bliss crossing into Ciudad Juárez "in civilian clothes. Numerous uniformed men of the armed forces en route through El Paso cross the International Bridge into Juarez." He considered these journeys into Mexico "real moral hazards" and warned that they "might lead to international complications due to friction between our men and the local inhabitants." He recommended that the surgeon general "disapprove of these crossings" and post military police at the bridge to enforce this ruling. Rather than implementing this drastic solution, the USPHS established the U.S. Mexico Border Health Organization Field Office with Mexico.[173] In El Paso and Laredo, the USPHS commandeered the typhus bathhouse and turned it into a very public VD treatment center.[174] The traffic in American men across the border into Mexico officially broke the American border quarantine model. This new border health model identified flexible ways to provide medical treatment and prevention that fit the desires and routines of American soldiers on their way to Los Angeles and San Diego. Other border communities' desire for equal schools, paved streets, sewage services, better jobs, open politics, and accessible treatment awaited their national politics and their border health projects.

Conclusion

This chapter explored the erosion of the connections that people on the border made between medical resistance and medical modernity in relation to epidemic diseases. Smallpox, yellow fever, and typhus appeared less frequently and had moderate consequences. The symbolic importance of these diseases receded from popular memory. Consequently, border-based USPHS officers started facing challenges to their relevance to the general health of people and communities at the border. The 1920s and 1930s inaugurated the era of separate Mexican schools in Texas, and most counties justified the unequal facilities through the medical danger "lousy" and "dirty" "Mexican" (American) children posed to American children. In Eagle Pass, the USPHS and the school district forced schoolchildren to go through the same experience as "dirty," "lousy" immigrants, and to do this every week of the school year. In El Paso, the city used the USPHS disinfection facilities to bathe prisoners and transients and to treat VD. This city-federal cooperation literally criminalized and sexualized working-class Mexican nationals through direct association.

Community-based medical authorities used political means to challenge the health effects of segregation. El Paso was the center of two such challenges: In 1925 Dr. Lawrence Nixon initiated the two-decade long NAACP campaign against the white primary in Texas; and in 1936 Juan Carlos Machuca and other medical professionals who were members of LULAC successfully beat back the attempt by the El Paso City-County Health Unit to reclassify and place Mexican and Mexican American residents in the "colored" category for vital statistics. By 1942, Dr. Hector Garcia envisioned a way for organized citizenship claims to transform the health conditions of Mexican

American communities.[175] In the process, the presence of TB, childhood mortality, and malnutrition came to stand in for the absence of good jobs, safe workplaces, decent housing, accessible childcare, education, and clean water. Public health reformers had shifted their attention away from typhus and the attendant mobility of communicable disease, but USPHS practice at the border focused on inspecting and certifying the fitness of laboring bodies crossing into the United States. American state medical borders challenged Mexican American and Mexican claims on American medical resources.

EPILOGUE

Moving between the Border Quarantine and the Texas-Mexico Borderlands

Public health professionals sought to explain the differences they identified in the Texas-Mexico borderlands in medical terms. When public health professionals connected medical issues to the nation, they helped make the nation real to their audiences in the United States, in Mexico, and at the border. The border—or, more precisely, the Rio Grande borderlands—provided an important place to make nations meaningful. Before 1848, the towns and ranches along the greater Rio Grande borderlands experienced the movement of Spanish, Mexican, Comanche, Cherokee, Texan, American, Confederate, French, and American borders. In this period of shifting borders and open imperial rivalries, forts, towns, cities, and states built their public health measures relatively independently from one another. The attitudes built around these measures provided the stage for medical encounters after 1848.

Men and women in the Texas borderlands sought ways to avoid the sudden devastation of epidemics and the less visible effects of everyday illness and death. The sanitary emphasis on the interaction between individual bodies and the local plants, bad airs, sanitation, sewerage, and local soil conditions made disease prevention a question of local civil engineering, sanitation, and disease. The royal importation of inoculation and smallpox vaccine to Texas in 1808 created the need for an additional medical link between Texas and urban centers like Mexico City and New Orleans. In fragmented and uneven ways, residents in northern Mexican towns like San Antonio and Monterrey pulled their children together and sought ways to protect their communities from epidemics of smallpox, cholera, and pneumonia. When towns were under military authority, town residents begged military authorities to find resources to address their medical crisis. When towns elected mayors and town councils, San Antonio and Laredo created boards of health, volunteer committees, petitioned to make vaccinations available to all residents and found ways to make illness everybody's responsibility. In Bexar (San Antonio), the participatory aspect of this political culture led to a decision that, because of limited medical resources, inoculation was just as legitimate a protection as smallpox vaccination. There was less agreement on the prevention measures for yellow fever, typhomalarial diseases, and influenza. People fled the particular conditions that brought on these illnesses and sought refuge in neighboring towns. This movement of people meant local initiatives had federal dimensions. Mexico and the state of Texas provided tax abatements for any funds spent treating and hosting the refugees from fevered places. In conjunction with the periodical need for new vaccine lymph, vibrant political and commercial relationships across American, Mexican, and Comanche domains were as important to the general public health as more available water, cleaner streets, and the existence of sewers.

Still, the majority of the public health initiatives were local in nature. In 1848, when the Treaty of Guadalupe Hidalgo officially joined Mexico and the United States, the Republic of Mexico and the United States of America did not have a public health corps charged with nation's health.[1] The American occupation forces in Matamoros felt the weight of the hot, humid, near tropic chaparral of the lower Rio Grande Valley. Samuel Curtis, the civilian director of the occupation in Matamoros, repeatedly mentioned that his soldiers seemed "rather languid and sallow in their complexion. I can see that the climate and exposure have made an impression on us."[2] Early American public health officers often found the weather, land, flora, fauna, and people at the Rio Grande border far too powerful and unpredictable to control. After suffering and witnessing a couple of months of fevers and intestinal distresses in Matamoros, Curtis felt that "the malignant diseases of this climate appear unconquerable."[3] Curtis and his military contemporaries believed that tropical conditions in Texas and Mexico threatened American bodies. This understanding made public health measures like fresh fruit, clean privies, and good sewers seem too small for the task. Even fifteen years later, during the Civil War, the U.S. Army was still unwilling to devote the resources to guarantee the health, or even the survival, of black or white troops at the mouth of the Rio Grande.[4] The army and volunteers did not have the desire to make the landscape or the people around the Rio Grande Valley healthier for the American occupiers. The medical situations along the Rio Grande lay outside the nation's military interests.

The social and industrial revolutions that followed the Civil War in the United States demonstrated that the nation-state and an active citizenry could begin to transform entrenched economic relationships in the South and the West.[5] In Mexico, the victory of liberal forces over Emperor Maximilian and his French and Mexican allies gave the victors the sense that they too could find ways to bring their nation ahead. Drawing from this new sense of nationhood, doctors, civil engineers, and social scientists convened and created the American Medical Association, the Asociación Médica Mexicana, and the American Public Health Association. Railroad workers, at great cost to themselves and great profit to their employers, had made travel across the United States possible in the winter, spring, and summer.[6] The projected advent of railroads across the Texas border changed the ways Mexican and American officials imagined the borders of their nation. These new visions, in turn, transformed the meaning of disease in the Rio Grande borderlands.

The 1878 Mississippi Valley yellow fever epidemic killed thousands of people, paralyzed the country, and challenged an early faith that Reconstruction measures had conquered yellow fever. The U.S. Congress established the National Board of Health (NBH), which sought ways to predict and contain the economic and human devastation of similar epidemics. When the NBH sent Dr. John Pope south and west of Houston to survey West Texas (South Texas and the lower Rio Grande Valley), he traveled with the confidence that political reforms and sanitary reforms went hand in hand. He had faith that a city could pass laws to transform the water, sewage, and housing stock available to the working majority in a given town. Pope feared the possible impact of another yellow fever epidemic. In the process of his conversations with local doctors, he realized that Mexicans suffered as much as Americans, if not more, from malaria and therefore yellow fever. Pope only advocated public health reforms to ensure that Texas-Mexican workers' queer (neighborly) attitudes toward illness and isolation would not jeopardize American consumers, but these were far-reaching reforms. He championed rent control, minimum housing standards inside and outside city jurisdiction, free municipal water, and accessible vaccination stock.[7] These suggestions directly challenged the politics behind the municipal infrastructure that diminished the quality of Mexican lives in the South Texas borderlands.[8] Pope minimized the medical challenge to the status quo by recommending that the local "best men" take the initiative to implement these public health reforms in each town.

The Mexican-Texas epidemic demonstrated that democratically led public health initiatives troubled the United States Marine Hospital Service (USMHS) and the state of Texas. The USMHS hired King Ranch cowboys to man a mounted quarantine guard along the Texas-Mexican railroad, draw a line across Texas, and contain the spread of yellow fever north from Brownsville and east from the Mexican Gulf Coast. Inside the quarantine, USMHS Surgeon Murray worked with local Mexican doctors, Anglo physicians, and Tejana nurses to create a free dispensary and a series of house calls to treat yellow fever and create confidence in the USMHS. Brownsville residents cooperated with this USMHS effort, modeling the benefits of including bilingual Tejana and Tejano staff in any national health initiative at the Mexico border. The mounted mobile quarantine on the Texas-Mexican railroad and the quarantine on the Rio Grande overshadowed and ultimately negated a successful federal innovation in the delivery of health services. The USMHS quarantine led to the drastic collapse of the local economy. This led to near starvation conditions in Brownsville. Once cases of yellow fever began to decrease, Brownsville authorities demanded access to the outside world and convened to a vote to make the USMHS quarantine illegal. Both the United States and the state of Texas publicly ignored this vote. Though still medically controversial, the USMHS insisted that the absence of yellow fever north of Corpus Christi and Laredo was proof that mounted quarantine guards could contain yellow fever and Mexican political disorder.[9] Therefore, the expansion of medical services and the removal of local conditions that fostered yellow fever in the United States were both politically unnecessary and fiscally inexpedient. The Mexican-Texas quarantine modeled two different approaches to an epidemic on the border, but the USMHS used the Mexican-Texas yellow fever quarantine guard to demonstrate the irrelevance of the NBH's emphasis on sanitary reforms. Congress subsequently defunded the NBH.

The success of the mounted quarantine around South Texas made quarantine a key element in subsequent state-building efforts. The debates over quarantine in Mexico City demonstrated the difficulty medical authorities had separating Mexican from American medical matters. Public health officials wanted political authority over quarantine but also wanted the other political bodies to acknowledge their responsibility for the presence of typhus, cholera, yellow fever, or smallpox. The debate over quarantine and the social origins of these communicable diseases brought two different transnational frameworks into view. State public health authorities in Texas, Mexico, and the United States emphasized a cognitive medical transnationalism, reading the movement of goods and people across borders to determine whether a given illness might cross state lines. [10] State building by public health authorities also followed a transnationalism grounded in social practices. They tracked the relationships of people affected by smallpox, cholera, or yellow fever to places outside their national territory. The border quarantines in the 1890s gave public health authorities the place and the resources to connect a cognitive medical transnationalism to the practice of a socially based medical transnationalism. When American and Texan authorities imagined that smallpox or yellow fever might appear in Texas, they envisioned that Mexicans were bringing this disease from Mexico, or that Mexicans of all nationalities were the reservoir for this disease in the United States. When Americans and Texan state officials grappled with smallpox or yellow fever and saw a Mexican face in the midst of the epidemic, this supposedly foreign presence allowed them to place their efforts to contain the germ-borne diseases within a transnational field, one without political implications for domestic public health policies. The national medical authorities in Mexico found this conflation of race and disease troubling in practice and intellectually appalling. Despite their distaste for the American politics of race and quarantine, Mexican medical authorities also claimed that quarantine stations helped model disease surveillance, interdiction, and sanitary measures for the general public. Even within the political spectacle in Mexico City in 1892, the participants at the APHA/Asociacion Medica Mexicana meeting agreed that quarantines provided health officers a place and a space to project medical progress.

The USMHS turned Eagle Pass into a demonstration site for medical progress. The detention of four hundred black American colonists for smallpox in Torreon, Coahuila, transformed a transnational labor dispute into an international medical problem. Their detention gave the USMHS access to a large group of unvaccinated people who had been exposed to smallpox. Surgeon General Walter Wyman asked two public health officers, J. J. Kinyoun and Milton Rosenau, to transfer the results of the latest medical thinking on smallpox antitoxin research into the politically vulnerable and racially visible bodies of noncitizens and American nationals in Mexico. The usmhs crossed borders to rescue American citizens in Mexico from smallpox and built borders around the same citizens in Eagle Pass, Texas, to keep people in Camp Jenner. The usmhs operated in a transnational social field. The colonists were American citizens in Mexico and American noncitizens in the United States. The transnational social field of the usmhs enabled medical exploitation and medical treatment to coexist at the Eagle Pass border.[11] The tragedy of the colonists in Mexico overwhelmed the institutional memory of a failed field trial of smallpox antitoxin serum as well the wider organizing effort to help colonists come back to the United States.[12] The mobility of usmhs officers Rosenau and George Magruder contributed to the general invisibility of Camp Jenner in institutional histories of the usphs.

American authorities in Eagle Pass were confident that smallpox would eventually disappear from Camp Jenner, as would their medical obligation to the detainees in Camp Jenner. The 1899 Laredo Smallpox Riot and the Laredo yellow fever quarantine in 1903 provide examples of a fleeting intervention in the lives of border residents. It may seem a little odd to frame the interventions in this manner, but the usmhs practiced a nearly fugitive medical transnationalism in Laredo. In 1899 William F. Blunt, Texas's state health officer, called in the Tenth Cavalry and the Texas Rangers because he deemed the assembly in Zacate Creek defending the rights of families with smallpox to be a military threat to the United States. In 1903, local memories of this violence haunted the usmhs demand for fuller cooperation with all yellow fever treatment and detention efforts. The occasionally violent insistence that medical authorities recognize the national claims of local residents brought identity and citizenship to bear on the actions of public health services at the border. As it was, the mobile nature of federal responses to epidemics across the United States and their possessions forestalled richer public health work within the poorer neighborhoods at the border. In Eagle Pass and Laredo, the transnational mobility of usmhs officers weakened the state-citizen relationship as it increased the public health service's profile across the United States. The service's new incarnation as the United States Public Health and Marine Hospital Service (usphmhs) afforded additional inspectors and border stations in Brownsville, Laredo, Eagle Pass, and El Paso, Texas.

Inspectors in these new border quarantine stations focused on the movement of disease across borders. The bridge station vantage point gave U.S. medical authorities a medical lens and a privileged view of the traffic across the Rio Grande. The responsibilities of this view prevented an examination of the situations and disease environments beyond the bridge in which people lived and worked. Health service officers did not go into South El Paso and Zacate Creek looking to better the conditions there. Their intense focus on people moving across the bridge turned the towns and cities on both sides of the river surrounding the inspection stations into potential sources for the next epidemic. The USPHS border quarantine responsibilities made it very difficult to build cooperative working relationships with the surrounding communities. The two typhus bath riots in El Paso emphasized this general discontent in the streets of Ciudad Juárez. The numerous legal challenges by citizens and consuls to the enforcement of forced and compulsory vaccination was additional proof that Mexicans and Mexican Americans used many means necessary, even the law, to challenge the sense of vulnerability, visibility, and humiliation. The diplomatic scandal in Mexico City over the vaccination of Mexican athletes on the way to the Los Angeles Olympics demonstrated how easily the Texas medical border could affect the work of other federal agencies.

Another wing of the federal government undermined the medical justification for a quarantine approach to border health. When the Bureau of the Census certified Texas as a vital statistics registration unit, county health units started tabulating more than 90 percent of the deaths in a given county.[13] The presence of vital statistics as a medical diagnostic tool in Texas began to transform the relationship of the USPHS to surrounding border communities. The numbers made it clear that TB, diarrhea, and the illnesses associated with pediatrics were a bigger threat than the possibility of typhus.[14] Like Curtis and Pope before them, county health officers determined that these diseases were a political outcome of the triracial caste system in the Southwest. Unlike Pope, they took these economic and political relationships for granted and simply sought ways to keep germs in Mexican living spaces.

The spatial segregation that kept streets, sewage, and sanitation services on the white Anglo sides of El Paso and Laredo meant that the reemergence of fevers, weakness (TB), and ague (intestinal troubles) at the border no longer threatened the American presence along the Rio Grande. Here, health officials like George Cox recommended means like health education to make "Latin Americans" intellectually responsible for not changing their housing and workplace situations. Their solutions—sealing milk containers, sweeping floors, covering cribs—paled in the face of the challenges. Even successful model public health projects like the Alamo housing projects in El Paso, which demonstrated the importance and viability of concrete (and plumbing) projects in difficult health situations, became an opportunity to model proper health behavior. On entry, one resident was told

> that we have certain rules and regulations that he must observe; that he must be considerate of his neighbors and treat them in the same manner he desires to be treated; that we expect him to be a law-abiding citizen, assist in the beautifying of his surroundings, take pride in his home and grounds; in fact, he should give his home the same attention that he would if he were the owner. *Also we impress upon him that the health of his family is a vital factor in the health of the community, and that he should use every precaution to see that a high sanitary and health standard is maintained* [my emphasis].[15]

Most people involved in political activities along the border would probably endorse these attitudes. The same activists also sought to shift the frame away from families to questions regarding the economic structures that shaped these public health outcomes. Labor activist Emma Tenayuca held city political structures responsible when she recalled, "My city had the dubious reputation for having the highest tuberculosis rates in the country."[16] George I. Sanchez indicted farmers, ranchers, and county code enforcers across South Texas when he noted in his photo survey the health resources missing from the photograph: "With the blazing sun, corrugated iron houses become hot houses. Notice the garbage scattered all over the grounds, no camp playgrounds, and no sanitary facilities of any nature."[17] Salvador Franco Urias made it clear that city officials were responsible for health outcomes in El Paso when he declared it "embarrassing that there should be a call for clean and paved streets in south El Paso, because the mud and the floods are a disgrace for any self-styled progressive city."[18] Civil rights reformers and community activists, when they faced the unpaved streets, the open sewers, the general absence of running water and clinics in the Mexican sections of towns across the Rio Grande border, knew that political decisions created these medical situations and that politics, not disease-specific medical interventions, would transform these medical situations.

The appearance of H1N1 in the United States brought Mexico back into American debates about politics and public health. As a historian of medicine, a Latino studies specialist, and a one-time epidemiologist, I was fascinated

and appalled by the easy way in which governments across the globe connected Mexicans in their nations to the sudden appearance of a difficult-to-
treat respiratory illness in Mexico City. News of quarantines abroad rendered
the existence of Mexican communities in China, the Southern Cone, and
France visible to North Americans like me. Moreover, anxiety over domestic
public policy complicated existing concerns over the promiscuous ways flu
viruses make their way across national borders.[19]

The American response to H1N1 provided a global lesson in the difficult
management of medicalized nativism—the use of medical language to justify
the exclusion of a minority population in the United States based on their alleged ties to another country.[20] Michael Savage surmised publicly that H1N1
could be part of a Mexican terrorist plot to destroy the United States, and
Rush Limbaugh blamed H1N1 on Mexico's national health system.[21] The *New
York Times* rejected the open discrimination but followed this racial framing, titling its discussion of the first confirmed death in the United States
"Mexican Child Visiting U.S. 1st to Die Here of Swine Flu."[22] Mexicans in
the United States and Mexico rejected this connection. At the popular level,
some people in Mexico and the United States started calling H1N1 "the NAFTA
flu" or "Naftosa" to counter this racial connection. Others, like Mike Davis,
connected H1N1 to the Smithfield Hams pig factories in rural Veracruz. Some
sought to defend their shared modernity with the United States. Julio Frenk,
Mexico's minister of public health from 2000 to 2006, argued in the *New
York Times* that the early flu surveillance network he implemented in Mexico
identified a new strain of influenza in time to save lives in Mexico and the
United States.[23] Frenk responded to the open climate of medical discrimination by demanding that Americans recognize Mexico's shared modernity.
Others simply tried to reject the link between flu and a specific race or nation. Both strategies echoed with previous attempts at the border to break the
racial connection between national identity and public health.

News of a potentially pandemic flu in Mexico arrived in a country already
debating the expansion of a meager distribution of health resources, the status of public schools, the rate of job loss, and the relative place of ethnic minorities in the political order.[24] The volatility of the presence of Mexicans in
the United States shaped the rhetoric of national health care reform. President
Barack Obama repeatedly stated in his September 2009 health care speech
to Congress that the Affordable Care Act would not cover unauthorized immigrants. Representative Joe Wilson's open unbelief that the Affordable Care

Act would refuse to provide care to everyone living and working the United States, especially unauthorized immigrants, led him to scream "You lie!" at President Obama.[25] Clearly, the shape of medicalized nativism had more to do with the politics of citizenship within borders than with the movement of peoples and goods across borders.

Mexicans, Mexican immigrants, and Mexican Americans should be included in the official history of medical exclusion in the United States. In the 1849 cholera epidemic, many Americans held the Irish responsible for the ongoing presence of cholera.[26] In 1886, anti-Chinese activists used the rumor of venereal disease among Chinese women in California to give the Chinese Exclusion Act a medical underpinning, and this racial exclusion lasted past the Second World War. The presence of typhus among Jewish families on the Lower East Side of New York City provided a rallying cry to pass the 1892 Immigration Act in order to cut the number of Eastern European Jews living in urban areas. In 1917, the USPHS started placing Mexican workers crossing into El Paso and Laredo in kerosene and vinegar baths to prevent the presence of lice—and typhus—in the United States, a policy that lasted through the 1930s. This vivid spectacle probably helped city authorities in El Paso justify separate Mexican and (white) American field hospitals to treat people suffering from the "Spanish" flu. The creation of separate and unequal schools to protect American children from "dirty," "lousy," "Mexican" children should be another reminder that unequal public policies will help shape the many separate experiences of illness in this country. Moreover, the presence of illness and the richness of our medical responses will depend on the same mundane factor: the quality of the contacts we have built to connect us to other people.

ACKNOWLEDGMENTS

Too many people have believed in this project.

In college, Steven Volk, William Hood, Patricia Mathews, Camille Guerin-Gonzalez, and William Norris encouraged me to pursue more time in school. I refused and went to Chicago instead. Francisco X. Dominguez and Dan Kiss encouraged me to consider telling stories about public health for a career after hearing me talk about work in the Cook County Department of Public Health. Amita Vasudeva, Ingrid Graf, Rani George, Joey Mogul, Dawn Moon, and Gawain deLeeuw shared my enthusiasm for Chicago. In graduate school, the faculty at the University of Michigan made coursework, prelims, and the dissertation a delight. Kathleen Canning, Sonya Rose, Jose Rabasa, Rebecca Scott, Earl Lewis, Sidney Chalhoub, Richard Candida Smith, Maria Montoya, Sueann Caulfield, Howard Markell, Michelle Mitchell, and Fred Cooper pushed me in ways I am still learning to appreciate. George J. Sánchez consistently modeled the joys of research and conversation. Martin S. Pernick encouraged me to think of epidemics in counterhegemonic fashions and asked me if bodies can lie. I still ponder their questions, and I hope they can see some of the best of themselves in this manuscript.

Graduate study would have been unthinkable without the financial and professional support of the Mellon Foundation through the Mellon Minority Foundation Fellowship at Oberlin College. The Rackham Graduate School provided the privilege of exclusive attention to the wonderful courses offered at the University of Michigan. Research and travel funds from the Office of Academic and Multicultural Initiatives, the International Institute, and Rackham Graduate School facilitated travel to Washington, D.C.; Chicago; San Juan, Puerto Rico; and Austin and El Paso, Texas. Romance Languages and the Department of History gave me the opportunity to teach in fascinating courses. The Graduate Employees Organization guaranteed that this work got the financial and professional recognition it deserved. The Social Science Research Council International Migration to the United States Dissertation Proposal Writing Workshop and the Latino Studies Graduate Student Fellowship at the Smithsonian Institution aided the transition into dissertation research. The 1998 Latino Initiatives at the National Museum of American History financially supported my time in Washington, D.C. An ssrc/Mellon Dissertation Summer Research grant in 2000 provided enough time to complete research for three chapters. The Department of History generously provided a Spring/Summer Fellowship to aid the completion of the dissertation. Mary Clark and Earl Lewis tapped the Rackham Discretionary Fund to support the final writing process. The Rockefeller Postdoctoral Fellowship at the University of Texas at Austin, a summer research assignment in 2007, a scholarly research assignment in the spring of 2008, and the Woodrow Wilson Junior Faculty Career Enhancement Fellowship provided the time and the funds to ground the manuscript in archival collections in Mexico City, Austin, Texas, and Washington, D.C.

The irreverent company of Niels Hooper, Andrew Diamond, Gianpaolo Baiocchi, Peter Shulman, Anthony Macías, Jeff Rangel, Cristina Perez, Greg Hunter, Riyad Koya, Alejandra Marchevsky, Cynthia Renfro, Kate Masur, Nancy Mirabal, Christopher Schmidt-Nowara, Alice Rim, Estevan Rael y Gálvez, and Rick Sperling made Ann Arbor a special place. I count Adrian Burgos, Graciela Hernandez, Wilson Valentin, Javier Morillo-Alicea, Cora Lagos, Natalia Molina, Parna Sengupta, Marya McQuirter, Jason McGill, Hugo Benavides, Rama Mantena, Tom Romero, Pablo Mitchell, Tom Guglielmo, Parna Sengupta, Andrew Needham, and Dylan Penningroth as friends and fellow travelers. Richard Eikstadt and Michael Van Lent made Ann Arbor a home. Nsenga Lee, Anna Pegler Gordon, Graciela Hernandez, Cynthia Wu, Pablo Ramirez, Kim Alidio, and Richard Kim—aka *the accountables*—made writing a dissertation with this group enjoyable. Nicole Stanton, Grace Wang, and Pablo Ramirez carried me over the finish line. Kim Alidio and Richard Kim made graduate school possible.

For my time in Washington, D.C., I would like to thank Odette Diaz Shuler, Susan Walter, Russell Cashdollar, Ramón Gutiérrez, Evelyn Hu-DeHart, Marvette Perez, Olivia Cadaval, Pete Daniel, Mary Dyer, and Fath Ruffins for their support at the National Museum of American History. Eduardo Contreras, Carey Hardin, Dahlia Aguilar, Graciela Berkovich, Grupo de Colores, Angela Chung, Chris Dege, Jeff Hunt, Dylan Penningroth, Catherine Christen, Garvin Heath, Nicole Stanton, Pat Vennebush, James Vigil, Gillian Coulter, and Kim Blakemore made D.C. swing. Cally Waite, Emma Taati, Jennifer Wilks, Hugo Benavides, Michelle Scott, and Nohemi Solorzano-Thompson helped me look forward to summer conferences. Jonathan Brown, Sarah Deutsch, Evelynn Hammonds, Ramón Gutiérrez, Margaret Humphreys, Jose Limon, Pablo Mitchell, Natalia Molina, Gunther Peck, Gina Perez, Raul Ramos, Ann Twinam, and Barbara Welke saw promise in smaller iterations of this project. Kate Masur always thought my work was relevant and gave my mother priceless advice on life after surgery.

In Tampa, Adriana Novoa was indispensable. At the University of South Florida, Golfo Alexopoulos, John Belohlavek, Giovanna Benadusi, Barbara Berglund, Madeline Camara, Norma Cano, Paul Dosal, Dawn Flood, Cristina Green, Sharon Hamilton Johnson, David Johnson, Phil Levy, Gary Mormino, William Murray, Fraser Ottanelli, Donna Perrino, Ward Stavig, Tomaro Taylor, Salvador Torres,

Graydon Tunstall, Tamara Zwick, and the Cuentos Project students went above and beyond to make Florida a warm and supportive community. In Texas, the Center for Mexican American Studies, the Department of History, the Lozano Long Institute of Latin American Studies, and the Department of American Studies have supported this work. Frank Guridy, Deborah Paredez, Jennifer Wilks, Meta Jones, Cherise Smith, Juliet Hooker, Jemima Pierre, Raul Ramos, Ramón Gutiérrez, Sonia Saldivar-Hull and Adriana Novoa provided invaluable feedback on various versions of this manuscript. Virginia Burnett, Madeline Hsu, Karl Miller, Nancy Stalker, Jose Limon, Richard Flores, Shannon Speed, Charlie Hale, Randy Diehl, Susan Dean-Smith, Ann Twinam, Bruce Hunt, Robert Abzug, Tracy Matysik, Emilio Zamora, Anne Martinez, Nicole Guidotti-Hernandez, Chris Ernst, Megan Seaholm, Ruramisai Charumbira, Carolyn Eastman, Nhi Lieu, Tatjana Lichtenstein, Shirley Thompson, Rebecca Torres, and Domino Perez for their unfailing enthusiasm. James Jenkins, Claudia Rueda, Irene Garza, Veronica Martinez-Matsuda, Valerie Martinez, Juandrea Bates, Katherine Boone, Allison Schottenstein, Neel Baumgardner, Jeff Parker, Samantha Serrano, Liz O'Brien, Tatiana Reinoza, Miguel Levario, David Villareal, Laura Padilla, and the students in my 2011 Borderlands seminar remind me that others also find life in research pleasurable. My Spring 2011 undergraduate Latino History seminar transformed my Monday evenings. Adrian Burgos, Jonathan Inda, Gilberto Rosas, Julie Dowling, Edna Viruell-Fuentes, and Arlene Torres stepped in at the right moment. Luis Carcamo-Huechante, Kelly Kerbow-Hudson, Christian Kelleher, Michael Heidenreich, Laurie Green, and Martin Summers have been wonderful coconspirators on some terribly distracting projects. Frank Guridy is, in Brecht's words, *imprescindible*. Courtney Berger's long faith in the project has been impressive. Eileen Quam, Christine Choi, and Ainee Athar found a myriad number of ways to improve the manuscript. Anitra Grisales provided guidance and enthusiasm at many difficult points in the writing process. I am also grateful to the two anonymous reviewers at Duke University Press for their insight and suggestions. Frank, Deb, Jen, and Cherise helped make family life seem imaginable here. And, in San Francisco, Jennifer Wilks made our family possible.

My immediate family inspires me. Solomon Cordova and Jennifer Feeley have been astonishingly supportive. Patricia and John Ciarleglio have been steadfastly generous throughout the years. Carlos and Islena Guerrero consistently lift my mom's spirits. Larry brought a funny and wise *cuñada*, Judy Mckiernan Jurado, into our family.

Larry and Eileen, *ustedes son parte del camino que hemos hecho al andar.*

Aleyda González Mckiernan, no hay palabras que puedan representar tu presencia en nuestras vidas. Sin ti, no sabría cómo ser una persona en este mundo. Espero saber más en el futuro, y poder vivir tu ejemplo en familia.

Cary Cordova, *de Café Tacuba to this day,* you have helped me build a far richer life than I ever imagined. That I can only do the same for you.

Feliciano Enrique Mckiernan Cordova: Sin ti, no hay paseo al andar.

NOTES

Notes on Places, Peoples, and Diseases

1. Gloria Anzaldúa, *Borderlands: The new Mestiza = la Frontera* (San Francisco: Aunt Lute Books, 2007), 25.

2. John Morán González, *Border Renaissance: The Texas Centennial and the Emergence of Mexican American Literature* (Austin: University of Texas Press, 2009).

3. Hernan Cortes, *Cartas y relaciónes de Hernan Cortés al emperador Carlos V.,* (Paris: A. Chaix y Ca., 1868), 168–69, 172. Recent scholarship has started correcting established spellings of Mexica and Talxcaltecan nobility. See Susan Schroeder, "The Mexico That Spain Encountered," in *The Oxford History of Mexico*, ed. William Beezly (New York: Oxford University Press, 2000), 75.

4. David Montejano, *Anglos and Mexicans in the Making of Texas, 1836–1986* (Austin: University of Texas Press, 1986), 5–6.

5. Interview with Señora X, December 6, 1979, conducted by Maria Nuckolss, University of Texas at El Paso, Institute of Oral History. From George Sánchez, *Becoming Mexican American: Ethnicity, Culture, and Identity in Chicano Los Angeles, 1900–1945* (New York: Oxford University Press, 1994), 56.

6. Dennis Váldes, "The Decline of Slavery in Mexico," *Americas* 44, no. 2 (October 1987): 167–94; Douglas Cope, *The Limits of Racial Domination: Plebeian Society in Colonial Mexico City* (Madison: University of Wisconsin Press, 1994), 49–67.

7. Ramón Gutiérrez, "Hispanic Identities in the Southwestern United States," in *Race and Classification in Mexican America* (Stanford: Stanford University Press, 2011), 174–94. I use the terms "Comanche," "Apache," "Navajo," "Pueblo," "Cherokee," and "Yaqui" for these Indian nations because they were the terms used in formal diplomatic negotiations. Each of these groupings of nations have other terms in their own languages to refer to themselves.

8. Charles Rosenberg, "Framing Disease: Illness, Society and History," *Framing Disease: Studies in Cultural History* (New Brunswick: Rutgers University Press, 1992), xii–xxvi.

9. Charles Briggs and Clara Mantini Briggs, *Stories in the Time of Cholera: Racial Profiling during a Medical Nightmare* (Berkeley: University of California Press, 2004).

10. Donald Hopkins, *Princes and Peasants: A History of Smallpox* (Chicago: University of Chicago Press, 1983).

11. Dale Smith, "The Rise and Fall of Typhomalarial Fever. II: Decline and Fall," *Journal of the History of Medicine and Allied Societies* 37, no. 3 (July 1982): 287–320.

12. Margaret Humphreys, *Yellow Fever and the South* (Baltimore: Johns Hopkins University Press, 1992), 5–7.

13. A faulty dose of yellow vaccine may have occasioned my cousin Milko Martinich González's death, may he rest in peace.

14. "Escasez de vacunas en Medellin," *El Colombiano*, www.elcolombiano.com /BancoConocimiento/H/hay_escasez_de_vacunas_contra_la_fiebre_amarilla/hay_ escasez_de_vacunas_contra_la_fiebre_amarilla.asp (accessed August 26, 2011).

Introduction

1. Gregorio Guiteras, "Report on the Epidemic of Yellow Fever of 1903 at Laredo, Minera and Cannel, Tx.," United States Public Health and Marine Hospital Service, ed., in *Annual Report of the United States Public Health and Marine Hospital Service for the Fiscal Year of 1903* (Washington, D.C.: Government Printing Office, 1904), 308.

2. Ibid., 308.

3. Mariola Espinosa, *Epidemic Invasions: Yellow Fever and the Limits of Cuban Independence* (Chicago: University of Chicago Press, 2009), 55–73. White and Mexican Laredo authorities may have also been reluctant to send black federal troops into white, Texas Mexican, and Mexican households in Laredo. James N. Leiker, *Racial Borders: Black Soldiers along the Rio Grande* (College Station: Texas A&M University Press, 2002), 118–44.

4. Miguel Barrera, resident of Sam Fordyce, Texas, reported, "In spite of having my residence on American Soil, the doctor refused to hear my arguments and vaccinated me. Filed in Rio Grande City, 09/18/1916." Record Group (RG) 59, Department of State Decimal Files, 1910–1920, 158.1208/13 Enclosure VI, National Archives and Records Administration, College Park, Md. (NACP).

5. J. P. Reynolds, "Final Report Regarding Complaints at Rio Grande City— J. P. Reynolds, 05/26/1917," in RG 59, Department of State, Decimal Files, 1910–1920, 158.1208/11, Enclosure VI, NACP.

6. Charles V, king of Spain, "Orden real sobre la vacuna," in *A Century of Medicine in San Antonio*, ed. Pat Ireland Nixon (San Antonio: Pat Ireland Nixon, 1936), 56.

7. Jaime Gurza, "Reporte sobre la bacuna" (1808), Bexar Papers Collection, Center for American History, Austin, Tex.

8. Priscilla Wald, *Contagious: Cultures, Carriers, and the Outbreak Narrative*, John Hope Franklin Center Books (Durham: Duke University Press, 2008). (Her first case study, imagined immunities: the epidemiology of belonging, pages 33–67, makes this point. The language is mine.)

9. Peter Andreas, "Borderless Economy, Barricaded Border," *North American Chronicle of Latin America* 33, no. 3 (1999): 16.

10. Claudia Huerkamp, "The History of Smallpox Vaccination in Germany: A First Step in the Medicalization of the General Public," *Journal of Contemporary History* 20, no. 4 (1985): 617–85. Amy Fairchild emphasizes the way public health inspections certified the productivity of American immigrant laborers to Americans in *Science at the Borders: Immigrant Medical Inspection and the Shaping of the Modern Industrial Labor Force* (Baltimore: Johns Hopkins University Press, 2003).

11. Huerkamp, "History of Smallpox Vaccination in Germany." For a succinct sketch of the challenges to medical authority, see Michel Foucault, "The Subject and Power," *Critical Inquiry* 8, no. 4 (1982): 777–95.

12. Natalia Molina, *Fit to Be Citizens? Race and Public Health in Los Angeles, 1880–1939* (Berkeley: University of California Press, 2007), 9–12.

13. Nayan Shah, *Contagious Divides: Epidemics and Race in San Francisco's Chinatown* (Berkeley: University of California Press, 2001), 8.

14. Linda Nash, *Inescapable Ecologies: A History of Environment, Disease, and Knowledge* (Berkeley: University of California Press, 2006), 5–12, 16–48. See also Sylvia Noble Tesh, *Hidden Arguments: Political Ideology and Disease Prevention Policy* (New Brunswick: Rutgers University Press, 1988), 3, 4, 11–15.

15. Charles Rosenberg, "The Therapeutic Revolution: Medicine, Meaning, and Social Change in Nineteenth-Century America," in *Explaining Epidemics: And Other Studies in the History of Medicine* (New York: Cambridge University Press, 1992), 12.

16. Ibid., 18. This is why doctors discussed the smells, pus, and excretions of, and the airs around, each patient.

17. Priscilla Wald makes the point that the act of representing a disease, of placing a microbe in a geographical representation of another place, is deeply caught in the process of designating who belongs and who threatens, and who can belong in a national community. Wald, *Contagious*, 1–28, 33, 67. See also Elizabeth Fenn, *Pox Americana: The Great Smallpox Epidemic of 1775–82* (New York: Hill and Wang, 2001), 259–72.

18. Thomas W. Kavanaugh, *Comanche Political History: An Ethnohistorical Perspective, 1706–1875* (Lincoln: University of Nebraska Press, 1996), esp. 294–387; Brian Delay, *War of a Thousand Deserts: Indian Raids and the U.S.-Mexican War* (New Haven: Yale University Press, 2008), 194–226; and Andres Resendez, *Changing National Identities at the Frontier: Texas and New Mexico, 1800–1850* (New York: Cambridge University Press, 2004).

19. Charles E. Rosenberg, *The Cholera Years: The United States in 1832, 1849, and 1866* (Chicago: University of Chicago Press, 1962), 121–31.

20. For a critique of the Paris school in the history of knowledge, see Michel Foucault, *Birth of the Clinic: An Archaeology of Medical Perception* (New York: Vintage,

1994). For the importance of the Paris school to American medical reform move-
ments, see John Harley Warner, *The Therapeutic Perspective: Medical Practice,
Knowledge, and Identity in America, 1820–1885* (Princeton: Princeton University
Press, 1997) and *Against the Spirit of System: The French Impulse in Nineteenth-
Century American Medicine* (Princeton: Princeton University Press, 1998).

21. Rosenberg, "Therapeutic Revolution," 18.

22. Resendez, *Changing National Identities*, 3.

23. Fenn, *Pox Americana*, 135–67.

24. Howard Markel, *When Germs Travel: Six Major Epidemics That Have Invaded
America and the Fears They Unleashed* (New York: Pantheon, 2004).

25. Sánchez, *Becoming Mexican American*, 51.

26. John Hunter Pope, "The Condition of the Mexican Population of Western
Texas in Its Relation to Public Health," in *Public Health Papers and Reports*, vol. 6,
ed. American Public Health Association (Boston: Franklin Press, Rand and Avery,
1881), 162.

27. The essay collection edited by Douglas Crimp, *AIDS: Cultural Analysis/Cultural
Activism*, offered a way to think of medicine and culture together. Paula Treichler's
"AIDS, Homophobia and Biomedical Discourse: An Epidemic of Signification" (31–
69) and Simon Watney's "The Spectacle of AIDS" (71–85) seemed the most relevant
to my work in the Public Health Department. Crimp, ed., *AIDS: Cultural Analysis/
Cultural Activism* (Cambridge: MIT Press, 1988). The term "GLBTQ" (gay/lesbian/
bisexual/transgender/queer) had not entered circulation yet. These essays are some-
times considered part of the emerging discipline of queer theory, but they still used
the formulation "gay and lesbian" to discuss GLBTQ practices in the 1980s.

28. See Ronald Bayer and Gerald Oppenheimer, *Voices from the Epidemic: An Oral
History* (New York: Oxford University Press, 2002), for the variety of ways physicians
learned to make their way in this landscape shaped by grassroots activism.

29. Steven Epstein's analysis of the ways engagement with medical authority transformed AIDS activists is particularly compelling. See Epstein, *Impure Science: AIDS,
Activism, and the Politics of Knowledge* (Berkeley: University of California Press,
1996), 246–50.

30. Marlon Riggs, *Black Is, Black Ain't* (Berkeley: California Newsreel, 1995). I found
Evelynn Hammonds's discussion of the ways the official record erased the experience
of black women with AIDS to be a compelling analysis of race and public health.
Hammonds, "Missing Persons: Black Women and AIDS," *Radical America* (April–
June 1990): 7–24.

31. Allan Brandt, *No Magic Bullet: A Social History of Venereal Diseases in the
United States since 1880* (New York: Oxford University Press, 1987); Crimp, *AIDS*;
Jeanne Watsutaki Houston, *Farewell to Manzanar* (Boston: Houghton Mifflin, 1973);
Allan Berube, *Coming Out under Fire: The History of Gay Men and Women in World
War Two* (Boston: New Press, 1992). I also found the collection edited by Elizabeth

Fee and Daniel Fox, AIDS: *The Making of a Chronic Disease* (Berkeley: University of California Press, 1992), to be very useful in my conversations about the implications of testing positive for HIV antibodies. For disease as a social diagnosis, framing mechanism, and biological event, see also Charles E. Rosenberg, "Framing Disease: Illness, Society and History," xi–xxii.

32. "Illinois Quick Links," Factfinder.gov, quickfacts.census.gov/qfd/states/17/1703 11k.html (accessed June 30, 2011).

33. Andrew Cliff, *Deciphering Global Epidemics: Analytical Approaches to the Disease Records of World Cities, 1888–1912* (New York: Cambridge University Press, 1998).

34. Collector of Customs William Fitch Report, "Camp Jenner," August 4, 1895, pp. 1–3, RG 90, United States Public Health Service Files, NC 34, Entry 11, Correspondence with Southern Quarantine Stations, Box 150, NACP.

35. H. J. Hamilton, "Report on the Prevalence of Smallpox on the Lower Mexican Border, 09/24/1911," RG 90, Subject Files No. 2796—Smallpox, United States Public Health Service Files, 1897–1923, NACP.

36. Richard S. Kim alerted me to the existence of this decimal file in 1999. He found them while researching Hawaii- and Mexico-based Korean exile nationalism in the National Archives in College Park. Mexico specialist Milton Gustafson was incredibly helpful, but both times I showed him my material, he found it hard to believe there was a decimal file called "complaints against quarantine" in the State Department files.

37. Mae Ngai, *Impossible Subjects: Illegal Aliens and the Making of Modern America* (Princeton: Princeton University Press, 2005), 2.

38. C. C. Pierce, "Cases of Typhus Fever in the City of El Paso, January 1–June 30, 1916," File No. 2126, Typhus, Box 207, File 1, RG 90, USPHS Central Files, 1897–1923, NACP. I presented a paper titled "The Typhus Bath Riots and the Invention of the Modern Mexican Border" at a National Museum of American History colloquium in April 1997. See Alexandra Minna Stern, "Buildings, Boundaries, and Blood: Medicalization and Nation-Building on the U.S.-Mexico Border, 1910–1930," *Hispanic American Historical Review* 79, no. 1 (1999): 41–81. David Dorado Romo, *Ringside Seat to a Revolution: An Underground Cultural History of El Paso and Ciudad Juarez* (El Paso: Cinco Puntos, 2005), 223–44.

39. "Order to Bathe Starts near Riot among Juarez Women. Auburn Haired Amazon at Santa Fe Street Bridge Leads Feminine Outbreak," *El Paso Morning Times*, January 29, 1917, 1.

40. Arnoldo De León, *They Called Them Greasers: Anglo Attitudes toward Mexicans in Texas, 1821–1900* (Austin: University of Texas Press, 1983), 99.

41. For an elegant set of articles on the impact of the American experience in Cuba, Puerto Rico, and the Philippines on the growth of the federal state, see Alfred W. McCoy and Francisco Scarano, eds., *Colonial Crucible: Empire in the Making of the Modern American State* (Madison: University of Wisconsin Press, 2009). For a

collection on the edge of exploring national and borderlands spaces together, see Samuel Truett and Elliott Young, eds., *Continental Crossroads: Remapping U.S.-Mexico Borderlands History* (Durham: Duke University Press, 2004).

42. Nicholas Trist and Manuel Peña y Peña, "The Treaty of Guadalupe Hidalgo," in *A Century of Lawmaking: U.S. Congressional Documents and Debates, 1774–1875* (Washington, D.C.: Library of Congress, 1848), 922–1065, esp. 923–24.

43. John Hamilton, "The Mexican-Texas Yellow Fever Epidemic," *Annual Report of the Supervising Surgeon General, USMHS, Department of the Treasury for the Fiscal Year of 1882* (Washington, D.C.: Government Printing Office, 1883), 310–45.

44. George Magruder, "Report on the Establishment and Administration of Camp Jenner, Eagle Pass, Tex.," *Weekly Abstract of Sanitary Reports* 10, no. 45 (October 25, 1895): 957–59.

45. Guiteras, "Report on the Epidemic of Yellow Fever of 1903 at Laredo," 303–20.

46. H. J. Hamilton, "Report of Investigation on Trip along Lower Mexican Border, September 18, 1911," RG 90, Subject Files No. 2796—Smallpox, United States Public Health Service Files, 1897–1923, NACP.

47. For a succinct description of the power of whiteness as an unmarked category, see Richard Dyer, *White: Essays on Race and Culture* (New York: Routledge, 1997), 1–40.

48. For Mariola Espinosa, this unequal geographic dynamic defines the relationship at the heart of nineteenth- and twentieth-century colonial medicine. Espinosa, *Epidemic Invasions*, 3, 5–8.

49. For the presence of an established working-class Mexican population, see Montejano, *Anglos and Mexicans*, 1–100. For land possession, see Armando Alonzo, *Tejano Legacy: Rancheros and Settlers in South Texas, 1734–1900* (Albuquerque: University of New Mexico Press, 1998). For land dispossession, see Montejano, *Anglos and Mexicans*, 101–28. For the rise of racially diverse, highly mobile regional labor forces, see Emilio Zamora, *The World of the Mexican Worker in Texas, 1880–1930* (College Station: Texas A&M University Press, 1996), and Neil Foley, *The White Scourge: Mexicans, Blacks, and Poor Whites in Texas Cotton Culture* (Berkeley: University of California Press, 1996). For the paradoxical importance of this Mexican middle class, see Montejano, *Anglos and Mexicans*, 83–99; David G. Gutiérrez, *Walls and Mirrors: Mexican Americans, Mexican Immigrants, and the Politics of Ethnicity* (Berkeley: University of California Press, 1995), and Leticia Magda Garza-Falcón, *Gente Decente: A Borderlands Response to the Politics of Dominance* (Austin: University of Texas Press, 1998).

50. Foucault uses the example of the Paris legislature, which appointed doctors to decide who deserved assistance and how much aid they deserved. Foucault called this the "decentralization of the means of assistance authorized a medicalization of its distribution" (*Birth of the Clinic*, 41). The first translation of this book into U.S. English appeared in 1973. The original publication was Foucault, *Naissance de la*

clinique: Une archeology du regard medical (Paris: Presses Universitaires de France, 1963).

51. Justo Cardenas, "Nuevo León cientifico: La viruela y la vacuna," *La Colonia Mexicana*, May 6, 1891, 1.

52. The scholarship on the promise and the exclusions of modern public health practice is vast and growing. Key texts include Foucault, *Birth of the Clinic*; Leslie Reagan, *When Abortion Was a Crime: Women, Medicine, and the Law* (Berkeley: University of California Press, 1997); Shah, *Contagious Divides*; Martin S. Pernick, *The Black Stork: Eugenics and the Death of "Defective" Babies in American Medicine and Motion Pictures since 1915* (New York: Oxford University Press, 1999). On quarantine in particular, see Howard Markel, *Quarantine! East European Jewish Immigrants and the New York City Epidemics of 1892* (Baltimore: Johns Hopkins University Press, 1999).

53. For a pathbreaking analysis of the multiple spaces in Los Angeles where the children of Mexican immigrants forged a shared sense of identity, see Sánchez, *Becoming Mexican American*, 11. For a discussion of the ways ethnic Mexican political activists experienced the difference between ethnic and national identities, see Gutiérrez, *Walls and Mirrors*.

54. Gutiérrez, *Walls and Mirrors*, 8.

55. Political responses to AIDS in the United States in the late 1980s and early 1990s helped generate communities of interest among people with AIDS and challenged the idea that people with AIDS shared the same identities, communities, and political goals. See Jennifer Brier, *Infectious Ideas: U.S. Political Responses to AIDS* (Chapel Hill: University of North Carolina Press, 2010), 6–9, 161–85.

56. Santos Benavides, "Swearingen Released under Protest," File 132, Box 301–118, Papers of Governor Oran Milo Roberts, Texas State Archives and Library (TSAL), Austin.

57. Ibid.

58. Robert M. Swearingen, "Please Exempt Me from Restrictions in Your Quarantine Proclamation," File 138, Box 301, Papers of Governor Oran Milo Roberts, TSAL.

59. Sam Claiborne deposition, "Failure of the Scheme for the Colonization of Negroes in Mexico" (1896), in 54th Cong., 1st sess., House of Representatives, Doc. 169, Enclosure 3, p. 3, National Archives Building (NAB), Washington, D.C.

60. James Joseph Kinyoun, "Preliminary Report on the Treatment of Variola by Its Antitoxin," in *Annual Report of the Supervising Surgeon General of the Marine Hospital Service of the United States for the Fiscal Year 1897*, ed. Walter Wyman (Washington, D.C.: Government Printing Office, 1899), 779.

61. Earl Lewis, "To Turn as on a Pivot: Writing African Americans into a History of Overlapping Diasporas," *American Historical Review* 100, no. 3 (June 1995): 765–87.

62. Erika Lee, *At the Gates: Chinese Immigration during the Exclusion Era, 1882–1942* (Chapel Hill: University of North Carolina Press, 2007), 162.

63. For California, see J. C. Geiger, "Investigation of an Outbreak of Smallpox at Banning: Special Report to James S. Cumming, Director, Bureau of Communicable Disease, California State Board of Health, 12/27/1916," p. 2, Smallpox Subject File No. 2796, RG 90, Central Files, United States Public Health Service, 1897–1923, Textual Records, Civilian Division, NACP. For New York see "Laredo y Nuevo Laredo: Se esta vacunando a los turistas," *La Prensa* (San Antonio), January 19, 1949.

64. Barbara Kruger, *Untitled (Your Body Is a Battleground) 1989 March on Washington Poster*, photographic silkscreen on vinyl, 112 inches by 112 inches. 1989.

One. From the Mexican Border to the Mexican-Texas Epidemic

1. For a fascinating analysis of the contradictions about expansion in American popular culture, see Shelley Streeby, *American Sensations: Class, Empire, and the Production of Popular Culture* (Berkeley: University of California Press, 2002).

2. Samuel Ryan Curtis, *Mexico under Fire*, ed. Joseph Chance (Fort Worth: Texas Christian University Press, 1994), 192.

3. Nicholas Trist, "The Treaty of Guadalupe Hidalgo," in *A Century of Lawmaking: U.S. Congressional Documents and Debates, 1774–1875*, ed. U.S. Congress, 924–1065 (Washington, D.C.: Library of Congress, 1848).

4. Ibid., 924.

5. The army recorded 12,355 deaths, of which 10,986 were by illness (88 percent). Slightly more than one out of every eight American soldiers died of illness in Mexico. The army also recorded close to 95,000 hospital visits, roughly equaling the number of soldiers who served in Mexico. See Vincent Cirillo, "More Fatal than Powder and Shot: Dysentery in the United States Army during the Mexican War, 1846–1848," *Perspectives in Biology and Medicine* 52, no. 3 (2009): 400–405.

6. In a treaty that demarcated boundaries of citizenship, race, and nation, only public health and reprisals against Indian raids dissolved the political boundaries connecting and separating the United States from Mexico. Giorgio Agamben, *State of Exception* (Chicago: University of Chicago Press, 2005), 3–5.

7. Curtis, *Mexico under Fire*, 60.

8. Romo, *Ringside Seat to the Revolution*, 229. Alexandra Minna Stern and Howard Markel, "Which Face? Whose Nation? Immigration, Public Health, and the Construction of Disease at America's Ports and Borders, 1891–1928," *American Behavioral Scientist* 42, no. 9 (1999): 1314–31. The placement of body politics at the end of the edited collection *Continental Crossroads* imply that body politics and medical authority at the border began with the Mexican Revolution, even though many of the contributors disagree with this narrative. Samuel Truett and Elliott Young, eds., *Continental Crossroads: Remapping U.S.–Mexican Borderlands History* (Durham: Duke University Press, 2004), iii–v.

9. For expansion and slavery, see Eric Foner, *Free Soil, Free Labor, Free Men: The*

Ideology of the Republican Party before the Civil War (New York: Oxford University Press, 1995). See also James McPherson, *Battle Cry of Freedom: The Civil War Era* (New York: Oxford University Press, 1988). For the centrality of slavery to the South, see James Oakes, *The Ruling Race: A History of American Slaveholders* (New York: W. W. Norton, 1998).

10. Pedro Santoni, *Mexicans at Arms: Puro Federalists and the Politics of War, 1845–1848* (Dallas: Texas Christian University Press, 1996). For an account that emphasizes the outsize role of personalities, see Enrique Krauze, *Mexico: Biography of Power: A History of Modern Mexico, 1810–1996* (New York: HarperCollins, 1997), 152–206. For the crucial importance of trade with the United States after the Civil War, see John Mason Hart, *Empire and Revolution: Americans in Mexico since the Civil War* (Berkeley: University of California Press, 2006), 9–45, 46–69.

11. James Vanderwood, "Betterment for Whom: The Reform Period, 1855–1875," in *The Oxford History of Mexico* (New York: Oxford University Press, 2010), 349–71.

12. Robert D. Murray, "The Mexican-Texas Epidemic," *Annual Report of the Supervising Surgeon General, usmhs, Department of the Treasury for the Fiscal Year of 1882* (Washington, D.C.: Government Printing Office, 1883), 271–320; quote on 271.

13. See Catherine Mark and Jose Rigau-Pérez, "The World's First Immunization Campaign: The Spanish Smallpox Vaccine Expedition," *Bulletin of the History of Medicine* 39, no. 2 (spring 2009): 63–94.

14. Fenn, *Pox Americana*, 135–66.

15. Michael Bennett, "Jenner's Ladies: Women and Vaccination in Early Nineteenth-Century Britain," *History* 93, no. 312 (January 2008): 498.

16. Jacques-Louis Moreau, *Tratado histórico y práctico de la vacuna*, trans. Francisco Xavier de Balmis (Madrid: Imprenta Real, 1803).

17. For a general overview, see Susana Ramirez, *La salud del imperio: Real expedición filantrópica de la vacuna* (Madrid: Fundación Jorge Juan, 2002). For the ways local political conflicts shaped the implementation of the vaccine in central Mexico, see Patricia Aceves Pastrana, "Conflictos y negociaciones en las expediciones de Balmis," *Estudios Novohispanos* 17 (2007): 171–200.

18. Marks and Rigau-Pérez, "The World's First Immunization Campaign," 63–94.

19. Charles V, king of Spain, "Orden real sobre la vacuna," in Nixon, *A Century of Medicine in San Antonio*, 18.

20. Viceroy Don Felix Maria Calleja, *Instrucción formada para ministrar la vacuna como único preservativo del contagio de las viruelas* (circular), in Don Mariano Ontiveros, Texana, Dolph Briscoe Center for American History (dbcah), the University of Texas at Austin.

21. Ibid. Unless otherwise noted, all translations from the original Spanish are mine.

22. Molina, *Fit to Be Citizens*, 5.

23. Calleja, *Instrucción formada para ministrar la vacuna*, 3.

24. Jaime Gurza, *Reporte sobre la bacuna*, Bexar Archives, 1770–1836, Dolph Briscoe Center for American History (DBCAH), Austin, Tex.

25. Don Antonio Cordero y Bustamante, "Sobre la bacuna," in Nixon, *A Century of Medicine in San Antonio*, 19–20.

26. Gurza, "Reporte sobre la bacuna," 2.

27. Antonio Cordero y Bustamante, *Llegaron 400 puntos* (April 1, 1809), Bexar Archives, 1770–1836, DBCAH.

28. Manuel Salcedo, "His Reports on Management of Hospital and Administration of Vaccine. 03/05/1808," Bexar Archives, 1770–1836, DBCAH.

29. Anonymous, "Petition to Mexican Authorities 02/1811," in Nixon, *A Century of Medicine in San Antonio*, 28.

30. Timothy Henderson, *A Glorious Defeat: Mexico's War with the United States* (New York: Hill and Wang, 2007), 49–73.

31. Jose María Sanchez, "A Trip to Texas in 1828," trans. Carlos Castañeda, *Southwestern Historical Quarterly* 29 (April 1926): 283, reprinted in Gutiérrez, *Walls and Mirrors*, 31.

32. Juan Antonio Padilla, "Epidemic and Employment of American Doctor, 11/14/1825," in Nixon, *A Century of Medicine in San Antonio*, 36–37.

33. Ramón Musquiz, *Atendiendo a que las viruelas naturales son una enfermedad epidémica*, January 31, 1831, 2001–168, Ramón Musquiz Collection, Austin, Tex. The members of the board were the police, priests, local merchants, and city council members: Vice Gobernador Juan Martin Berazmendi, Jefe de Policías Ramón Musquiz, Excelentísimo Jose Maria Salinas, Cura Párroco Don Refugio de la Garza, Don Francisco Maynes, Capitán Alejandro Trevinio, Teniente Ygnacio Rodriguez, Manuel Menchaca, Regidor Jose Cariano, Sindia Procurador Felipe Musquiz, Jose Maria Balmaceda, Jose Antonio Garza, Juan Macmulen, Alejandro Vidal, Regidor Ygnacio Chavez, Gaspar Flores, Jose Rosas, Vicente Gortari, Fernando Cabeza, and Juan Maria y Salvador Torres.

34. Musquiz, *Atendiendo a que las viruelas*, 2001–168.

35. Ibid.

36. Ibid.

37. Ibid.

38. Raul Ramos, *Beyond the Alamo* (Chapel Hill: University of North Carolina Press, 2008), 23–50.

39. These political responses to the challenge of public health in an epidemic reflect Musquiz's prominent role as a federalist and nationalist in Mexico. He defended trade with the United States as a way to strengthen Mexican Texas. At the same time he opposed attempts, like the constitution of 1836, to centralize power in Mexico City. Unlike Juan Seguin and other Tejano leaders, these commitments did not lead him to join the insurrection in Texas that ultimately became the Texas Revolution.

Andres Resendez, "Ramón Múzquiz: The Ultimate Insider," in *Tejano Leadership in Mexican and Revolutionary Texas*, ed. Jesús de la Teja (College Station: Texas A&M University Press, 2010), 131–35.

40. Walter White, "Vacuna de Nueva Orleans. 05/28/1831," Bexar Archives, 1770–1836, DBCAH.

41. Jesús de la Teja, "Juan Nepomuceno Seguin: Rebel. Patriot. Exile," ed. Jesús de la Teja, *Tejano Leadership*, 225.

42. The historiography of the Texas Revolution is vast. This synthesis comes from three recent texts: Ramos, *Beyond the Alamo*; Resendez, *Changing National Identities*; and Henderson, *A Glorious Defeat*.

43. "President James K. Polk, "War Message to Congress, May 11, 1846," in *The U.S. War with Mexico*, ed. Ernesto Chavez (New York: Bedford St. Martin's, 2008), 74.

44. Frederick Douglass, "The War with Mexico," 78–80 and Henry David Thoreau, "On Civil Disobedience," 82–83, in Chavez, *The U.S. War with Mexico*. See also Henderson, *A Glorious Defeat*, 133–57.

45. Patricia Nelson Limerick, *The Legacy of Conquest: The Unbroken Past of the American West* (New York: W. W. Norton, 1987), 179–351. McPherson, *Battle Cry of Freedom*, 3–4, 47–115.

46. Curtis, *Mexico under Fire*, 192.

47. Ibid., 61.

48. Ibid., 209.

49. Ibid.

50. "Vaccine Matter," *American Flag*, June 12, 1846, 1.

51. Curtis, *Mexico under Fire*, 182.

52. Ibid., 192.

53. Gobernador Serapio Vargas, "Se solicitan vidrios de pus vacuna. 04/18/1852," Grupo Documental 127, Gobernación, Archivo General de la Nación (AGN), Mexico City.

54. Serapio Vargas (governor of Coahuila), *Suplicase se le remita vitrales con pus vacuna*, 04/19/1852, memorandum request of Gobernación, GD 127 Gobernación, AGN.

55. M. Anaya (governor of Baja California), *Avisa haber certificado y recibido un paquete de pus vacuno*, GD 127 Gobernación, Caja 405, Expediente 6, AGN.

56. Nathan Sturges Jarvis, "Reports from Texas: Article II—Report on the Rise, Progress, and Decline of Epidemic Cholera in the Valley of the Rio Grande" (1850), in Texana, DBCAH.

57. Ibid.

58. Rafael Espinoza, "Por extraordinaria violencia comunico a usted los efectos que estaba comenzando a hacer la epidemia del cólera morbus que condujo el bergamino ingles Gazelle, al puerto de San Lucas," in GD 127 Gobernación, Caja 391, Expediente 1, December 10, 1850, AGN.

59. Rafael Espinoza, "El jefe politico de la Baja California emitiendo los estragos

del numero de muertos que hubo en Don Jose del Cabo por el cólera morbo," in GD 127 Gobernación, Caja 391, Expediente 1, March 6, 1851, AGN.

60. Gobernación, "Observando el pedido del jefe publico de Baja California," in GD 127 Gobernación, Caja 405, Expediente 12, Mexico City, August, 17,1852, AGN.

61. Charles E. Rosenberg, *The Cholera Years: The United States in 1832, 1849, and 1866* (Chicago: University of Chicago Press, 1962), 72–98.

62. Jose María Reyes (El Srio del Consejo Central de Salubridad), "Criterio para el jueves 17 a la una de la tarde y aviso a la prefectura," in GD 127 Gobernación, Caja 1, Folio 2, Expediente 10, January 11, 1867, AGN, 1867.0111.

63. Margaret Humphreys, *Intensely Human: The Health of the Black Soldier in the American Civil War* (Baltimore: Johns Hopkins University Press, 2008), 119–21.

64. Jose María Reyes, "Higiene pública: Cuatro palabras sobre las cuarentenas," in *Gaceta médica: Periódico de la academia de medicina de México*, ed. Academia de Medicina de Mexico (Mexico City: Imprenta de Miguel Escalante, 1883), 8–9.

65. The original citation is "White to the Editor," *Christian Recorder*, September 19, 1865, in Humphreys, *Intensely Human*, 127–28.

66. U.S. Census, *Twelfth Census of the United States Taken in the Year 1900*, ed. Charles Merriam (New York: Norman Ross, 1997), 40–42.

67. Leiker, *Racial Borders*, 70.

68. General Sherman to Secretary of War, July 7, 1875, AGO-LR, M666, RG 94, NAMP, roll 19y. The citation comes from Leiker, *Racial Borders*, 72.

69. For the American West, see Elliott West, *The Contested Plains: Indians, Gold-seekers, and the Rush to Colorado* (Lawrence: University Press of Kansas, 1998). For North and South, see Eric Foner, *Reconstruction: America's Unfinished Revolution* (New York: W. W. Norton, 1988), and Edward Ayers, *The Promise of the New South: Life after Reconstruction* (New York: Oxford University Press, 1992).

70. Khalid Bloom, *Mississippi Valley's Great Yellow Fever Epidemic of 1878* (Baton Rouge: Louisiana State University Press, 1993).

71. William H. Allen, "The Rise of the National Board of Health," *Annals of the American Academy of Political and Social Science* 15 (1900): 61.

72. Ibid., 66.

73. Ibid., 67.

74. Ibid.

75. Ibid., 68.

76. John Hunter Pope, "The Condition of the Mexican Population of Western Texas in Its Relation to Public Health," in *Public Health Papers and Reports*, vol. 6, ed. American Public Health Association (Boston: Franklin Press, Rand and Avery, 1881), 159.

77. Making the tropical world safe for white northerners—for American and European colonial administrators—animated much of nineteenth-century colonial politics. Philip D. Curtin, *Death by Migration: Europe's Encounter with the Tropi-*

cal World in the Nineteenth Century (New York: Cambridge University Press, 1989), 1–39. For the Anglo-centered reforms in India, see Mark Harrison, *Public Health in British India: Anglo-Indian Preventive Medicine, 1859–1914* (New York: Cambridge University Press, 1994), 3–7. Jo Ann Carrigan said as much in *The Saffron Scourge: A History of Yellow Fever in Louisiana, 1796–1905* (Lafayette: Center for Louisiana Studies, University of Southwestern Louisiana, 1994), 82–96. John Ellis argued that public health reforms emphasized the importance of keeping cross-regional commerce safe from the vagaries of southern diseases. John Ellis, "Businessmen and Public Health in the Urban South during the Nineteenth Century: New Orleans, Memphis, and Atlanta," *Bulletin of the History of Medicine* 44, no. 3 (1977): 197–212, 346–71. Margaret Humphreys emphasized the signal importance of yellow fever to the early prominence of southern state health officers after Reconstruction. Humphreys, *Yellow Fever and the South.*

78. The perception of racial difference and relative immunity framed much of the debate over yellow fever.

79. Pope, "The Condition of the Mexican Population," 158.

80. Ibid., 158.

81. Agrippa N. Bell, "The Relations of Certain Filth Diseases to Cold Weather: Pneumonia, Diphtheria, Croup and Measles," *Public Health Papers and Reports* 7 (1881): 154–57.

82. Pope, "The Condition of the Mexican Population," 158. As far as I can tell, Pope used perceptions of property ownership and education, not citizenship, to draw distinctions between upper- and lower-class Mexicans in the region.

83. Ibid., 159. A *jacal* should refer to huts with wooden walls and straw roofs. However, Anglos in Texas used the term to refer to any Mexican working-class residence.

84. Ibid., 160.

85. Ibid., 162.

86. Arnoldo de León and Kenneth Stewart, *Tejanos and the Numbers Game: A Socio-Historical Interpretation of the Federal Censuses, 1850–1900* (Albuquerque: University of New Mexico Press, 1989), 3–9. De León and Stewart argue that urban centers like Brownsville, Laredo, and San Antonio were the main locations of Mexican population growth and that this growth came from the settlement of previously rural migrants in urban areas.

87. The term comes from Curtin, *Death by Migration.*

88. Marcos Cueto, *El regreso de las epidemias: Salud y sociedad en el Perú del siglo XX* (Lima: Instituto de Estudios Peruanos, 1997), esp. chap. 5. See Miguel Bustamante, *La fiebre amarilla en México y su origen en América*, Monografía Numero 2 (Mexico City: Secretaria de Salubridad y Asistencia: Instituto de Salubridad y Enfermedades Tropicales, 1958).

89. Aviva Chomsky, *West Indian Workers and the United Fruit Company in Costa Rica, 1870–1940* (Baton Rouge: Louisiana State University Press, 1997), 89–109.

90. Christine Stansell, *City of Women: Sex and Class in New York, 1789–1860* (Urbana: University of Illinois Press, 1988); Timothy Gilfoyle, *City of Eros: New York City, Prostitution, and the Commercialization of Sex, 1750–1920* (New York: W. W. Norton, 1994).

91. Pope, "The Condition of the Mexican Population," 162.

92. Ibid.

93. Ibid. "Good virus" refers to wet or dry vaccine lymph that is in good enough condition to bring on an immune response after vaccination.

94. Ibid., 163.

95. Ibid.

96. Ibid.

97. Ibid., 159.

98. Ibid., 163.

99. Thomas Ochiltree, "Quarantine Must Be Maintained, 9.23.1882," in *Annual Report of the Supervising Surgeon General of the USMHS for the Year of 1882* (Washington, D.C.: Government Printing Office, 1883), 282. Evidently, this appeal helped him win a seat in the Forty-eighth Congress (1883–1885) as an independent representative from Galveston. Born in Alabama, he was a Texas Ranger, a colonel in the Confederacy, and a prisoner of the Union Army. Ochiltree also supported Grant's candidacy in 1868 and stood publicly for the "fair" treatment of freedpeople. From 1870 to 1902, he spent a great deal of time promoting Texas to British and European investors in his work as advocate for the cable, telegraph, and mining interests of J. W. Mackay. See Texas State Historical Association, "Ochiltree, Thomas P.," in The Online Handbook of Texas, www.tshaonline.org/handbook/online/articles/foco1 (accessed February 22, 2012).

100. "Threatened Scourge: Fears That Yellow Fever May Become Epidemic in Texas," *Washington Post*, August 10, 1882, 1.

101. Newspaper headline cited in Bess Furman and Ralph C. Williams, *A Profile of the USPHS, 1798–1848* (Washington, D.C.: Government Printing Office, 1973), 186.

102. Margaret Warner, "Local Control versus National Interest: The Debate over Southern Public Health," *Journal of Southern History* 50, no. 3 (August 1984): 407–28.

103. Foner, *Reconstruction*, 211.

104. R. M. Swearingen, "Possible Yellow Fever Case in Brownsville," August 7, 1882, Papers of the Collection of Governor Oran Milo Roberts, TSAL; "Austin: Telegraph from Brownsville," *San Antonio Express*, August 8, 1882, 1.

105. "Corpus Christi: Citizens Organize," *San Antonio Express*, August 9, 1882, 1.

106. Charles Fowler, "Who Should I Believe about Yellow Fever in Brownsville? Is It Actually Yellow Fever?," August 15, 1882, Papers of the Governor Oran Milo Roberts, Texas State Archives and Library (TSAL), Austin.

107. "Austin: Corpus Christi Mayor Requests Quarantine," *San Antonio Express*, August 13, 1882, 1.

108. "Austin: Quarantine Proclamation," *San Antonio Express*, August 14, 1882, 1.

109. Jo Ann Carrigan discussed the motivation the residents of rural towns had in "shotgun" quarantines. Based on fragmentary evidence, town residents would be more likely to know someone with yellow fever than the statistics that dramatized deaths in urban areas. She coupled this fear with a distrust and resentment of city mores and dominant economic position vis-à-vis rural economies. Carrigan, *The Saffron Scourge*, 149–54, 163–66.

110. Fowler, "Who Should I Believe about Yellow Fever."

111. R. M. Swearingen, "I Am Now in Quarantine in Rio Grande City," August 16, 1882, Papers of Governor Oran Milo Roberts, TSAL.

112. R. M. Swearingen, "I Am Now in Roma," August 21, 1882, Papers of Governor Oran Milo Roberts, TSAL.

113. Porfirio Benavides, "Dr. Swearingen Released under Protest," August 23, 1882, Papers of Governor Oran Milo Roberts, TSAL.

114. Ibid.

115. A. P. Tugwell, "The Boat Is Threatened by an Armed Mob. My Life Is in Danger," August 23, 1882, Papers of Governor Oran Milo Roberts, TSAL.

116. James Luby, "Starr County Quarantine against Brownsville," August 12, 1882, Papers of Governor Oran Milo Roberts, TSAL.

117. A. G. Bordin, "Re: Establishing Quarantine at the Nueces River at the Three Ferries," August 14, 1882, Papers of Governor Oran Milo Roberts, TSAL.

118. Thomas Hickey, "We Have Quarantined against Brownsville, the Rio Grande and All Mexican Ports on the Gulf," August 18, 1882, Papers of Governor Oran Milo Roberts, TSAL.

119. H. F. French, "USMHS Will Pay Expenses in Brownsville and Quarantine Guards," August 19, 1882, Papers of Governor Oran Milo Roberts, TSAL.

120. Howard Atwood Kelly, "Robert Drake Murray," *A Cyclopaedia of American Medical Biography, Comprising the Lives of Eminent Deceased Physicians and Surgeons, 1610–1910* (Philadelphia: W. B. Sanders, 1912), 209–10.

121. Ford Dixon, "Roberts, Oran Milo," in Texas State Historical Association, The Online Handbook of Texas, www.tshaonline.org/handbook/online/articles/fro18 (accessed August 26, 2011).

122. John Hamilton, "The Mexican-Texas Yellow Fever Epidemic," *Annual Report of the Supervising Surgeon General, USMHS, Department of the Treasury for the Fiscal Year of 1882* (Washington, D.C.: Government Printing Office, 1883), 310–45.

123. E. H. Goodrich, "Telegram 8.11.1882," in *Preliminary Report on the Yellow Fever Epidemic of 1882 in the State of Texas* (Washington, D.C.: Government Printing Office, 1883), USMHS, Department of the Treasury File Document no. 341, RG 90, NC 34, Entry 11.1, NAB.

124. Ibid.

125. Ibid.

126. Arthur E. Spohn, "Report on Preliminary Cordon. 08/22/1882," RG 90, USPHS Central Files, NC 34, Entry 11.1, Correspondence with Southern Quarantine Camps, Box 150, NACP.

127. Ibid.

128. Ibid.

129. Hart, *Empire and Revolution*, 87.

130. Murray, "The Mexican-Texas Epidemic," 296.

131. Ibid.

132. According to John Hart, James Stillman—the son of Charles Stillman, the owner of the Kenedy Ranch—had controlling interest in the steamship line connecting Tampico to Bagdad, the Monterrey & Mexican Gulf Railroad, and the Kenedy Ranch. His financial decisions led to the capital investments that restructured South Texas, yet again. See Hart, *Empire and Revolution*, 81–91.

133. Murray, "The Mexican-Texas Epidemic," 296.

134. R. H. Wood, "Due to Considerable Mexican Population, We Urge Quarantine," August 11, 1882, Papers of Governor Oran Milo Roberts, TSAL.

135. Ibid.

136. August Spohn, "Report on the Corpus-Christi Laredo Cordon," in *Annual Report of the Supervising Surgeon General, 1882*, 335.

137. Robert Murray, "Citizens Organize against Yellow Fever," *San Antonio Express*, August 10, 1882, 1.

138. Arthur E. Spohn, "Quarantine Guards Needed, 9/16/1882," RG 90, USPHS Central Files, NC 34, Entry 11.1, Correspondence with Southern Quarantine Camps, Box 150, NACP.

139. Ibid.

140. Andrés Tijerina, *Tejano Empire: Life on the South Texas Ranchos* (College Station: Texas A&M University Press, 1998), 91–107.

141. Montejano, *Anglos and Mexicans*, 50–75.

142. "Austin" (telegraph), *Dallas Herald*, October 10, 1881.

143. Cecil Kirk Hutson, "Texas Fever in Kansas, 1863–1930," *Agricultural History* 68, no. 1 (winter 1994): 74–106.

144. E. Wheeler (Special Office, Customs), "Supplemental Payroll for Quarantine Guards for the Month of August, 1882," RG 90, USPHS, Entry 11, Correspondence with Southern Quarantine Camps, Box 150, NACP.

145. Ibid. Only one of the nearly one hundred Corpus Christi residents or King Ranch hands Spohn employed as quarantine guards carried an ethnic Mexican surname. Miguel Solis, a forty-two-year-old laborer for the Rancho Kineño (King Ranch) was lucky to find employment to help maintain his wife and three children, two of whom were counted as shepherds.

146. For the concept of illegality, see Nicholas De Genova, *Working the Boundaries:*

Race, Space, and "Illegality" in Mexican Chicago (Durham: Duke University Press, 2005), 276.

147. Joanna Nicolls, "The United States Marine Hospital Service: Something of Its History, Work, and Officers," *Frank Leslie's Popular Monthly* 44 (1897): 282–96, esp. 276.

148. Ibid., 276.

149. For a discussion of the medical origins of the border patrol at the end of the Mexican revolution, see Alexandra Minna Stern, "Nationalism on the Line: Masculinity, Race, and the Creation of the U.S. Border Patrol," in Truett and Young, *Continental Crossroads*, 299–324. For the close connection between the Rangers and large property holders in Texas, see Andrew Graybill, *Policing the Frontier: Rangers, Mounties, and the North American Frontier* (Lincoln: University of Nebraska Press, 2007).

150. W. C. Fisher, "Report," *Annual Report of the Supervising Surgeon General for 1882*, 323–24.

151. Augustus E. Spohn, "Report," *Annual Report of the Supervising Surgeon General for 1882*, 335.

152. Robert Drake Murray was born in Ohlton, Ohio, in 1845. He enlisted in the U.S. Army at sixteen and fought in Cedar Mountain, Virginia, and Antietam. He was honorably discharged in November 1862 for a rifle wound. He reenlisted, was wounded four times, and spent four months as a prisoner of war. After the war, he started medical school, finally graduating from Jefferson Medical College in 1871. The USMHS offered him an assistant surgeonship in 1872. He served in all the major yellow fever ports through 1903, until he died from injuries in Laredo during the 1903 yellow fever epidemic. His reports on the 1875 Key West epidemic show a great deal of sympathy with the local Hispanos and Latin Americans in these borderlands regions. Henry Wilson, *Itinerary of the Seventh Ohio Volunteer Infantry* (New York: Neale Publishing Company, 1907), 477–78.

153. Thomas Carson, "Destitution by Quarantine, 8.17.1882," *Preliminary Report on the Yellow Fever Epidemic of 1882 in the State of Texas* (Washington, D.C.: Government Printing Office, 1883), USMHS, Department of the Treasury File Document No. 341, RG 90, Entry 11.1, NAB, p. 14.

154. John B. Hamilton, "08/26/1882. Department Cannot Feed Any Except Sick," *Preliminary Report on the Yellow Fever Epidemic of 1882 in the State of Texas* (Washington, D.C.: Government Printing Office, 1883), USMHS, Department of the Treasury File Document No. 341, RG 90, Entry 11.1, NAB.

155. "Open Air Free Grocery," *San Antonio Express*, September 10, 1882, 2. Robert Murray, "No English Doctors Needed," *Preliminary Report on the Yellow Fever Epidemic of 1882 in the State of Texas* (Washington, D.C.: Government Printing Office, 1883), USMHS, Department of the Treasury File Document no. 341, RG 90, Entry 11.1, NAB.

156. Murray, "The Mexican-Texas Epidemic," 297.

157. Ibid., 296.

158. Ibid.

159. Amy Dru Stanley, *From Bondage to Contract: Wage Labor, Marriage, and the Market in the Age of Slave Emancipation* (New York: Cambridge University Press, 1998), 60–96. This understanding of contract comes from two sections in this book, "The Labor Question and the Sale of Self" and "Beggars Can't Be Choosers," on the rise of vagrancy laws in Massachusetts and other self-styled bastions of contract freedom in the northeastern United States.

160. Murray, "The Mexican-Texas Epidemic," 297.

161. Ibid., 298.

162. Bloomberg and Raphael gave future Mexican revolutionary Catarino Garza his first accounting position. See Garza, "La lógica de los hechos" (1890), 42, Nettie Lee Benson Rare Books Collection and Library, Austin, Tex.

163. This is from one of the more fascinating documents from this epidemic, an article from the *New York World* on September 7, 1882, reprinted in the *San Antonio Express* on September 17, 1882, 1.

164. G. Klein, "Two Hundred Dollar Check Drawn on Hanover National Bank," October 11, 1882, Papers of Governor Oran Milo Roberts, TSAL.

165. "Mexicans and the Free Grocery," *San Antonio Express*, September 20, 1882, 1.

166. Murray, "The Mexican-Texas Epidemic," 297.

167. Robert Murray, "9.22.1882. Letter to Deputy Collector, Sam Stewart, Rio Grande City," *Annual Report of the Supervising Surgeon General, USMHS, Department of the Treasury for the Fiscal Year of 1882* (Washington, D.C.: Government Printing Office, 1883), 285.

168. Ibid.

169. "Squabble in Brownsville," *San Antonio Express*, September 19, 1882, 1.

170. Ibid.

171. T. Carson, "Since Disease Has Run Its Course, Quarantine Should Not Be Sustained," September 20, 1882, Papers of Governor Oran Milo Roberts, TSAL.

172. Robert Murray, "9.20.1882 Guard Arrested for Stopping Ferry," *Annual Report of the Supervising Surgeon General, USMHS, Department of the Treasury for the Fiscal Year of 1882* (Washington, D.C.: Government Printing Office, 1883), 283.

173. A. Brito, "We Fear Our Excited Populace Cannot Be Contained from Forcing Quarantine," September 20, 1882, Papers of Governor Oran Milo Roberts, TSAL.

174. E. H. Goodrich, "920.1882. Quarantine Guards Arrested by City Authorities," *Annual Report of the Supervising Surgeon General, Department of the Treasury for the Fiscal Year of 1882* (Washington, D.C.: Government Printing Office, 1883), 283.

175. Robert Murray, "9.20.1882. City Full of Matamoros People," *Annual Report of the Supervising Surgeon General, USMHS, Department of the Treasury for the Fiscal Year of 1882* (Washington, D.C.: Government Printing Office, 1883), 283.

176. "Brownsville—Great Indignation," *San Antonio Express*, September 20, 1882, 1.

177. Murray, "9.20.1882. City Full of Matamoros People."

178. Ibid.

179. Robert Murray, Surgeon, and C. B. Combe, Health Officer, "9.19.1882. Guarding of River Will Prevent Ingress of Paupers and New Material," *Annual Report of the Supervising Surgeon General, USMHS, Department of the Treasury for the Fiscal Year of 1882* (Washington, D.C.: Government Printing Office, 1883), 283.

180. Ibid.

181. Brito, "We Fear Our Excited Populace Cannot Be Contained."

182. "Mayor Carson Downed," *San Antonio Express*, September 26, 1882, 1.

183. Robert Murray, "9.20.1882. Forcible Breaking of Quarantine," *Annual Report of the Supervising Surgeon General for 1882*, 283; Murray, "9.20.1882. City Full of Matamoros People," 283.

184. Robert Murray. "9.22.1882. Letter to Deputy Collector, Sam Stewart, Rio Grande City," *Annual Report of the Supervising Surgeon General, USMHS, Department of the Treasury for the Fiscal Year of 1882* (Washington, D.C.: Government Printing Office, 1883), 285.

185. Murray, "9.21.1882. Ferry Traffic," *Annual Report of the Supervising Surgeon General for 1882*, 284.

186. Ibid.

187. Fitzhugh Mullan, *Plagues and Politics: The Story of the United States Public Health Service* (New York: Basic Books, 1989), 22.

188. O. M. Roberts, "My Written Opinion on the Efficacy of the Cordon," in *Annual Report, 1882* (Washington, D.C.: Government Printing Office, 1883), 55.

189. Bess Furman, *A Profile of the USPHS, 1798–1848* (Washington, D.C.: Government Printing Office, 1973), 186.

190. Nicolls, "The United States Marine Hospital Service," 291.

191. Jovita Gonzalez, *Life on the Border: A Landmark Tejana Thesis* (Houston: Arte Publico Press, 2006), 74.

192. U.S. Census, *Twelfth Census of the United States*, Table 34, 783–89.

193. "Threatened Scourge," *Washington Post*, August 10, 1882, 1.

194. Murray, "The Mexican-Texas Epidemic," 271.

195. John B. Hamilton, "Preliminary Report on the Yellow Fever Epidemic of 1882 in the State of Texas" (Washington, D.C.: Government Printing Office, 1882), 4, USMHS: Department of the Treasury Document No. 341, RG 90, USPHS, NC 34, Entry 11.1, Correspondence with Southern Quarantine Camps, NAB.

196. Ibid.

197. Garza, "La lógica de los hechos," 47 (my translation).

198. Ibid.

199. For a comprehensive look at Garza's career, see Elliott Young, *Catarino Garza's Revolution on the Texas-Mexico Border* (Durham: Duke University Press, 2004).

200. Kelly, "Robert Drake Murray," 209–10.

Two. The Promise of Progress

1. Bell, A. N. "Proceedings of the Tenth Annual Meeting," *American Public Health Association Reports and Papers* 8 (1882): 262.

2. Jose María Reyes, "Higiene pública: Cuatro palabras sobre las cuarentenas," in *Gaceta médica: Periódico de la academia de medicina de México*, Academia de Medicina de Mexico (Mexico City: Imprenta de Miguel Escalante, 1883), 9.

3. Hamilton, "Preliminary Report on the Yellow Fever Epidemic of 1882," 310–45.

4. Shah, *Contagious Divides*, 5.

5. For medical identity see Warner, *The Therapeutic Perspective*. For Koch's postulates in American culture, see Susan Lederer, *Subjected to Science: Human Experimentation in American before the Second World War* (Baltimore: Johns Hopkins University Press, 1995).

6. Mullan, *Plagues and Politics*, 35, 36, 37; Cliff, *Deciphering Global Epidemics*, xxiii, 53–55.

7. Cliff, *Deciphering Global Epidemics*, xxiii, 53–55.

8. Bert Hansen, "New Images of a Medicine: Visual Evidence for the Widespread Popularity of Therapeutic Discoveries in America after 1885," *Bulletin of the History of Medicine* 73, no. 4 (1999): 629–78.

9. Martin S. Pernick, "Eugenics and Public Health in American History," *American Journal of Public Health* 87, no. 11 (1997): 1767–72; Evelynn Hammonds, *Childhood's Deadly Scourge: The Campaign to Control Diphtheria in New York City, 1880–1930* (Baltimore: Johns Hopkins University Press, 1998).

10. "Surgeon John Guiteras Reports on Yellow Fever in Veracruz, Mexico," *New Orleans Republican*, Caja 28, Expediente 40, GD 3000, Relaciones Exteriores, Siglo XIX, Consulado de New Orleans, AGN.

11. Mariola Espinosa, "The Threat from Havana: Southern Public Health, Yellow Fever, and the U.S. Intervention in the Cuban Struggle for Independence, 1878–1989," *Journal of Southern History* 72, no. 3 (August 2006): 541–68.

12. Sánchez, *Becoming Mexican American*, 19–23.

13. Cyrus Edson, "The Microbe as Social Leveler," *North American Review* 161, no. 467 (October 1895): 421–30.

14. Ibid., 423.

15. Nancy Tomes, *The Gospel of Germs: Men, Women, and the Microbe in American Life* (Cambridge: Harvard University Press, 1998), 206.

16. See Alexander Keyssar, *The Right to Vote: The Contested History of Democracy in the United States* (New York: Basic Books, 2000), esp. 79–171. The 1890s, in his analysis, marked the high point of voting restriction.

17. For the southern politics of restriction, see Ayers, *The Promise of the New South*, esp. 35–53.

18. For local campaigns around *Plessy*, see Rebecca Scott, *Degrees of Freedom:*

Louisiana and Cuba after Slavery (Cambridge: Harvard University Press, 2005). For a Supreme Court–based account of this process, see Lawrence Goldstone Jr., *Inherently Unequal: The Betrayal of Equal Rights by the Supreme Court, 1865–1903* (New York: Walker & Company, 2011).

19. See *Lochner v. New York*, 198 U.S. 45 (1905).

20. Nell Painter, *Standing at Armageddon: A Grassroots History of the Progressive Era* (New York: W. W. Norton, 2008).

21. For the northern border, see Melissa L. Meyer, *The White Earth Tragedy: Ethnicity and Dispossession at a Minessota Annishinaabe Reservation* (Lincoln: University of Nebraska Press, 1999). For Salt Lake and the Great Basin, see Ned Blackhawk, *Violence over the Land: Indians and Empires in the Early American West* (Cambridge: Harvard University Press, 2008). For Texas, see Pekka Hammalainen, *The Comanche Empire* (New Haven: Yale University Press, 2008).

22. An Act to Provide for the Allotment of Lands in Severalty to Indians on the Various Reservations (General Allotment Act or Dawes Act), Statutes at Large 24, 388–91, NADP Document A1887, www.ourdocuments.gov/doc.php?flash=old&doc=50 (accessed November 2, 2010).

23. For a drastic example of the ways members of an Indian Nation negotiated the Dawes Act see Melissa Meyer, "'We cannot get a living as we used to': Dispossession and the White Earth Anishinaabeg, 1889–1920," *American Historical Review* 96, no. 2 (1991): 368–95.

24. Russell Thornton, *American Indian Holocaust and Survival: A Population History since 1492* (Norman: University of Oklahoma Press, 1987), esp. 91–134. Gregory Ellis Smoak, *Ghost Dances and Identity: Prophetic Religion and American Indian Identity* (Berkeley: University of California Press, 2008), esp. 154–71.

25. John Gregory Bourke, "The American Congo," *Scribner's Magazine* 15 (May 1894): 590–610.

26. Mauricio Tenorio-Trillo, *Mexico at the World's Fair: Crafting a Modern Nation, 1876–1911*, New Historicism: Studies in Cultural Poetics (Berkeley: University of California Press, 1996), 141–55; Claudia Agostoni, *Monuments of Progress: Modernization and Public Health in Mexico City, 1876–1910* (Boulder: University of Colorado Press, 2003).

27. Alex Saragoza, *The Monterrey Elite and the Mexican State, 1910–1940* (Austin: University of Texas Press, 1990); Juan Mora-Torres, *The Making of the Mexican Border: The State, Capitalism, and Society in Nuevo León, 1848–1910* (Austin: University of Texas Press, 2001); Margarita Larrazolo, *Coahuila 1893: Una respuesta a la centralización política* (México: Instituto Nacional de Estudios Históricos de la Revolución Mexicana), 1997.

28. Claudia Agostoni, *Monuments of Progress: Modernization and Public Health in Mexico City, 1876–1910,* (Boulder: University of Colorado Press, 2003), esp. 117–55.

29. Paul Ross, "Mexico's Superior Health Council and the American Public Health Association: The Transnational Archive of Porfirian Public Health, 1887–1910," *Hispanic American Historical Review* 89, no. 4 (2009): 573–603.

30. John Coatsworth, *Growth against Development: The Economic Impact of Railroads in Porfirian Mexico* (DeKalb: Northern Illinois University Press, 1981).

31. Delia Salazar Anaya, ed., *Xenofobia y Xenofilia en Mexico del Siglo XIX y XX* (Mexico City: SEP INAH, 2006). See also Teresa Alfaro Velckamp, *So Far from Allah, So Close to Mexico: Middle Eastern Immigrants in Modern Mexico* (Austin: University of Texas Press, 2007).

32. For a wide overview based in records in Gobernación in Mexico City, see Jonathan Brown, "Trabajadores nativos y extranjeros en el Mexico Porfiriano," *Siglo XIX: Cuadernos de Historia* 3, no. 9 (1994): 7–49. For Chinese laborers in Mexico, see Evelynn Hu-deHart, *At America's Gates: Chinese Immigration during the Exclusion Era* (Chapel Hill: University of North Carolina Press, 2003), 151–86. For Korean workers, see Richard S. Kim, *Quest for Statehood: Korean Immigrant Nationalism and U.S. Sovereignty, 1905–1945,* (New York: Oxford University Press, 2011), 26–45.

33. Raul Perez Lopez Portillo, *Una historia breve de Mexico* (Mexico City: Ediciones Silex, 2002), 195. See also Hector Diaz Zermeno, *Mexico: De la reforma y el imperio* (Mexico: Unam, 2005), 289.

34. Justo Cardenas, "Nuevo Leon cientifico: La viruela y la vacuna," *La Colonia Mexicana* (Laredo), May 6, 1891, 1.

35. Ibid.

36. Ibid.

37. Ibid.

38. Justo Cardenas, "Medios higienicos de prevenir la viruela y su propagacion," *El Correo de Laredo*, August 18, 1891, 1–2.

39. Ibid.

40. Tomes, *Gospel of Germs*, 48–67.

41. Frederick Jackson Turner, "The Significance of the Frontier in American Life," www .learner.org/workshops/primarysources/corporations/docs/turner.html (accessed March 6, 2012).

42. Faustino Sarmiento, *Facundo, or Civilization and Barbarism* (New York: Penguin, 1998), xv–xvii, 12, 21–24. The first American edition was *Life in the Argentine Republic in the Time of the Tyrants, or Civilization and Barbarism* (New York: Hurd and Houston, 1868). The earliest publication date in the Nettie Lee Benson Library is Domingo Faustino Sarmiento, *Civilización y barbarie: I aspect fisico, costumbres y ábitos de la Republica Arjentina* (Santiago: Imprenta del Progreso, 1845). The first volume in Spanish published in the United States was *Facundo* (New York: William Jackson, 1900).

43. The literature on modern ideology and the Porfiriato is vast. For a good overview, see Charles Hale, *The Transformation of Liberalism in Late Nineteenth-Century*

Mexico (Princeton: Princeton University Press, 1990). For an overview of the culture of modernity in Mexico, see William French and Robert Buffington, "The Culture of Modernity," in *The Oxford History of Mexico*, ed. William Beezly (New York: Oxford University Press, 2000), 397–431.

44. See John Kenneth Turner, *Barbarous Mexico* (Austin: University of Texas Press, 1984).

45. See Young, *Catarino Garza's Revolution*, 81, 86, 88, 92, 95, 202, 205.

46. See ibid. See also Elliott Young, "Imagining Alternative Modernities: Ignacio Martinez' Travel Narratives," in Truett and Young, *Continental Crossroads*, 151–81.

47. Young, "Imagining Alternative Modernities."

48. Justo Cardenas, "Nuevo Leon cientifico: La viruela y la vacuna," *La Colonia Mexicana* (Laredo, Tex.), May 6, 1891, 1.

49. Bourke, "The American Congo," 590–610. For an extended discussion of the ways middle- and working-class Tejanos, Mexicans, and Mexican Americans mobilized in Texas to gain the benefits of progress, see Zamora, *The World of the Mexican Worker in Texas*.

50. T. J. Bennett, "Report at APHA: R. M. Swearingen on 'the Sanitary Relations between Texas and Mexico,'" *Texas Sanitarian* 2, no. 2 (1892): 68–69.

51. Ibid.

52. Ibid.

53. Ibid.

54. Ross, "Mexico's Superior Health Council," 573–603.

55. Bennett, "Report at APHA."

56. Bennet, "Report at APHA," 68.

57. Tenorio-Trillo, *Mexico at the World's Fair*.

58. Agostoni, *Monuments of Progress*.

59. Ross, "Mexico's Superior Health Council."

60. Bennett, "Report at APHA."

61. Ibid., 68.

62. For a sober look at clean hands, see Atul Gawande, *Better: A Surgeon's Notes on Performance* (New York: Metropolitan Books, 2007), 13–27.

63. W. M. Yandell, "Contagious Diseases on the Rio Grande Border," *Texas Sanitarian* 2, no. 2 (1892): 63.

64. Ibid.

65. Ibid.

66. U.S. Bureau of the Census, *Twelfth Census of the United States Taken in the Year 1900*, vol. 2, ed. Charles Merriam (New York: Norman Ross, 1997), 521–28.

67. Young, *Catarino Garza's Revolution*.

68. Ibid.

69. Leiker, *Racial Borders*.

70. Ross, "Mexico's Superior Health Council," 589.

71. Irving A. Watson, "The Republic of Mexico—Medicine Curative and Preventive," *Sanitarian* 29 (July–December 1892): 122. The quote comes from Ross, "Mexico's Superior Health Council," 574.

72. Bennett, "Report at APHA."

73. Ibid.

74. Texas established its first statewide compulsory vaccination statute in 1923. The Supreme Court decided that compulsory vaccination statutes were legal in Texas in *Zucht v. King*, 260 U.S. 174 (1922).

75. Bennett, "Report at APHA," 69.

76. Ibid., 68.

77. Humphreys, *Yellow Fever and the South*.

78. R. M. Swearingen, "The Sanitary Relations of Texas and Mexico, and the Official Correspondence Relating Thereto," *Public Health Papers and Reports* 18 (1892): 323. Source comes from Ross, "Mexico's Superior Health Council."

79. T. J. Bennett, "The Health System of Texas," *Texas Sanitarian* 2, no. 2 (1892): 31. See also Robert M. Swearingen, "Please Exempt Me from Restrictions in Your Quarantine Proclamation," August 17, 1882, in Papers of Governor Oran Milo Roberts, TSAL.

80. Bennett, "The Health System of Texas," 32.

81. Ibid.

82. T. J. Bennett, "State vs. National Control of Quarantines," *Texas Sanitarian* 2, no. 5 (1893): 165.

83. Ibid., 164.

84. T. J. Bennett, "The National Sin of Omission," *Transactions of the Texas State Medical Association* (1894): 291–97.

85. Bennett, "The Health System of Texas," 32–33.

86. Bennett, "The National Sin of Omission," 291–92.

87. T. J. Bennett, "The Necessity of a National Bacteriological Institute," *Texas Sanitarian* 2, no. 2 (1892): 136.

88. E. Liceaga, "Defense of the Ports and Frontier Cities of Mexico against the Epidemic of Cholera That Invaded Europe and Was on the Point of Invading the United States This Year," *Texas Sanitarian* 2, no. 2 (1892): 58.

89. Ibid., 51.

90. Michael Meyer and William Sherman, *The Course of Mexican History* (New York: Oxford University Press, 2010), 446.

91. Liceaga, "Defense of Ports," 51.

92. Ibid.

93. Ibid.

94. Bennett discussed Eduardo Liceaga's proposal to prevent any person diagnosed with tuberculosis from getting married. See Bennett, "The National Sin of Omission," 291.

95. Stern and Markel, "Which Face? Whose Nation?"

96. William Yandell, "Contagious Diseases on the Rio Grande Border," *Texas Sanitarian* 2, no. 2 (1892): 63.

Three. The Appearance of Progress

1. William Ellis, "Arrivals in Tlahualilo," February 25, 1895, House of Representatives Doc. (H.R. Doc.) No. 169, NAB, p. 50.

2. Ibid.

3. The journey south has absorbed historians of various stripes over the last ninety years. See J. Fred Rippy, "A Negro Colonization Project in Mexico, 1895," *Journal of Negro History* 6, no. 1 (1921): 66–73. For a meditation on the many meanings Mexico and this labor recruitment project held for African Americans in the nineteenth-century United States, see Karl Jacoby, "Between North and South: The Alternative Borderlands of William Ellis and the African American Colony of 1895," in Truett and Young, *Continental Crossroads*, 209–39.

4. Mullan, *Plagues and Politics*, 35–37.

5. Cliff, *Deciphering Global Epidemics*, xxiii, 53–55.

6. Markel, *Quarantine!*, 9.

7. Tomes, *Gospel of Germs*, 5–18. See Fairchild, *Science at the Borders*, 3–11.

8. George Magruder, "Report on the Establishment and Administration of Camp Jenner, Eagle Pass, TX," *Weekly Abstract of Sanitary Reports* 10, no. 45 (October 25, 1895): 957–59.

9. For a discussion of the medical gaze and the disciplining of mostly European and Asian migrant bodies, see Fairchild, *Science at the Borders*, 83–117, 190–249. On racialized African American segregation and the ideology of germ theory, see John Cell, *The Highest Stage of White Supremacy: The Origins of Segregation in South Africa and the American South* (Cambridge: Cambridge University Press, 1982); Tera Hunter, *To 'Joy My Freedom: Black Southern Women's Lives and Labor in the South after the Civil War* (Cambridge: Harvard University Press, 1996), 187–219; Samuel Roberts, *Infectious Fear: Politics, Disease, and the Health Effects of Segregation* (Chapel Hill: University of North Carolina Press, 2008).

10. Compare this to the 16-day individual detentions and the 352 patients treated in the three different USMHS camps in Birmingham, Alabama, in 1898. Michael Willrich, *Pox: an American History* (New York: Penguin, 2011), 68.

11. On the West Coast, Chinese migrants and Asian Americans challenged the anti-Asian dimensions of urban quarantine policies. See Lucy Salyer, *Laws Harsh as Tigers: Chinese Immigrants and the Shaping of Modern Immigration Law* (Chapel Hill: University of North Carolina Press, 1995). See also Shah, *Contagious Divides*, and Molina, *Fit to Be Citizens*. In the South, state boards of health openly challenged the USMHS prerogative to declare yellow fever quarantines on their key seaports. However, movement across the Mexican border turned these national challenges into transnational disputes.

12. Sanchez, *Becoming Mexican American,* 38–62.

13. William K. Meyers, "Politics, Vested Rights, and Economic Growth in Porfirian Mexico: The Company Tlahualilo in the Comarca Lagunera," *Hispanic American Historical Review* 57, no. 3 (1977): 435.

14. Karl Jacoby, "From Plantation to Hacienda: The Mexican Colonization Movement in Alabama," *Alabama Heritage,* no. 35 (1995): 34–43.

15. There are two exemplary monographs that treat this nineteenth-century migration: Nell Painter, *Exodusters: Black Migration to Kansas after Reconstruction* (New York: W. W. Norton, 1992), and Edwin Redkey, *Black Exodus: Black Nationalist and Back-to-Africa Movements, 1890–1910* (New Haven: Yale University Press, 1970).

16. "Special correspondent, Ciudad Porfirio Díaz," *San Antonio Express,* July 26, 1895, 4.

17. For a general portrait, see William K. Meyers, *Forge of Progress: Popular Politics in the Comarca Lagunera, 1880–1920* (Albuquerque: University of New Mexico Press, 1991). For the individual transactions, see Jacoby, "Between North and South," 215.

18. William K. Meyers, "La Comarca Lagunera: Work, Protest, and Popular Mobilization in North Central Mexico," in *Other Mexicos: Essays on Regional Mexican History, 1876–1911,* ed. Thomas Benjamin and William McNeelie, 243–74 (Albuquerque: University of New Mexico Press, 1984).

19. Ibid.

20. Meyers, *Forge of Progress,* 51.

21. Ibid.

22. Ibid.

23. "Compania Agricola Tlahualilo and William H. Ellis," 54th Cong., 1st sess., H.R. Doc. No. 169, p. 47. Judging by the congressional record and the newspaper accounts, administrative control seems to have shifted by 1885, not 1903, as claimed by Meyers in *Forge of Progress,* 51.

24. For a blow-by-blow portrait, see Alfred W. Reynolds, "The Alabama Negro Colony in Mexico, 1894–1896," *Alabama Review* 5, no. 4 (1952): 244–68.

25. Keith Wailoo, *Dying in the City of Blues: Sickle Cell Anemia and the Politics of Race and Health* (Chapel Hill: University of North Carolina Press, 2001), 9.

26. "Compania Agricola Tlahualilo and William H. Ellis," 54th Cong., 1st sess., H.R. Doc. No. 169, Enclosure 2 in No. 78, p. 46.

27. Ibid.

28. Pablo Piccato, *City of Suspects: Crime in Mexico City, 1900–1931* (Durham: Duke University Press, 2001), 67–72, especially the fear of working-class mestizo and indigenous residents of cities.

29. This recalls the passage in *Up from Slavery* where Washington writes, "My observations convinced me that workers were worse off at the end of the strike. Before the days of strikes, I knew miners who had plenty of savings in the bank, but as soon as the professional agitators got control, the savings of even the more thrifty

ones began to disappear." See Washington, *Up from Slavery* (New York: Bedford St. Martin's, 2002), 61.

30. *El Tiempo* (Mexico City), February 14, 1895. From Reynolds, "The Alabama Negro Colony," 260.

31. Ibid.

32. Ibid.

33. "Tuscaloosa Circular," in "Arrivals in Tlahualilo, February 25, 1895," 54th Cong., 1st sess., H.R. Doc. No. 169, 50.

34. Ibid.

35. For a direct discussion of free U.S. black settlement in Mexico before the Civil War, especially in Matamoros, Tamaulipas, see Rosalie Schwartz, *Across the Rio to Freedom: U.S. Negroes in Mexico* (El Paso: Texas Western Press, 1974). For Mexico as a possibility for emigration, see "Address of the Colored Convention," *Weekly Louisianan* (New Orleans), April 26, 1879. The possibility of emigration under Ellis's auspices had been in conversation in Alabama since 1889. See "Bill to Grant Concession," *Huntsville Gazette*, November 2, 1889, 2. See also Jacoby, "Between North and South."

36. R. Williams, "Arrivals in Tlahualilo, February 25, 1895," 54th Cong., 1st sess., H.R. Doc. No. 169, p. 50.

37. Ibid.

38. Ayers, *The Promise of the New South*, 154–58.

39. Ibid.

40. For an evocation of the life of women in a sharecropping household in the 1880s, see Jacqueline Jones, *Labor of Love, Labor of Sorrow: Black Women, Work, and the Family from Slavery to the Present* (New York: Basic Books, 2010).

41. Major Dwyer, 54th Cong., 1st sess., H.R. Doc. No. 169, Enclosure No. 12.

42. Mr. Sparks to Mr. Uhl, June 22, 1895, 54th Cong., 1st sess., H.R. Doc. No. 169, Enclosure No. 8, p. 7.

43. Ibid.

44. James Scott, *Weapons of the Weak: Everyday Forms of Peasant Resistance* (New Haven: Yale University Press, 1987).

45. The railroad manifest indicates the arrival of the four-member Claiborne family. Consular records indicate that Sam Claiborne petitioned Consul Burk in Chihuahua. Medical records in Camp Jenner indicate that Sam and Emma Claiborne, ages four and two, respectively, passed away in the camp. The 1913 telephone directory for Tuscaloosa, Alabama, noted that Sam Claiborne was a reverend and Emma Claiborne a schoolteacher.

46. Sam Claber deposition, May 21, 1895, 54th Cong., 1st sess., H.R. Doc. No. 169, Enclosure 12, p. 3.

47. Mr. Burke to Mr. Uhl, May 28, 1895 (received June 4, 1895), 54th Cong., 1st sess., H.R. Doc. No. 169, Enclosure 12, p. 2.

48. Ibid., 3.

49. Mr. Sparks to Mr. Uhl, June 22, 1895, 54th Cong., 1st sess., H.R. Doc. No. 169, Enclosure No. 8, p. 6. The numbers of fleeing colonists vary between depositions and news reports.

50. Mr. Bankhead to Mr. Olney, July 9, 1895, 54th Cong., 1st sess., H.R. Doc. No. 169, p. 10.

51. Ibid.

52. Mr. Watson to Mr. Bankhead, June 26, 1895, 54th Cong., 1st sess., H.R. Doc. No. 169, p. 11.

53. Ibid.

54. Ibid., 3.

55. C. Vann Woodward, *Tom Watson: Agrarian Rebel* (New York: Macmillan, 1938), 216–44.

56. Ibid.

57. Mr. Sparks to Mr. Uhl, June 21, 1895, 54th Cong., 1st sess., H.R. Doc. No. 169, p. 6.

58. Daniel Margolies, *Spaces of Law in American Foreign Relations: Extradition and Extraterritoriality in the Borderlands and Beyond* (Athens: University of Georgia Press, 2011), 5–28.

59. Ibid., 7.

60. 54th Cong., 1st sess., H.R. Doc. No. 169, p. 9.

61. Ibid.

62. "Tlahualilo," June 11, 1895, 54th Cong., 1st sess., H.R. Doc. No. 169, pp. 9–10.

63. Mr. Sparks to Mr. Uhl, July 20, 1895, 54th Cong., 1st sess., H.R. Doc. No. 169, p. 10.

64. Mr. Adee to Mr. Sparks, July 20, 1895, 54th Cong., 1st sess., H.R. Doc. No. 169, p. 11.

65. Ibid.

66. "Negroes Are in a Bad Fix: Numbers Have Breached the Mexican Border," *Houston Post*, July 26, 1895, 2.

67. Ibid.

68. "The Negroes in Mexico," *Houston Post*, July 22, 1895, 6.

69. Mr. Burke to Mr. Uhl, May 28, 1895 (received June 4, 1895), 54th Cong., 1st sess., H.R. Doc. No. 169, Enclosure No. 12, p. 2.

70. President Cleveland to Mr. Adee, July 26, 1895 54th Cong., 1st sess., H.R. Doc. No. 169, p. 13.

71. "The Negroes in Mexico," *Houston Post*, July 26, 1895, 6.

72. Saidiya V. Hartman, *Scenes of Subjection: Terror and Self-Making in Nineteenth-Century America* (New York: Oxford University Press, 1999), 149; Stanley, *From Bondage to Contract*, 1–59.

73. Hart, *Empire and Revolution*, 97–102.

74. Jonathan Brown has ably described the ways American railroad workers' wages

and benefits in Mexico provided a template for Mexican railroad workers' demands. See Brown, "Trabajadores nativos y extranjeros en el Mexico Porfiriano," *Siglo XIX: Cuadernos de Historia* 3, no. 9 (1994): 7–49, esp. 27–31.

75. Markel, *Quarantine!*, 3–5.

76. Paul Kens, *Judicial Power and Reform Politics: The Anatomy of Lochner v. New York* (Lawrence: University of Kansas Press, 1998). From 1895 to 1905, most state and federal courts found the Bakeshop Act to be constitutional. In 1905, the U.S. Supreme Court found the act to be an unconstitutional restriction on the substantive due process right to enter into contracts without extramarket restrictions.

77. "Deluded Colonists: A Railroad Official Feeding the Negroes—Smallpox Victims," *Los Angeles Times*, July 30, 1895, 3.

78. "Will Feed the Negroes," *Houston Post*, July 28, 1895, 2.

79. "Quarantine for Colonists," *Houston Post*, July 31, 1895, 2.

80. Redkey, *Black Exodus*, 188.

81. In *Gonzalez v. Williams* the Supreme Court could find no constitutional justification for excluding Puerto Ricans who were also American nationals. The Tlahualilo colonists had an even stronger claim for belonging in the United States. Sam Erman, "Meanings of Citizenship in the U.S. Empire: Puerto Rico, Isabel Gonzalez, and the Supreme Court, 1898 to 1905," *Journal of American Ethnic History* 27, no. 4 (2008): 5–33.

82. Collector William Fitch to Surgeon General Wyman, August 4, 1895, RG 90, USPHS, NC 34, Entry 11, Correspondence with Southern Quarantine Stations, Box 150, Textual Records, Civilian Division, NACP.

83. Ibid.

84. Ibid.

85. Ibid.

86. Fitch, "Smallpox among Negro Refugees from Mexico," *Weekly Abstract of Sanitary Reports* 10, no. 31 (August 3, 1895): 619–20.

87. "Camp Jenner," Collector of Customs William Fitch Report, August 4, 1895, pp. 1–3, RG 90, USPHS Files, NC 34, Entry 11, Correspondence with Southern Quarantine Stations, Box 150, NACP.

88. Ibid.

89. Ibid.

90. Ibid.

91. "Fitch Wins All," *San Antonio Express*, October 17, 1895, 1.

92. William Fitch was on record as opposing the appointment of Jack Evans as the state quarantine officer in Eagle Pass. William Fitch, "Report, August 4, 1895," p. 4, RG 90, USPHS, NC 34, Entry 11, Correspondence with Southern Quarantine Stations, Box 150, NACP.

93. George Magruder, August 4, 1895, RG 90, USPHS, NC 34, Entry 11, Correspondence with Southern Quarantine Stations, Box 150, NACP. See also "Failure of the

Scheme for the Colonization of Negroes in Mexico," 54th Cong., 1st sess., 1895–1896, H.R. Doc. No. 169, p. 44.

94. George Magruder, August 4, 1895, RG 90, USPHS, NC 34, Entry 11, Correspondence with Southern Quarantine Stations, Box 150, NACP.

95. T. J. Bennett, "Report at APHA," *Texas Sanitarian* 2, no. 2 (1892): 68–69.

96. Look at the use of superstition and black folk medication among health practitioners who advocated both specific reductionist and social environmental explanations for disease among African Americans. See Gertrude Jacinta Fraser, *Dialogues of Birth, Race, and Memory: African American Midwifery in Green County, Virginia* (Cambridge: Harvard University Press, 1998), 4–70. For a discussion of various African American medical responses to urban epidemics in the twentieth century, see David McBride, *From TB to AIDS: Epidemics among Urban Blacks since 1900* (Albany: State University of New York Press, 1991).

97. Robert Baker, "African Americans and Organized Medicine: Origins of a Racial Divide," *Journal of the American Medical Association,* jama.ama-assn.org/content/300/3/306.full (accessed January 20, 2011).

98. Sharla Fett, *Working Cures: Healing, Health and Power in Southern Slave Plantations* (Chapel Hill: University of North Carolina Press, 2002), 61–82, esp. 72, 74; for the change in status, see 143–67. Bernard Vogel, *American Indian Medicine* (Norman: University of Oklahoma Press, 1970); Todd Savitt, "Black Health on the Plantation: Masters, Slaves, and Physicians," in *Sickness and Health in America: Readings in the History of Medicine and Public Health,* 3rd ed., rev., ed. Judith Walzer Leavitt and Ronald Numbers (Madison: University of Wisconsin Press, 1997), 351–68.

99. George Magruder, August 4, 1895, RG 90, USPHS, NC 34, Entry 11, Correspondence with Southern Quarantine Stations, Box 150, NACP.

100. Ibid.

101. George Magruder, August 4, 1895, p. 1, RG 90, USPHS, NC 34, Entry 11, Correspondence with Southern Quarantine Stations, Box 150, NACP.

102. George Magruder, August 8, 1895, RG 90, USPHS, NC 34, Entry 11, Correspondence with Southern Quarantine Stations, Box 150, NACP.

103. Ibid., 1.

104. Ibid., 4.

105. Ibid.

106. George Magruder, "August 14, 1895," p. 4, RG 90, USPHS, NC 34, Entry 11, Correspondence with Southern Quarantine Stations, Box 150, NACP.

107. Rosenau, "Report on the Camp Jenner Epidemic, Eagle Pass, Texas," 234; "Telegram, R. M. Swearingen to Surgeon General Walter Wyman, August 10, 1895," *Annual Report of the Supervising Surgeon General* (Washington, D.C.: Government Printing Office, 1895), 234.

108. "Variola" is medical Latin for "smallpox." J. J. Kinyoun, "Serum Therapy of Variola and Vaccinia: Preliminary Report on the Treatment of Variola by Antitoxin,"

edited by Walter Wyman, *Annual Report of the Supervising Surgeon General of the United States Marine Hospital Service of the United States Treasury for the Fiscal Year 1897* (Washington, D.C.: Government Printing Office, 1899), 779.

109. Ibid., 767.

110. Ibid., 772.

111. Ibid., 773.

112. George Miller Sternberg, *Immunity, Protective Inoculation in Infectious Diseases and Serotherapy* (New York: William and Wood, 1895), v.

113. Ibid., iv.

114. See "Anti-Toxine and Dr. Kinyoun," *Daily Charlotte Observer*, December 22, 1894, 2.

115. J. J. Kinyoun, "Smallpox Serum Remedy Tested," *New York Times*, January 23, 1895, 4.

116. Kinyoun, "Serum Therapy of Vaccinia and Variola," 775.

117. The *New York Times* editorial board was guardedly optimistic about the results of this clinical trial. They demanded larger tests before Kinyoun could claim that smallpox would yield to serum therapy. Kinyoun, "Smallpox Serum Remedy Tested," 4.

118. Ibid.

119. Ibid.

120. Kinyoun, "Serum Therapy in Vaccinia and Variola," 779.

121. Ibid.

122. Ibid.; Associated Press, "Help for the Prodigals," *The State* (Columbia, S.C.), August 9, 1895, 1.

123. Kinyoun, "The Application of Serotherapy in Vaccinia and Variola," 779.

124. "A Government Scientist Sent to Texas on an Important Mission," *New Orleans Picayune*, August 7, 1895.

125. Associated Press, "Help for the Prodigals," *The State* (Columbia, S.C.), August 9, 1895, 1.

126. Milton Rosenau to Walter Wyman, August 14, 1895, RG 90, USPHS, NC 34, Entry 11, Correspondence with Southern Quarantine Camps, Box 150, NACP.

127. "Roux's Diphtheria," *Daily Charlotte Observer*, October 20, 1894, 2.

128. We would consider this procedure similar to the injection of antibodies; however, the term they used to describe the active principle in this serum was "antitoxin." See Sternberg, *Immunity*, v; quote on 167.

129. Ibid., 372.

130. "Mr. Eccles Brings News of His Trip," *Daily Charlotte Observer*, August 25, 1895, 1.

131. George Magruder, "Smallpox at Eagle Pass, Texas among Negro Colonists Returning from Mexico," *Annual Report of the Supervising Surgeon General* (Washington, D.C.: Government Printing Office, 1895), 370–73.

132. Milton Rosenau, "Photos of Camp Jenner" (1895), Folder 15, Series 2: Letter books, M. J. Rosenau Papers, 1871–1940, University of North Carolina, Chapel Hill.

133. "Camp Jenner and Negro Colonists," *Leslie's Weekly*, October 13, 1895, 5.

134. Ibid.

135. Milton Rosenau, "Smallpox—Some Peculiarities of Camp Jenner Epidemic—a Clinical Study of One Hundred and Thirty Seven Cases," edited by Walter Wyman, *Annual Report of the Surgeon General of the United States Marine Hospital Service for the Fiscal Year 1896*, (Washington, D.C.: Government Printing Office, 1896), 237–44.

136. Milton Rosenau, "Smallpox—Some Peculiarities of Camp Jenner Epidemic," 234.

137. Susan Lederer, "'The Sacred Cord': Doctors, Patients, and Medical Research," in *Subjected to Science: Human Experimentation in America before the Second World War* (Baltimore: Johns Hopkins University Press, 1995), 1–25, esp. 20–25; Warner, *The Therapeutic Perspective*, 235–50.

138. Rosenau, "Smallpox—Some Peculiarities of Camp Jenner Epidemic," 235.

139. E. H. Wilson, "A Contribution to the Serum Therapy of Smallpox," in *Annual Report of the Supervising Surgeon General of the United States Marine Hospital Service for the Fiscal Year 1897*, ed. Walter Wyman, 776–79 (Washington, D.C.: Government Printing Office, 1899). "A Serum Remedy for Smallpox," *New York Times*, January 23, 1895, 4.

140. Milton Rosenau (1869–1946) became the director of the National Hygienic Laboratory from 1896 to 1909, professor of preventive medicine and hygiene at Harvard University (1909–1935), chief of Division of Biologics Laboratories for the Massachusetts Board of Health (1914–1921), and professor of epidemiology at the University of North Carolina Chapel Hill (1935–1946). His book, *Preventive Medicine and Hygiene*, went into multiple editions. "Obituary," AJPH, v. 36, no. 5 (May 1946), 530–531.

141. "Negroes Who Have Been Cooped Up in Camp Jenner to Be Sent Back to Alabama," *Dallas Morning News*, September 23, 1895, 1.

142. "Birmingham Quarantine against Negro Colonists," *Houston Post*, October 15, 1895, 2.

143. "Negroes Who Have Been Cooped up in Camp Jenner to Be Sent Back to Alabama," *Dallas Morning News*, September 23, 1895, 1.

144. Birmingham News, "Ungrateful Are the Negroes Brought Back to Alabama," *Tuscaloosa Times*, October 8, 1895.

145. "Clippings from the Eagle Pass Guide Newspaper, November 3, 1895," in Consular Despatches, State Department Records, Mexico, Piedras Negras, NACP.

146. George Magruder, "Discharge of Refugees from Camp Jenner, Eagle Pass," *Weekly Abstract of Sanitary Reports* 10, no. 43 (1895): 901.

147. Clippings from the Eagle Pass Guide Newspaper, November 3, 1895, in State Department Records, Mexico, Piedras Negras, NACP.

148. Redkey, *Black Exodus*.

149. Eric Burin, "Rethinking Northern White Support for the African Colonization Society: The Pennsylvania Colonization Society as an Agent of Emancipation," *Pennsylvania Magazine of History and Biography* 127, no. 2 (April 2003): 197–229.

150. Fitch, "Smallpox among Negro Refugees from Mexico," *Weekly Abstract of Sanitary Reports* 10, no. 3 (August 3, 1895): 619–20.

151. Ibid.

152. "The Negro Colonists: Eighteen Cases of Smallpox among the Refugees," *Los Angeles Times*, August 2, 1895, 2.

153. A. P. Tugwell, "Refugees Coming Up from Brownsville," August 2, 1882, Papers of Governor Oran Milo Roberts, TSAL.

154. Kate Masur, "A Rare Phenomenon of Philological Vegetation: The Word 'Contraband' and the Meanings of Emancipation in the United States," *Journal of American History* 93, no. 4 (2007): 1050–84.

155. Ibid.

156. Markel, *Quarantine!*, 2–3.

157. "A Government Scientist Sent to Texas on an Important Mission," *New Orleans Picayune*. From the *Houston Post*, August 7, 1895, 4.

158. "The Inability of the Negro," *Memphis Commercial Appeal*, August 7, 1895.

159. George Magruder, August 4, 1895, RG 90, USPHS, NC 34, Entry 11, Correspondence with Southern Quarantine Stations, Box 150, NACP. See also "Failure of the Scheme for the Colonization of Negroes in Mexico," 54th Congress, 1st sess., 1895–1896, H.R. Doc. No. 169, p. 44.

160. Rosenau, "Some Peculiarities of Smallpox during the Camp Jenner Epidemic," 234.

161. Sternberg, *Immunity*, xv, 266.

162. "Ellis Back from Mexico," *San Antonio Express*, August 11, 1895, 4.

163. Ibid.

164. Ibid.

165. "Hardly Any Punishment Would Be Too Severe," *Memphis Commercial Appeal*, August 11, 1895.

166. "Ellis in El Paso," *San Antonio Express*, July 5, 1895, 3.

167. "Hundred of Us Here Starving," *Houston Post*, July 26, 1895, 2.

168. "Church Meeting," *Houston Post*, July 26, 1895.

169. "Negroes Giving Suppers," *Houston Post*, August 17, 1895.

170. Hart, *Empire and Revolution*, 250.

171. Romana Falcón, "Force and the Search for Consent: The Role of the *Jefaturas Políticas* of Coahuila in National State Formation," in *Everyday Forms of State Formation: Revolution and the Negotiation of Rule in Modern Mexico*, ed. Gilbert M. Joseph and Daniel Nugent (Durham: Duke University Press, 1994), 107–36.

172. These generalizations apply to the Kickapoo colony and the black Seminole colony in Mexico. Kevin Mulroy, *Freedom on the Border: The Seminole Maroons*

(Lubbock: Texas Tech University Press, 1993); Felipe Latorre, *The Mexican Kickapoo* (New York: Dover, 1991).

173. Dwyer, "Report of the Doctor of the Tlahualilo Company," 54th Cong., 1st sess., H.R. Doc. No. 169, Enclosure 1, in No. 78, p. 45.

174. Ibid.

175. Ibid.

176. "The Negro as a Pioneer," *San Antonio Express*, July 28, 1895, 4.

177. J. T. Harris, "The Mexican Failure," *Birmingham Herald*, August 24, 1895, 3.

178. Alfred W. Reynolds, "The Alabama Negro Colony in Mexico, 1894–1896: Part II," *Alabama Review* 6, no. 1 (1953): 31–59; quote on 57.

179. Knight Render, "Letter to Editor," *San Antonio Express*, August 17, 1895, 4.

180. Texas State Historical Association, "Stillman, James," in The Handbook of Texas Online, http://www.tshaonline.org/handbook/online/articles/fstbp (accessed March 6, 2012).

181. L. L. Campbell, "The Statesman Calls for Colored Help," *Austin Herald*, August 3, 1895, 2.

182. Jerrold Michael and Thomas R. Bender, "Fighting Smallpox on the Texas Border: An Episode from PHS's Proud Past," *Public Health Reports* 99, no. 6 (1984): 579–82.

Four. The Power of Progress

1. Ciudadanos, Justo Saunders Penn, "Protest against Forcible Vaccination. Translated for the Benefit of the Readers of the Times," *Laredo Times*, March 18, 1899, 3.

2. Ibid.

3. Ibid.

4. Associated Press, "Mexican Mayor at Laredo," *Los Angeles Times*, April 5, 1899, 2.

5. "Crisis Is Reached: Troops from Fort Mcintosh Quickly Change Things. Gatling Gun and Ambulance Corps Do the Rest," *Los Angeles Times*, March 21, 1899, 2.

6. Harrison Gray Otis, "Laredo a new riot center," *Los Angeles Times*, March 21, 1899, 8.

7. Harrison Gray Otis, "Vaccinated with a Gatling Gun," *Los Angeles Times*, March 22, 1899, 3.

8. "Fever at Laredo: Poorer Classes of Mexicans Have No Faith in Doctor's Efforts," *Dallas Morning News*, September 30, 1903.

9. For open Filipino resistance to American medical measures in the Philippines, see Reynaldo Ileto, "Cholera and the Origins of the American Sanitary Order," in *Imperial Medicine and Indigenous Societies*, ed. David Arnold (Manchester: Manchester University Press, 1988), 125–48. For Cuba, see Espinosa, *Epidemic Invasions*, 46–67.

10. Shah, *Contagious Divides*, 78–82. Shah coined the phrase "queer domesticity" to highlight the ways American reformers considered Chinese bachelor households, plural marriages, and mixed-status families to be irreducibly different, but these

households maintained other forms of emotional and intimate arrangements that could be threatening to heterosexual nuclear families.

11. Walter Prescott Webb, *The Texas Rangers: A Century of Frontier Defense* (Austin: University of Texas Press, 1965), 450–51.

12. De Leon, *They Called Them Greasers*, 130.

13. James Leiker, *Racial Borders: Black Soldiers along the Rio Grande* (College Station: Texas A&M University Press, 2002), 118–45.

14. Joanna Nicolls, "The United States Marine Hospital Service: Something of Its History, Work, and Officers," *Frank Leslie's Popular Monthly* 44 (1897): 296.

15. Espinosa, *Epidemic Invasions*, 55–73.

16. Ibid., 31–49.

17. Humphreys, *Yellow Fever and the South*, 158.

18. Ibid., 160.

19. Espinosa, *Epidemic Invasions*, 71.

20. U.S. Census Bureau, *Twelfth Census of the United States*, 601–4.

21. Elliott Young, "Red Men, Princess Pocahontas, and George Washington: Harmonizing Race Relations in Laredo at the Turn of the Century," *Western Historical Quarterly* 29, no. 1 (1998): 48–85.

22. For presence in the elite, see "Businessmen's Club: Message from the President," *Laredo Daily Times*, March 11, 1899, 1. For a more autobiographical account see Leonor Villegas de Magnon, *La rebelde* (Houston: Arte Publico Press, 1994). For Mexican membership in the Anglo elite, see Justo Penn, "Initial Dance at the Pansy Social Club," *Laredo Daily Times*, August 16, 1903, 3.

23. Leiker, *Racial Borders*, 93–118.

24. This is a clear indication that the Laredo City Council sought to act in a way that allayed suspicions in Texas that border Mexicans had more tolerant attitudes toward the presence of smallpox and other illnesses. Shah described the process of respectability among Chinese Americans in the 1940s; see *Contagious Divides*, 204–7.

25. Justo Penn, "New System Adapted," *Laredo Times*, February 1, 1899, 2.

26. Laredo City Council, "Health Inspectors," *Laredo Times*, February 2, 1899, 3.

27. "Smallpox," *Chaparral*, February 18, 1899, 1–3.

28. "The Streets of Laredo Are Nastier Than Ever," *Chaparral*, March 4, 1899.

29. "Society Is at a Standstill," *Laredo Times*, March 8, 1899.

30. "Sociedad Josefa Ortiz de Dominguez Celebrated Seventh Anniversary," *Laredo Times*, March 10, 1899, 3.

31. C. W. McNeil, "Motion to Red Men," *Laredo Times*, March 17, 1899, 3.

32. "Smallpox," *Chaparral*, February 18, 1899, 1–3.

33. "Smallpox," *Laredo Times*, February 2, 1899, 3.

34. "Patients Escape from Pesthouse. Two Colored Girls," *Laredo Times*, February 29, 1899.

35. Cecilia Coleman, Heritagequest Online, census records, 1900, Texas, Series T623,

Roll 1678, p. 234, http://www.heritagequestonline.com/hqoweb/library/do/index (accessed March 8, 2012).

36. For the substantially larger amount of property among Anglo households in Mexican majority counties in 1900, see Stewart, *Not Room Enough: Mexicans, Anglos and Socio-Economic Change in Texas, 1850–1900* (Austin: University of Texas Press, 1993), 51.

37. Three sample news articles: "Negro Surgeon Discharged," *Laredo Times*, March 11, 1899, 1; "Colored Troops Out Exercising Horses," *Laredo Times*, March 20, 1899, 3; "White Brakemen Reinstated," *Laredo Times*, March 11, 1899, 1. See Leiker, *Racial Borders*, 1–3.

38. "Governor of Tamaulipas Entertained at Austin," *Laredo Times*, March 11, 1899, 1.

39. "Businessmen's Club: Message from the President," *Laredo Times*, March 11, 1899, 1.

40. Ibid.

41. J. M. McKnight, "Current of Smallpox Cases—Telegraph Response to W. F. Blunt," March 9, 1899, in Laredo Smallpox Epidemic, Box 301-175, Governor Sayers Collection, TSAL.

42. "Meeting Yesterday. City Council and Representative Citizens Met and Discussed the Smallpox Situation," *Laredo Times*, March 14, 1899, 1.

43. The City of Laredo, "Proclamation to the Inhabitants of Laredo," *Laredo Times*, March 14, 1899, 3.

44. Ibid.

45. Ibid.

46. "Smallpox: Active Work of Physicians," *Laredo Times*, March 16, 1899, 3. Heritagequest seems to indicate that Davila and Gongora were both born in Mexico, and Kross was born in Texas. See Heritage Quest Online, http://www.heritagequeston line.com/hqoweb/library/do/index (accessed March 8, 2012).

47. "Active work of physicians," 3.

48. "Espirideon Hernandez Arrested and Released," *Laredo Times*, March 14, 1899, 3.

49. "Herlinda Hernandez Caught Coming Out of Infected House," *Laredo Times*, March 14, 1899, 3.

50. Walter Fraser Blunt, "Quarantine Request for Webb County, March 9, 1899," in Box 301-175, Governor Joseph Sayers Collection, TSAL.

51. J. O. Nicholson, "Request for Governor to Take Charge of Smallpox Epidemic, March 14, 1899," in Laredo Smallpox Epidemic, Box 301-175, Governor Sayers Collection, TSAL.

52. Joseph D. Sayers, "Telegraph to the Surgeon General Marine Hospital Service," in Laredo Smallpox Epidemic, Box 301-175, Governor Sayers Collection, TSAL.

53. J. Gilliam, "Volunteer Personal Letter from Physician," in Laredo Smallpox Epidemic, Box 301-175, Governor Sayers Collection, TSAL.

54. Alfred G. Abdelal, "Texas Is My Adoptive State," in Laredo Smallpox Epidemic,

Box 301-175, Governor Sayers Collection, TSAL. The census states that he was born in France. See Alfred Abdelal, 1900 Census, Kansas, Series T623, Roll 479, p. 74. HeritageQuest Online, http://www.heritagequestonline.com/hqoweb/library/do/index (accessed March 8, 2012).

55. "Dr. Blunt Assumes Charge: Large Meeting in Market Hall," *Laredo Times*, March 17, 1899, 1.

56. "Dr. Blunts Work—Preparations Rushed and Are Now Ready to Move Patients to Hospital," *Laredo Times*, March 17, 1899, 3.

57. James Saunders (Justo) Penn, "Little Locals—Colored Soldiers," *Laredo Times* (March 17, 1899), 3.

58. James Saunders (Justo) Penn, "Little Locals—Announcement," *Laredo Times*, March 17, 1899, 3.

59. James Saunders (Justo) Penn, "Little Locals—Refusing to Be Vaccinated," *Laredo Times*, March 17, 1899, 3.

60. "Dr. Blunts Work—Preparations Rushed," 3.

61. Judge J. M. Rodriguez, "Cover Letter of Protest from Citizens of Mexican Origin, March 18, 1899," in Laredo Smallpox Epidemic, Box 301-175, Governor Sayers Collection, TSAL.

62. Penn, "Protest against Forcible Vaccination," 3.

63. Carlos Diaz et al., "Protest against Forcible Vaccination," *Laredo Times*, March 18, 1899, 1.

64. East European Jewish immigrants resented the *lel-leit* (spoon-people), the Yiddish word for doctors who entered households and forced their spoons down children's throats. Markel, *Quarantine!*, 70, 217.

65. For legal strategies against quarantines, see Charles McClain, *In Search of Equality: The Chinese Struggle against Discrimination in Nineteenth-Century America* (Berkeley: University of California Press, 1994), 234–77.

66. The links between social control, ethnic social movements, and vaccination resistance movements jump to the literature on colonialism and medicine. For vaccination as social control, see David Arnold, *Colonizing the Body: State Medicine and Epidemic Disease in Nineteenth-Century India* (Berkeley: University of California Press, 1993), 116–58. See also Harrison, *Public Health in British India*, 3–15.

67. Ibid.

68. De Leon, *They Called Them Greasers*, 99.

69. John Hamilton, "Laredo," *Weekly Abstract of Sanitary Reports* 14, no. 11 (March 31, 1899): 423–25.

70. De Leon narrated this incident as if the marshals and the medical officers were Anglo. The Texas Online Handbook marks Sheriff Ortiz as an ethnic Mexican. Until Raymond Martin built a political machine at the beginning of the twentieth century, Tejanos held the majority of elected offices in Laredo. See Alonzo, *Tejano Legacy*, 273. The quotes come from de Leon, *They Called Them Greasers*, 99.

71. De Leon, *They Called Them Greasers*, 99.

72. Ibid.

73. "Laredo's Bloody Day," *San Antonio Express*, March 21, 1899.

74. "Another Account: How the Gatling Gun Overawed the Riotous Mob in Laredo," *San Antonio Express*, March 21, 1899.

75. Ibid.

76. This discussion is based on the primary sources cited in de Leon, *They Called Them Greasers*.

77. Webb, *Texas Rangers*, 450.

78. Utley, *Lone Star Justice*, 270. Anti-Mexican attitudes among Mexican immigrant communities are important to understand. Otherwise, communities like El Paso can enthusiastically elect border patrol agents and maintain anti-immigrant attitudes and this will continue to surprise academics. See Gutiérrez, *Walls and Mirrors* and Pablo Vila, *Crossing Borders, Reinforcing Borders: Social Categories, Metaphors, and Narrative Identities on the U.S.-Mexico Frontier* (Austin: University of Texas Press, 2000).

79. Gutiérrez, *Walls and Mirrors*, 161, 193, 217.

80. *Población flotante* is a derogatory term used by middle classes in Chihuahua and Nuevo León to refer to a seasonal migrant labor pool who did not appear anchored in respectable property. See William E. French, *A Peaceful and Working People: Manners, Morals, and Class Formation in Northern Mexico* (Albuquerque: University of New Mexico Press, 1996).

81. Young, "Red Men, Princess Pocahontas, and George Washington," 41–85.

82. "Dolores Gamboa Charged with Conspiracy to Incite a Riot," *Chaparral*, April 1, 1899, 2.

83. "Clash against Mexicans," *New York Times*, March 20, 1899, 7.

84. "Laredo," *Los Angeles Times*, March 21, 1899, 8.

85. Harrison Gray Otis, "Vaccinated with a Gatling Gun," *Los Angeles Times*, March 22, 1899, 3.

86. "Esy Christen," Heritagequest, 1st Ward, Webb County, Texas, 1900, Series T623, Roll 1678, p. 100 Heritage Quest Online, http://www.heritagequestonline.com/hqoweb/library/do/index (accessed March 4, 2008).

87. This violent suppression of Native American, Mexican, Cuban, Filipino, and Puerto Rican resistance and dissent with American reformist measures does seem to mark federal policy in the Western states, the Mexican borderlands, and the recently occupied islands of Cuba, the Philippines, and Puerto Rico in the 1890s.

88. Associated Press, "Mexican Mayor at Laredo," *Los Angeles Times*, April 5, 1899, 2.

89. For an analysis of local resistance and racializing public health precautions during American occupation, see Ileto, "Cholera and the Origins of the American Sanitary Order," 125–48. For the surprising resonance, see "Uprising Planned: Important Secret Document Gives Time the Snap Away," *Los Angeles Times*, March

26, 1899, A2. "It Is a Long Way Off: What American Officers Say about Pacification. Those in Field Think It Will Take Two to Six Years to Quell Guerrilla Epidemic," *Los Angeles Times*, February 28, 1900, 18b.

90. Calvin Chase, "Riots on the Rio Grande: Texans Objected to Having Arms Scratched with Vaccine Virus," *Washington Bee*, May 25, 1899, 3.

91. Ibid.

92. "The New Mayor of Laredo," *Chaparral*, April 15, 1899.

93. "Quarantine Raised at Laredo," *San Antonio Express*, June 28, 1899.

94. Thomas Fleming, "Pershing's Island War," *American Heritage* 19, no. 5 (1968): 32–104.

95. "Will Continue Tests for Yellow Fever: Of Eight Persons Bitten by Infected Mosquitoes, Three Have Died," *New York Times*, August 27, 1901, 2.

96. "Havana Purged of Fever: Major Gorgas Regards 'Yellow Jack' as a Back Number." The Anti-mosquito Plan's Success," *New York Times*, February 16, 1902, 5.

97. Humphreys, *Yellow Fever and the South*, 158. According to Humphreys, most state health officers supported a national department of health with heavy state representation.

98. Comments of Henry Clayton, 57 Cong. Rec. 7758. From Humphreys, *Yellow Fever and the South*, 159.

99. Comments of Samuel Richardson, 57 Cong. Rec. 7756 (July 1, 1902). From Humphreys, *Yellow Fever and the South*, 159.

100. Wyman to G. M. Guiteras, September 25, 1903, *Annual Report of the Marine Hospital Service*, 255. From Humphreys, *Yellow Fever and the South*, 159.

101. "Are Ordered to Shoot. Death Will Be Penalty for People from Yellow Fever Points Trying to Enter Monterey, Mex.," *Dallas Morning News*, September 4, 1903.

102. Justo Penn, "Yellow Jack Reported at City of Monterey," *Laredo Daily Times*, August 11, 1903, 1.

103. Justo Saunders Penn, "Clean the City," *Laredo Daily Times*, August 15, 1903, 2.

104. Ibid.

105. Penn, "Yellow Jack Reported at City of Monterey."

106. "Border Is Guarded. No Trains Are Allowed to Cross the Rio Grande," *Dallas Morning News*, September 17, 1903, 1.

107. H. J. Hamilton, Acting Assistant Surgeon, "Yellow Fever Quarantine in Laredo," *Weekly Abstract of Sanitary Reports* 23 (September 25, 1903): 1582.

108. John Guiteras, "Yellow Fever Quarantine in Laredo," *Weekly Abstract of Sanitary Reports* 23 (October 2, 1903): 1620–47.

109. "Fever at Laredo: Worse across River," *Dallas Morning News*, October 3, 1903, 3.

110. Ibid.

111. James Saunders (Justo) Penn, "Laredo Needs More Oil to Pour Upon the Waters," *Laredo Times*, November 3, 1903, 3.

112. Justo Saunders Penn, "Little Locals," *Laredo Daily Times*, October 11, 1903, 2.

113. "Fever at Laredo: One Death among the Poorer Class of Mexicans in the Border City," *Dallas Morning News*, October 12, 1903, 3.

114. William Nesbitt, "The Latest Mosquito Joke," *Laredo Daily Times*, October 9, 1903, 2.

115. "Fever at Laredo: Worse across River."

116. Justo Saunders Penn, "Twenty Seven New Cases of Yellow Fever, Making 300. Two Deaths, Sixteen All Told," *Laredo Daily Times*, October 13, 1903, 3.

117. "Fever at Laredo: Poorer Classes of Mexicans Have No Faith in Doctor's Efforts," *Dallas Morning News*, September 30, 1903.

118. Edward C. Butler, "Yellow Jack's Dread March," *Los Angeles Times*, November 30, 1903, 5.

119. Ibid.

120. James Saunders (Justo) Penn, "Twenty Five Cases Reported Yesterday. The Banner Day of the Fever since It Lodged in This City," *Laredo Daily Times*, October 9, 1903, 1.

121. "Fever at Laredo: Poorer Classes of Mexicans Have No Faith in Doctor's Efforts," 2.

122. Penn, "Twenty Seven New Cases of Yellow Fever, Making 300," 3.

123. "Fever at Laredo: One Death Among the Poorer Class of Mexicans in the Border City," *Dallas Morning News*, October 12, 1903, 1.

124. Tabor, "The Advance of Medical Science," *San Antonio Daily Express*, October 21, 1903, 4.

125. Robert D. Murray, "The Mexican-Texas Epidemic," *Annual Report of the Supervising Surgeon General for the Year 1882*, ed. John Hamilton (Washington, D.C.: Government Printing Office, 1883), 271–334.

126. James Saunders (Justo) Penn, "Asking for Help. A Petition to the City Council from Fifty Seven Women," *Laredo Daily Times*, October 19, 1903, 3.

127. Guiteras, "Report on the Epidemic of Yellow Fever of 1903," 304.

128. Ibid.

129. See Brian McCallister-Linn, *Guardians of Empire: The U.S. Army and the Pacific, 1902–1940* (Chapel Hill: University of North Carolina Press, 1997), 60–61.

130. "Moving Troops to Texas," *Dallas Morning News*, August 16, 1903, 3.

131. "To Protect the Soldiers," *Dallas Morning News*, September 17, 1903, 3.

132. James Saunders (Justo) Penn, "Absolute Quarantine," *Laredo Daily Times*, October 10, 1903, 3.

133. James Saunders (Justo) Penn, "A Cool Wave Lends Encouragement," *Laredo Daily Times*, November 6, 1903, 1.

134. Gregorio Guiteras, "Concerning Yellow Fever in Laredo," *Weekly Abstract of Sanitary Reports* 18, no. 49 (November 27, 1903): 2132–38.

135. Ibid.

136. Edmond Souchon, "Not a Firm Belief in the Mosquito Theory," *Dallas Morning News*, December 28, 1903, 6.

137. C. W. Trueheart, "Common Sense Quarantine Methods," *Texas Medical Journal* 23 (1907): 495–99.

138. Guiteras, "Report on the Epidemic of Yellow Fever of 1903," 304.

139. Ibid., 304.

140. Ibid., 310.

141. Ibid.311.

142. Ibid., 319.

143. Ibid., 320.

144. Penn, "A Cool Wave Lends Encouragement," 1.

145. Guiteras, "Report on the Epidemic of Yellow Fever of 1903," 320.

146. According to the 1900 census, the Mexico-born population in Webb County was 10,755 of 22,766, which is less than 50 percent of the population. U.S. Census Bureau, *Twelfth Census of the United States*, 789.

147. For his family's work for Cuban independence, see "Cuba: Progress of the Revolution," *New York Herald*, June 5, 1869. For his work as an exile, see "How the Three Friends Met the Dons: Graphic Description of the Brush Which the Alleged Filibuster Had with Warships," *Philadelphia Inquirer*, December 26, 1896. For employment as USMHS surgeon from 1888 to 1910, see "Las novedades," *Novedades*, August 16, 1888, and "Dr. Juan Guiteras, Cuba," *Belleville News Democrat*, August 10, 1909, 2.

148. Guiteras, "Report on the Epidemic of Yellow Fever of 1903," 303–20.

149. Milton Rosenau, "Consideration of Measures against Yellow Fever in Association with Texas-Mexico Inspection Service," *Annual Report of the Surgeon General of the United States Public Health and Marine Hospital Service*, ed. Walter Wyman (Washington, D.C.: Government Printing Office, 1904), 302.

150. Ruth Dodson, *Don Pedrito Jaramillo, Curandero* (San Antonio: Casa Editorial Lozano, 1934), 14, 18, 52, 58, 114, 110.

151. Jose E. Limón, *Dancing with the Devil: Society and Cultural Poetics in Mexican-American South Texas* (Madison: University of Wisconsin Press, 1994), 196.

152. Villegas de Magnon, *La rebelde*, 101.

Five. Domestic Tensions at an American Crossroads

1. The inspector may have racialized another aspect of Mrs. Quinn's appearance: "Because I was blond and had green eyes, the village all treated me like something special. I felt really loved by them." Anthony Quinn, *The Original Sin: A Self Portrait by Anthony Quinn* (Boston: Little, Brown, 1972), 19.

2. Ibid., 20.

3. Alexandra Minna Stern, "Buildings, Boundaries, and Blood: Medicalization and

Nation-Building on the U.S.-Mexico Border, 1910–1930," *Hispanic American Historical Review* 79, no. 1 (1999): 41–81.

4. Markel and Stern, "Which Face? Whose Nation?," 1314–31.

5. Pablo Mitchell, *Coyote Nation: Sexuality, Race, and Conquest in Modernizing New Mexico, 1880–1920* (Chicago: University of Chicago Press, 2004).

6. For a cynical framing of community "harmonizing," see Young, "Red Men, Princess Pocahontas, and George Washington," 48–85. For a discussion of the struggles to have "ethnic Mexicans" elected representatives of this kind of public in El Paso, see Mario Garcia, *Mexican Americans: Leadership, Ideology, and Identity, 1930–1960* (New Haven: Yale University Press, 1991), 113–45. For analogous struggles faced by "ethnic Mexican" political organizations across the United States, see Gutiérrez, *Walls and Mirrors*. For the discipline imposed by the perception of ethnic Mexicans as permanent immigrants, see David Leal and Luis Fraga, "Playing the 'Latino Card': Race, Ethnicity, and National Party Politics," *Du Bois Review: Social Science Research on Race* 1, no. 2: (September 2004): 297–317.

7. For eloquent accounts of the taken-for-granted American/Mexican divide, see Romo, *Ringside Seat to a Revolution*, 219–33. See also Stern, "Buildings, Boundaries, and Blood"; Alexandra Minna Stern, *Eugenic Nation: Faults and Frontiers of Better Breeding in Modern America* (Berkeley: University of California Press, 2005), 57–82.

8. See A. Gabriel Melendez, *The Poetics of Print in Nuevomexicano Communities, 1875–1916* (Albuquerque: University of New Mexico Press, 1997), 81–84.

9. U.S. Census Bureau, "Composition and Characteristics of the Population, for Counties: 1920," in *Fourteenth Census of the Population Taken in 1920* (Washington, D.C.: Government Printing Office, 1921), 997. See also Conrey Bryson, *Dr. Lawrence Nixon and the White Primary* (El Paso: Texas Western Press, 1974).

10. Darlene Clark Hine, *Black Victory: The Rise and Fall of the White Primary in Texas* (Columbia: University of Missouri Press, 2003), 20–35.

11. Ibid.

12. Mullan, *Plagues and Politics*, 30–70.

13. Espinosa, *Epidemic Invasions*.

14. Warwick Anderson, "Colonial Pathologies: American Medicine in the Philippines" (Ph.D. diss., University of Pennsylvania, 1992).

15. Brandt, *No Magic Bullet*, 40–41.

16. Markel, *Quarantine!*, 166–93.

17. Lucy Salyer argues that it took approximately forty years for exclusionists to design an effective legislative and administrative response that would withstand these constitutional challenges. See Salyer, *Laws Harsh as Tigers*, 139–210.

18. See Anna Pegler Gordon's *In Sight of America* on the conflicts over the meaning of photographs for Chinese exclusion, including *Reisterer v. Lee Sum*, where the judge decided the indistinct photograph did not challenge Lee Sum's claim for residency: Pegler Gordon, *In Sight of America: Photography and the Development of U.S. Immi-*

gration Policy (Berkeley: University of California Press, 2010), 71, esp. 70–95. See also Salyer, *Laws Harsh as Tigers.*

19. For nuisance laws and the nineteenth-century regulation of individual liberties, see William J. Novak, *The People's Welfare: Law and Regulation in Nineteenth-Century America* (Chapel Hill: University of North Carolina Press, 1996).

20. The argument regarding the legal boundary between doctors and patients in medical decision making comes directly from Martin S. Pernick, "The Patient's Role in Medical Decisionmaking: A Social History of Informed Consent in Medical Therapy," in *Making Health Care Decisions: The Ethical and Legal Obligations of Informed Consent in the Patient-Practitioner Relationship,* vol. 3: *Appendices Studies on the Foundation of Informed Consent,* ed. Morris Abram (Washington, D.C.: Government Printing Office, 1982), 1–37, especially 3, 31–32.

21. Espinosa, *Epidemic Invasions,* 73–84.

22. Judith Walzer Leavitt, *Typhoid Mary: Captive to the Public's Health* (Boston: Beacon, 1996), 39–69; Keith Wailoo, *Drawing Blood: Technology and Disease Identity in Twentieth-Century America* (Baltimore: Johns Hopkins University Press, 1997), 14–16; Hammonds, *Childhood's Deadly Scourge,* 7–10.

23. Leavitt, *Typhoid Mary,* 70–96, 96–120.

24. Hammonds, *Childhood's Deadly Scourge,* 7–10. See also Paul Weindling, "From Medical Research to Clinical Practice: Serum Therapy for Diphtheria," *Medical Innovations in Historical Perspective,* ed. John Pickstone (New York: St. Martin's, 1992), 72–82.

25. James Joseph Kinyoun, "Preliminary Report on the Treatment of Variola by Its Antitoxin," ed. Walter Wyman. *Annual Report of the Supervising Surgeon General of the Marine Hospital Service of the United States for the Fiscal Year 1897* (Washington, D.C.: Government Printing Office, 1899), 772–73.

26. Brandt, *No Magic Bullet,* 123–29. Pierce was named the national coordinator of this campaign after his work on the Mexican border and in France.

27. For an analysis of how the U.S. military waged eradication campaigns against Filipino folk practices that "maintained" cholera, see Ileto, "Cholera and the Origins of the American Sanitary Order," 125–48.

28. Rex Taylor and Annelie Rieger, "Medicine as Social Science: Rudolf Virchow on the Typhus Epidemic in Upper Silesia," *International Journal of Health Services* 15, no. 4 (1995): 547–59. For a longer look at the links between social medicine advocates and social democratic politics in nineteenth-century Germany, see Paul Weindling, *Health, Race, and German Politics between National Unification and Nazism, 1870–1945* (New York: Oxford University Press, 1989), 3–7, 37–49.

29. Ibid.

30. See Paul Weindling, *Epidemics and Genocide in Eastern Europe, 1890–1945* (New York: Oxford University Press, 2000), 39–42.

31. The scholarship on exclusion is vast, growing, and fascinating. For an overview

of these immigration policies in the United States, see Markel and Stern, "Which Face? Whose Nation?" Two canonical works with a focus on European immigrants are John Higham, *Strangers in the Land: Patterns of American Nativism, 1860–1925,* 2nd ed. (New Brunswick: Rutgers University Press, 1988), and Alan Kraut, *Silent Travelers: Germs, Genes, and the Immigrant Menace* (Baltimore: Johns Hopkins University Press, 1995). For a deeper examination of the experience of Chinese exclusion, see Erica Lee, *At America's Gates: Chinese Immigration during the Exclusion Era* (Chapel Hill: University of North Carolina Press, 2007). For Germany, see Weindling, *Epidemics and Genocide.* For Britain, see Thomas Jordan, "'An Awful Visitation of Providence': The Irish Famine of 1845–49," *Journal of the Royal Society of Health* 117, no. 4 (1997): 216–27, and Hazel Waters, "The Great Famine and the Rise of Anti-Irish Racism," *Race and Class* 37, no. 1 (July–September 1995): 95–108. For Canada, see Lisa Rose Mar, *Brokering Belonging: Chinese in Canada's Exclusion Era, 1885–1945* (New York: Oxford University Press, 2010). For Australia, see Warwick Anderson, *The Cultivation of Whiteness: Science, Health and Racial Destiny in Australia* (Melbourne: Melbourne University Press, 2005).

32. Weindling, *Epidemics and Genocide,* 39–42.

33. Ibid., 59–72.

34. T. J. Bennett, "Typhus in Mexico," *Texas Sanitarian* 2, no. 2 (1892): 136.

35. Clarence Warfield, "Clinical Notes on Typhus Fever of Northern Mexico," *Transactions of the Texas State Medical Association* (1894): 122–32; quote on 123.

36. Ibid., 126.

37. Ibid., 132.

38. Markel, *Quarantine!,* 15–16.

39. For an enthusiastic account of this movement, see Paul De Kruif, *Microbe Hunters* (New York: Harcourt, Brace & World, 1966).

40. Ludwik Gross, "How Charles Nicolle of the Pasteur Institute Discovered That Epidemic Typhus Is Transmitted by Lice: Reminiscences from My Years at the Pasteur Institute in Paris," *Proceedings of the National Academy of Sciences of the United States of America* 93, no. 10 (October 1, 1996): 539–40.

41. John F. Anderson and Joseph Goldberger, "The relation of so-called Brill's disease to typhus fever," *Public Health Reports,* v. 27, no. 5 (December 1912), 149–52. State Medical Association of Texas, "Lead Editorial," *Texas State Journal of Medicine* 8 (March 1912): 1.

42. H. L. McNeil, "A Case of Typhus," *Texas State Journal of Medicine* 12 (September 1916): 234.

43. C. C. Pierce, "Typhus Fever, Prevention and Control," *Texas State Journal of Medicine* 12 (August 1916): 182–88.

44. Ibid.

45. *Jacobson v. Commonwealth of Massachusetts,* 197 U.S. 11 (1905). For a contextual analysis, see James Colgrove, *States of Immunity: The Politics of Vaccination in*

Twentieth-Century America (Berkeley: University of California Press, 2006), 1–67. See also Michael Willrich, *Pox: An American History* (New York: Basic Books, 2010), 285–330.

46. *Schloendorff v. Society of New York Hospital*, 211 N.Y. 125; 105 N.E. 92; 1914. For a fascinating commentary, see Pernick, "The Patient's Role in Medical Decisionmaking," 1–37. For the backlash against the female doctor who performed the surgery, see Regina Markell Morantz Sanchez, *Conduct Unbecoming a Woman: Medicine on Trial in Turn-of-the-Century Brooklyn* (New York: Oxford University Press, 1999).

47. Friedrich Katz, *The Life and Times of Pancho Villa* (Stanford: Stanford University Press, 1998).

48. For a discussion of the Mexican elite in El Paso, see Romo, *Ringside Seat to a Revolution*, 168–81.

49. U.S. Census Bureau, *Fourteenth Census of the United States, 1920*, vol. 2: *1920 Population: General Report and Analytical Tables* (New York: Norman Ross Publishing, 2001), 993, 1000.

50. Shawn Lay argues that the El Paso Klan had strong roots among the arriving white lawyers and doctors in El Paso; according to Lay, Tom Lea was a Klan member. See Lay, *War, Revolution, and the Ku Klux Klan: A Study of Intolerance in a Border City* (El Paso: Texas Western Press, 1985), 78–85. Lay maintains that the general fear of Mexicans as a growing southern and midwestern constituency in El Paso made any political contact with the Mexican American voters toxic to the white majority in El Paso.

51. For exclusion for being unlikely to become a single male industrial laborer, see Fairchild, *Science at the Borders*, 3–10. For the ways inspectors learned to read sexuality from the 1940s to the present, see Eithne Luibheid, *Entry Denied: Controlling Sexuality at the Border* (Minneapolis: University of Minnesota Press, 2002).

52. For contrasting styles of inspection on different borders, see Markel and Stern, "Which Face, Whose Nation?" *American Behavioral Scientist*, 42, no. 9 (1999): 1314–31. For Chinese exclusion as the organizational basis and institutional precedent for immigrant inspection in El Paso, see Lee, *At America's Gates*, 151–89, and Clifford Perkins, *With the Border Patrol: With the U.S. Immigration Service on the Mexican Boundary* (El Paso: Texas Western Press, 1978). For anxieties about the fixity of racial identities among Mexican border-crossers, see Lee, *At America's Gates*, 162, and Pegler Gordon, *In Sight of America*, 179–82. For anxieties about the professionalism of medical inspectors in El Paso, see Ann Gabbert, "El Paso, a Sight for Sore Eyes: Medical and Legal Aspects of Syrian Immigration," *Historian* 65 (September 2002): 15–42. For the importance of the LPC category, see Sánchez, *Becoming Mexican American*, 51–58; Vicki Ruiz, *Out of the Shadows: Mexican Women in Twentieth-Century America* (New York: Oxford University Press, 2006), 9; Fairchild, *Science at the Borders*, 5, 13–14. For U.S. anxieties about the emerging "racial" identities of Eurasian immigrants, see Mathew Frye Jacobson, *Whiteness of a Different Color: European*

Immigrants and the Alchemy of Race (Cambridge: Harvard University Press, 1998). For initial discussion of "bodies out of place," see Mary Douglas, *Purity and Danger* (London: Routledge and Kegan Paul, 1969), 44–50.

53. C. C. Pierce, "Cases of Typhus Fever in the City of El Paso, January 1–June 30, 1916," File No. 2126, Typhus, Box 207, File No. 1, RG 90, USPHS Central Files, 1897–1923, NACP.

54. U.S. Census Bureau, "Composition and Characteristics of the Population, for Counties: 1920," in *Fourteenth Census of the Population Taken in 1920*, 997. These numbers are very hard to interpret. The census counted 26,414 people (out of a total population of 101,877) who were "Native white of native parentage," some of whom, like Felix Martinez, could trace their line of descent to long-standing Hispano and Mexicano communities in New Mexico.

55. Montejano, *Anglos and Mexicans*, 3.

56. The rhetoric of an "American standard of living" was impossible to maintain, as it depended on the exclusion of Asian and Mexican labor and the presence of labor below an American standard of living. See "Jap Importation," *El Paso City and County Labor Advocate*, September 26, 1916. For the importance of this racist claim on the labor movement, see Alexander Saxton, *The Indispensable Enemy: Labor and the Anti-Chinese Movement in California* (Berkeley: University of California Press, 1971). For public health discourse on this matter, see the chapter on white labor and the American standard of living in Shah, *Contagious Divides*, 158–77.

57. "Girl Provides Life Savings for Buttner Memorial Fund," *El Paso Morning Times*, March 8, 1916, 8.

58. Ibid.

59. Sarah Deutsch, *Women and the City: Gender, Space and Power in Boston, 1870–1940* (New York: Oxford University Press, 2000), 3.

60. Public Health Service officers used detainees in prison facilities in occupied Cuba and the Philippines to test communicable disease theories. See Susan Lederer, *Subjected to Science: Human Experimentation in America before the Second World War* (Baltimore: Johns Hopkins University Press, 1995), 75–76, 131–36.

61. "Jury Probes Explosion: Investigation into Cause of El Paso Jail Explosion Begins: Coroner's Findings Withheld," *El Paso Morning Times*, March 9, 1916, 8.

62. "Cigarette Starts Jail Fire, Causing Death and Rioting; Eighteen Burn in El Paso Jail—Twenty Six Injured—Americans Fired Upon," *San Antonio Express*, March 9, 1916, 1.

63. *El Paso Morning Times*, March 9, 1916, 1.

64. "Cigarette Starts Jail Fire, Causing Death and Rioting."

65. See the *El Paso Morning Times*, March 8, 1916, 1; *El Paso Herald*, March 8, 1916, 1; *San Antonio Express*, March 9, 1916, 1.

66. "Prayers for Dead and Suffering Victims of Jail Holocaust Are Offered by Laymen's Convention," *El Paso Morning Times*, March 8, 1916, 8.

67. "Jury Ordered to Probe Explosion. Strong Instructions Given by Judge Jackson; Death List Reaches 18. Coroner Holds Inquest," *San Antonio Express*, March 8, 1916, 1.

68. *San Antonio Express*, March 9, 1916, 1.

69. Ibid. "Mexicans from the interior" is not a neutral term in northern Mexico. Pablo Vila claims that Juarenses (long-term residents of Ciudad Juárez) debate whether "darker, more Indian" Mexican immigrants from the interior should be part of the Chihuahua landscape. See Vila, *Crossing Borders, Reinforcing Borders*, 45–49, 167–91. For legacies of this attitude, see Rosalinda Fregoso, *MeXicana Encounters: The Making of Social Identities in the Borderlands* (Berkeley: University of California Press, 2003), Lourdes Portillo, *Mujer Extraviada* (New York: Women Make Movies, 2001), and Cecilia Balli, "La ciudad de la muerte," *Texas Monthly*, June 2003.

70. *San Antonio Express*, March 9, 1916, 1.

71. See the *El Paso Herald*, March 8, 1916, 1. *San Antonio Express*, March 8, 1916, 1. *El Paso Morning Times*, March 8, 1916, 1, for first-hand accounts of the disturbances in Ciudad Juárez and their political aftermath.

72. "Judge Jackson's Instructions," *El Paso Morning Times*, March 9, 1916, 7.

73. "Evidence Is Being Gathered at Hearing for Grand Jury," *El Paso Morning Times*, March 9, 1916, 1.

74. Ibid., 3.

75. In 1914, Woodrow Wilson thought Pancho Villa would be America's best ally in Mexico. By 1916, as subsequent events will show, Villa went on to be vilified in the press, though he still had allies across the United States. See Christopher Wilson, "Plotting the Border: John Reed, Pancho Villa, and *Insurgent Mexico*," in *Cultures of United States Imperialism*, ed. Amy Kaplan and Donald Pease (Durham: Duke University Press, 1993), 340–65. See also Katz, *The Life and Times of Pancho Villa*.

76. See Alexandra Minna Stern, "Eugenics beyond Borders" (Ph.D. diss., University of Chicago, 1998), 131–38.

77. See Katz, *The Life and Times of Pancho Villa*, 548–60.

78. See Stern, "Eugenics beyond Borders," 135.

79. Mario García, *Desert Immigrants: The Mexicans of El Paso, 1880–1920* (New Haven: Yale University Press, 1981), 193. Mauricio Cordero claimed he escaped mob violence by convincing them he was African American and therefore not "Mexican." Mauricio Cordero Transcript, 41, Institute of Oral History collection, University of Texas–El Paso.

80. See Stern, "Eugenics beyond Borders," 131–39.

81. Vila, *Crossing Borders, Reinforcing Borders*.

82. "Mexicans Connect Jail Horror with Columbus Outrage," *El Paso Morning Times*, March 21, 1916, 2.

83. "Disinfection to Be Used against Typhus Fever," *El Paso Morning Times*, March 18, 1916.

84. Ibid. Also see, C. C. Pierce, "Cases of Typhus Fever in the City of El Paso,

January 1–June 30, 1916," File No. 2126, Typhus, Box 207, File No. 1, RG 90, USPHS Central Files, 1897–1923, NACP.

85. Editorial, *El Paso Morning Times*, March 14, 1917, 2.

86. C. C. Pierce, "Cases of Typhus Fever in the City of El Paso, January 1–June 30, 1916," File No. 2126, Typhus, Box 207, File No. 1, RG 90, USPHS Central Files, 1897–1923, NACP.

87. Quinn, *Original Sin*, 47.

88. Ibid., 48.

89. Markel and Stern, "Which Face? Whose Nation?," *American Behavioral Scientist* 429 (1999): 1314–31.

90. Pierce, "Typhus fever cases in El Paso, January 1–June 30, 1916" RG 59, Decimal Records of the State Department, 1910–1920, File No. 158.129/52, NACP.

91. "Local News," *El Paso City and County Labor Advocate*, January 5, 1917, 8.

92. Pierce, "Typhus fever cases in El Paso, January 1–June 30, 1916," RG 59, Decimal Records of the State Department, 1910–1920, File No. 158.129/52, NACP.

93. Memorandum to Rupert Blue for employees, June 30, 1917, USPHS general files, 1897–1923, RG 90, File No. 1248, Folder No. 4, NACP; *El Paso Morning Times*, January 28, 1917, 1.

94. *El Paso Morning Times*, January 28, 1917, 1.

95. Irene Ledesma, "Texas Newspapers and Chicana Workers' Activism, 1919–1974," *Western Historical Quarterly* 26, no. 3 (1995): 309–31; quote on 309.

96. "Quarantine Riots in Juárez: Women Lead Demonstration against American Regulation," *El Paso Morning Times*, January 28, 1917, 1.

97. *New York Times*, January 29, 1917, 4.

98. See the 1858 illustration of a mob marching on a yellow fever detention facility in Mullan, *Plagues and Politics*, 27. See also the "Mob at Fire Island" illustration in Markel, *Quarantine!*, 117; Rosenberg, *Cholera Years*.

99. "Quarantine Riots in Juarez: Women Lead Revolt against American Regulation," *New York Times*, January 28, 1917, 4.

100. "Anti-American Riot Led by Red Haired Chief of Woman Mob," *San Antonio Express*, January 29, 1917, 1.

101. *El Paso Morning Times*, January 29, 1917, 1.

102. *El Paso Morning Times*, January 28, 1917, 2.

103. Ibid.

104. *San Antonio Express*, January 28, 1917, 1. The *El Paso Morning Times* and the *El Paso Herald* reported that rioters broke the streetcar windows; they did not report burning streetcars.

105. *El Paso Morning Times*, January 28, 1917, 2.

106. Ibid.

107. Ibid., 1.

108. *Los Angeles Times*, January 29, 1917, 1.

109. *El Paso Morning Times*, January 28, 1917, 2.

110. Ibid.

111. See Michael Adas, *Machines as the Measure of Men: Science, Technology, and Ideologies of Western Dominance* (Ithaca: Cornell University Press, 1989), and Mathew Jacobson, *Barbarian Virtues: The United States Encounters Foreign Peoples at Home and Abroad* (New York: Hill and Wang, 2000).

112. See Kristin Hoganson, *Fighting for American Manhood: How Gender Politics Provoked the Spanish-American and Philippine-American Wars* (New Haven: Yale University Press, 1998), and Nancy K. Bristow, *Making Men Moral: Social Engineering during the Great War* (New York: New York University Press, 1997).

113. *El Paso Morning Times, Edición en Español*, January 29, 1917, 1. See also Ana María Alonso on settlers and Chihuahuan political authorities between 1850 and 1910: Alonso, *Thread of Blood: Colonialism, Gender, and Revolution on Mexico's Northern Frontier, 1800–1920* (Tucson: University of Arizona Press, 1995), 10, 177–213.

114. See *Edición en Español, El Paso Morning Times*, January 29, 1917, 1. On shifting perceptions of Pancho Villa, see Wilson, "Plotting the Border," 340–41.

115. "Precautions Taken against Epidemics of Deadly Disease," *El Paso Morning Times*, March 18, 1916, 7. Given the general absence of open armed conflict between Pershing's Expeditionary Force and Villa's forces, Pierce was probably correct that more soldiers faced illness in Fort Bliss and El Paso and Chihuahua than bullets in Mexico.

116. *San Antonio Express*, January 29, 1917, 1.

117. *Edición en Español, El Paso Morning Times*, January 29, 1917, 1.

118. Ibid.

119. For the rise of this crab-like definition of a nation's borders, see John Torpey, *The Invention of the Passport: Surveillance, Citizenship and the State* (New York: Cambridge University Press, 2000), 93–100.

120. Briggs and Briggs, *Stories in the Time of Cholera*.

121. Nancy Tomes, "The Private Side of Public Health: Sanitary Science, Domestic Hygiene, and the Germ Theory, 1870–1900," *Bulletin of the History of Medicine* 64, no. 4 (1990): 509–39. See also Pierrette Hondagneu-Sotelo, *Domestica: Immigrant Workers Cleaning and Caring in the Shadow of Affluence* (Berkeley: University of California Press, 2001); Tomes, *The Gospel of Germs*.

122. Hunter, *To 'Joy My Freedom*, 74–96.

123. *El Paso Times Edicion en Español*, January 30, 1917, 1.

124. *El Paso Times, Edición en Español*, February 15, 1917, 8.

125. Ibid.

126. Ibid.

127. Interview with Charles Armijo, January 30, 1973, conducted by Leon C. Metz, University of Texas El Paso, Institute of Oral History [UTEP-IOH], No. 106, pp. 2–3. From Sánchez, *Becoming Mexican American*, 51.

128. Interview with Conrado Mendoza, December 4, 1976, conducted by Mike Acosta, No. 252, UTEP-IOH, From *Becoming Mexican American*, 51.

129. Of the fifteen images of El Paso in the Blenkle Postcard collection at the Archives Center, five featured the streetcar and the bridge. Blenkle was a German immigrant who settled in Indiana and decided to collect postcards. The bulk of his collection is European and midwestern. His friends, however, seem to have sent him cards from their trips to the Southwest. Conversation, n.d., Fath Ruffins, Historian, Archives Center, National Museum of American History, http://collections.si.edu/search/results.jsp?q=blenkle+el+paso&image.x=0&image.y=0 (accessed March 9, 2012).

130. *El Paso Labor Advocate*, March 15, 1916. See also García, *Desert Immigrants*, 104.

131. Colgrove, *States of Immunity*, 46–52.

132. *San Antonio Express*, March 9, 1916, 1. For an extended description and analysis of American gambling, fighting, and bullring attendance, see Oscar J. Martinez, *Border Boomtown: Ciudad Juarez since 1848* (Austin: University of Texas Press, 1978).

133. C. C. Pierce, "Typhus Fever, Prevention and Control," *Texas State Medical Journal* 12 (1916): 182.

134. C. C. Pierce, "USPHS Explains How to Get Rid of Typhus," *El Paso Morning Times*, March 23, 1916, 7.

135. García, *Desert Immigrants*, 104–10; for Los Angeles, see William Francis Deverell, *Whitewashed Adobe: The Rise of Los Angeles and the Remaking of its Mexican Past* (Berkeley: University of California Press, 2004), 172–85.

136. Mexican women predominated in the Laundry Worker's Union between 1910 and 1920. García, *Desert Immigrants*, 104–10.

137. Evelynn Nakano Glenn, *Unequal Freedom: How Race and Gender Shaped American Citizenship and Labor* (Cambridge: Harvard University Press, 2002), 144–98.

138. Mario Garcia, "The Chicana in American History: The Mexican Women of El Paso, 1880–1920: A Case Study," *Pacific Historical Review* 49, no. 2 (May 1980): 315–37.

139. Pierrette Hondagneu-Sotelo, "Regulating the Unregulated? Domestic Workers' Social Networks," *Social Problems* 41 (February 1994): 50–64; Mary Romero, *Maid in the USA* (New York: Routledge, 1992).

140. The full statement: "El Paso citizens who have servants residing in Juarez are urged to have them patronize the disinfecting plant." To further seal Anglo-Americans in El Paso off from the labor they relied on, Pierce hired a "Mexican Nurse" for Mexican women. See "Disinfection to Be Used against Typhus," *El Paso Morning Times*, March 18, 1916, 12.

141. See Tomes, *The Gospel of Germs*, 229–33; Hunter, *To 'Joy My Freedom*, iii–xv.

142. See Ledesma, "Texas Newspapers and Chicana Workers' Activism," esp. 311–19.

143. For Chicana and Mexican American understandings in the 1930s and 1940s

of the importance of dressing up for a picket line, see Vicki Ruiz, "The Flapper and the Chaperone: Historical Memory among Mexican-American Women," in *Seeking Common Ground: Multidisciplinary Studies of Immigrant Women in the United States*, ed. Donna Gabaccia, 143–57 (Westport, Conn.: Greenwood, 1992). For the importance of public space to Chicana workers, see Vicki Ruiz, *From Out of the Shadows: Mexican Women in Twentieth-Century America* (New York: Oxford University Press, 2008), esp. 72–98. The coalition to pass maximum hours successfully used the example of working women's long hours to convince the Supreme Court to allow maximum hours legislation. Working women protesting in the streets were part of the First World War public scene. For the legislative campaign see Nancy Woloch, *Muller v. Oregon: A Brief History with Documents* (New York: Bedford St. Martin's, 1996), i–xxii. See Nancy Cott, *The Grounding of Modern Feminism* (New Haven: Yale University Press, 1989), for a discussion of working women's participation in the suffrage movement.

144. Ledesma, "Texas Newspapers and Chicana Workers' Activism," 312.

145. Ibid., 313. The quote comes from *El Paso Labor Advocate*, October 31, 1919.

146. Ibid., 314.

147. García, *Desert Immigrants*, 104–10. For sample articles, see "Erect No Adobes," *El Paso City and County Labor Advocate*, October 22, 1915, 2. See also "The South End of El Paso," *El Paso City and County Labor Advocate*, October 3, 1915.

148. "Craze to Examine Workers Denounced," *El Paso City and County Labor Advocate*, September 3, 1915.

149. "A Visit to the South End of El Paso," *El Paso City and County Labor Advocate*, September 3, 1915, 4.

150. Tomes, "The Private Side of Public Health."

151. Quinn, *One Man Tango*, 47–48.

152. Sánchez, *Becoming Mexican American*, 51.

153. Ibid.

154. Debbie Nathan, "The Eyes of Texas Are Upon You," in *Women and Other Aliens* (Houston: Arte Publico Press, 1993), 5–18.

Six. Bodies of Evidence

1. J. R. Monroe, "Requests Congressional Aid from John Garner," August 17, 1911, RG 90, Subject Files No. 2796—Smallpox, USPHS Files, 1897–1923, NACP.

2. H. J. Hamilton, "Report of Investigation on Trip along Lower Mexican Border," September 18, 1911, pp. 1–7, RG 90, Subject Files No. 2796—Smallpox, USPHS Files, 1897–1923, NACP.

3. H. J. Hamilton, "Report of Investigation on Trip along Lower Mexican Border," September 18, 1911, RG 90, Subject Files No. 2796—Smallpox, USPHS Files, 1897–1923, NACP.

4. H. J. Hamilton, "Report on the Prevalence of Smallpox on the Lower Mexican

Border," September 24, 1911, RG 90, Subject Files No. 2796—Smallpox, USPHS Files, 1897–1923, NACP.

5. H. J. Hamilton, "Regarding Smallpox Epidemic Past Winter and Spring," August 24, 1915, p. 7, RG 90, Subject Files No. 2796—Smallpox, USPHS Files, 1897–1923, NACP.

6. Despatch No. 1105 from Piedras Negras Regarding Issuance of Order by Texas Health Officer and United States Marine Hospital Service Officer Stationed at Eagle Pass, Texas, for Vaccination of All Persons Entering United States through Port of Eagle Pass, January 18, 1916, Piedras Negras, Consular Despatches, RG 59, State Department Decimal Files, 812.00/17134, NACP.

7. J. P. Reynolds, "Letter to Spivey, in Reference to Certain Charges Brought Against Me by Mexican Consul, by Dr. John H. Hunter," RG 59, State Department Decimal Files, 1910–1920, Enclosure VII, 158.1208/11, NACP.

8. Cardenas, "Nuevo Leon Cientifico," *La Colonia Mexicana*, May 6, 1891, 1. Raymundo Benavides García, *Historia de la salud pública en Nuevo León, 1820–1950* (Monterrey: Universidad Autonoma de Nuevo León, 1998).

9. H. J. Hamilton, "Regarding Smallpox Epidemic Past Winter and Spring," August 24, 1915, p. 7, RG 90, Subject Files No. 2796—Smallpox, USPHS Files, 1897–1923, NACP.

10. Dr. W. A. Sawyer, "Smallpox in Mexican Quarter in Banning," September 27, 1915, RG 90, Subject Files No. 2796—Smallpox, USPHS Files, 1897–1923, NACP.

11. Ibid. In response to the epidemic in Chattanooga, the Chattanooga chamber of commerce mounted a compulsory vaccination campaign.

12. Ibid.

13. J. C. Geiger, "Investigation of an Outbreak of Smallpox at Banning, Special Report to James S. Cumming, Director, Bureau of Communicable Disease, California State Board of Health," December 27, 1916, p. 2, RG 90, Subject Files No. 2796—Smallpox, USPHS Files, 1897–1923, NACP.

14. Dr. Sawyer, "Smallpox in Banning," November 9, 1916, RG 90, Subject Files No. 2796—Smallpox, USPHS Files, 1897–1923, NACP.

15. There are two book-length surveys of Mexican consular advocacy in the United States between 1910 and 1940: F. Arturo Rosales, *¡Pobre Raza! Violence, Justice, and Mobilization among México Lindo Immigrants, 1900–1936* (Austin: University of Texas Press, 1999), and Gilbert González, *Mexican Consuls and Labor Organizing: Imperial Politics in the American Southwest* (Austin: University of Texas Press, 1999). For a suggestive account of the contradictions of Mexican national formation in Los Angeles's greater Mexican community, see Sánchez, *Becoming Mexican American*, 107–29.

16. Surgeon R. H. Creel, "Re: Communication from Confidential Agent of Defacto Government of Mexico Requesting Modification of Quarantine Restrictions at Rio Grande City against Incoming Travel on the Mexican Border," August 17, 1916," RG 59, State Department Decimal Records, Mexico, 1910–1920, Decimal Files, 158.129/31, NACP.

17. Hamilton, "Report of Investigation on Trip along Lower Mexican Border," 1–7.

18. For cogent discussions of Chihuahua between 1910 and 1914, see William Beezley, *Insurgent Governor: Abraham Gonzalez and the Mexican Revolution in Chihuahua* (Lincoln: University of Nebraska Press, 1973); and Katz, *The Life and Times of Pancho Villa.*

19. This long summary comes from the following three monographs: Friedrich Katz, *The Secret War in Mexico: Europe, the United States, and the Mexican Revolution* (Chicago: University of Chicago Press, 1981); Katz, *The Life and Times of Pancho Villa*; and Beezley, *Insurgent Governor.*

20. Katz, *Secret War*; Katz, *The Life and Times of Pancho Villa*; Beezley, *Insurgent Governor*; Sánchez, *Becoming Mexican American*, 17–37; Montejano, *Anglos and Mexicans*, 118–25.

21. H. J. Hamilton, Acting Assistant Surgeon, "Report from Dr. Elizondo Received," December 3, 1911, RG 90, Subject Files No. 2796—Smallpox, USPHS Files, 1897–1923, NACP; Eduardo Idar, "Rumor infundo," *Evolución*, July 15, 1899, 3.

22. Edward Flannery, Inspector, Rio Grande City Station, "Enclosure: Board of Special Inquiry Regarding the Exclusion of Juana Garza and Her Two Children, Epemenia Solis, Female, Age 5 and Ophelia Solis, Female, Age 3," September 24, 1916, RG 59, State Department Decimal Files, 1910–1920, Enclosure X, 158.1208/11, NACP.

23. Ibid.

24. Ibid.

25. George J. Harris, Acting Supervising Inspector, El Paso Station, "Final Report on Alleged Abuses at Rio Grande City Immigration Station," June 2, 1917, RG 59, State Department Decimal Files, 1910–1920, Enclosure X, 158.1208/11, NACP.

26. Miguel Barrera, Resident of Sam Fordyce, Texas, "In Spite of Having My Residence on American Soil, the Doctor Refused to Hear My Arguments and Vaccinated Me," Filed in Rio Grande City, September 18, 1916, RG 59, State Department Decimal Files, 158.1208/13, Enclosure VI, NACP.

27. J. P. Reynolds, Chief Inspector, Brownsville Station, "Deposition Taken from Leoncio P. Revelas Regarding Complaints at Immigration Station by Chief Inspector J. P. Reynolds, Brownsville District," May 23, 1917, RG 59, State Department Decimal Files, 1910–1920, Enclosure V, 158.1208/11, NACP.

28. Sánchez, *Becoming Mexican American*, 51–55.

29. Fairchild, *Science at the Borders*, 122, from figure 4.3: "Number of immigrants deported on arrival for all causes by region, 1891–1930."

30. Ibid., 23–53.

31. Ibid., 119–23.

32. For Mexican nationals, see Sánchez, *Becoming Mexican American*, 25–50. For Chinese migrants, see Erika Lee, "Enforcing the Borders: Chinese Exclusion along the U.S. Borders with Canada and Mexico, 1882–1924," *Journal of American History* 89, no. 1 (2002): 54–87; Ann Gabbert, "El Paso, a Sight for Sore Eyes: Medical and Legal Aspects of Syrian Immigration, 1906–1907," *Historian* 65, no. 1 (2002): 15–42.

33. Benjamin Hebert Johnson, *Revolution in Texas: How a Bloody Insurrection Turned Mexicans into Americans* (New Haven: Yale University Press, 2003), 111–20. See also Montejano, *Anglos and Mexicans*, 106–29.

34. Johnson, *Revolution in Texas*.

35. Leavitt, *Typhoid Mary*, 70–96.

36. Reynolds, "Deposition Taken from Leoncio P. Revelas."

37. Rosales, *¡Pobre Raza!*, 35–37.

38. Ibid., 39 n. 34.

39. For further exploration of the terror that targeted Mexicans between 1915 and 1920 in South Texas, see Montejano, *Anglos and Mexicans*, 106–29.

40. Two monographs on Mexican consular activism in the United States have highlighted opposing images of Mexican consular activities in the United States. Gilbert González, in his examination of consular activities in farm labor disputes in California, argued that consuls, because of their middle-class origins and Mexican affiliation, emphasized forms of institutional cooperation between agrobusiness interests and labor organizers in California. F. A. Rosales argues that consuls defended "the Mexican race" through individual advocacy of specific claims of injustice between 1900 and 1930. See González, *Mexican Consuls and Labor Organizing*, 39, and Rosales, *¡Pobre Raza!*

41. Patricia Williams, "The Pain of Word Bondage," in *The Alchemy of Race and Rights* (Cambridge: Harvard University Press, 1991), 147–50.

42. Eliseo Arredondo, "Smallpox Quarantine against Camargo Unnecessary and Causing Much Hardship," January 28, 1916, RG 59, State Department Decimal Records, Mexico, 1910–1920, Subject Files, 158.125/68, NACP.

43. Eliseo Arredondo, "Mexican Embassy. Protests Sanitary Restrictions against Camargo. Believes Vaccination Indiscriminately Practiced," April 18, 1916, RG 59, State Department Decimal Records, Mexico, 1910–1920, Subject Files, 158.125/79, NACP.

44. United States Consul, Piedras Negras, "Two Deaths from Smallpox and Orders Vaccination of All Persons Entering United States from Mexico at That Point," January 16, 1916, RG 59, State Department Decimal Records, Mexico, 1910–1920, Subject Files, 158.125/63, NACP.

45. Piedras Negras, United States Consul, "Similar Orders to American Quarantine Issued against Americans Entering Mexico. Situation Serious," March 6, 1916, RG 59, State Department Decimal Records, Mexico, 1910–1920, Subject Files, 158.125/71, NACP.

46. Piedras Negras, United States Consul, "Quarantine Regulations Issued on Both Sides of the Border," March 7, 1916, RG 59, State Department Decimal Records, Mexico, 1910–1920, Subject Files, 158.125/76, NACP.

47. Ibid.

48. Piedras Negras, United States Consul, "Quarantine Raised and Differences

Amicably Settled," March 7, 1916, RG 59, State Department Decimal Records, Mexico, 1910–1920, Subject Files, 158.125/72, NACP.

49. Katz, *The Life and Times of Pancho Villa*, 545–615.

50. Eliseo Arredondo, "Mexican Embassy. Protests Sanitary Restrictions Against Camargo. Believes Vaccination Indiscriminately Practiced," April 18, 1916, RG 59, State Department Decimal Records, Mexico, 1910–1920, Subject Files, 158.125/79, NACP.

51. Ambassador R. H. Creel, "Re: Communication from Confidential Agent of De-facto Government of Mexico Requesting Modification of Quarantine Restrictions at Rio Grande City against Incoming Travel on the Mexican Border," August 17, 1916, RG 59, State Department Decimal Records, Mexico, 1910–1920, Decimal Files, 158.129/31, NACP.

52. Ibid.

53. Eliseo Arredondo, "Deposition Taken in Mexico from Coroner and Witnesses Regarding Cause of Montelongo's Death," August 19, 1916, RG 59, State Department Decimal Files, Mexico, 1910–1920, 158.008/12, NACP.

54. Eliseo Arredondo, "Death of Jose Montelongo Because 'All Mexicans Caught in the Act of Entering the United States Surreptitiously Should Be Returned to the Mexican Side by Water,'" August 21, 1916, RG 59, State Department Decimal Files, Mexico, 1910–1920, 158.008/11, NACP.

55. Judge H. C. Ramirez, "Deposition Taken in Mexico from Coroner and Witnesses Regarding Cause of Montelongo's Death," August 19, 1916, RG 59, State Department Decimal Files, Mexico, 158.008/12, NACP.

56. Ibid.

57. Ibid.

58. Arredondo, "Death of Jose Montelongo."

59. Texas Quarantine Officer Dr. H. C. Hall, "Report Regarding Unfortunate Drowning Death of Mexican," August 19, 1916, RG 59, State Department Decimal Files, Mexico, 1910–1920, 158.008/13, NACP.

60. Arredondo, "Death of Jose Montelongo."

61. John Wroe, Secretary to Texas Governor Ferguson, "The Montelongo Complaint Is Registered with the Department for the Purpose of Injuring Dr. Hall and of Encouraging the Law Breakers along the Border," September 11, 1916, RG 59, State Department Decimal Files, Mexico, 1910–1920, 158.008/13, NACP.

62. Ibid.

63. Office of the Solicitor, Department of State, "Solicitor Recommends Prosecution of Dr. Hall under Texas Statute, 'Excusable Homicide,'" October 12, 1916, RG 59, State Department Decimal Files, Mexico, 1910–1920, 158.008/14, NACP.

64. Secretary John Wroe, "In re—Death of Jose Montelongo," RG 59, State Department Decimal Files, 1910–1920, 158.008/15, NACP.

65. John Walls, D.A., "Report to the Governor on Grand Jury Finding re: Drowning of Mexican Citizen named Jose Montelongo," December 1, 1916, RG 59, State Department Decimal Files, 1910–1920, 158.008/17, NACP.

66. For a far more in-depth discussion of the racial-national contradictions of federal and state jurisdiction, see Leiker, *Racial Borders*, esp. 93–118.

67. Wroe, "Report to the Governor on Grand Jury Finding re: Drowning of Mexican Citizen named Jose Montelongo."

68. Melquiades Garcés, "Translation of Letter to Ygnacio Bonillas, Ambassador to the United States," April 23, 1917, RG 59, State Department Decimal Files, 1910–1920, 158.1208/3, Enclosure 1, NACP. I have the copy of the letter in English.

69. Ibid.

70. Ibid.

71. Ibid.

72. Dr. H. C. Hall, Texas State Health Officer, Quarantine Service, Laredo, "Re: Mexican Complaints about Vexations of Quarantine Guards," RG 59, State Department Files, Mexico, Decimal Files, 1910–1920, 158.1208/3, NACP.

73. Ibid.

74. Ibid.

75. Ibid.

76. Ibid.

77. Ibid.

78. Ibid.

79. Ibid.

80. Gurza, "Vacuna, August 27, 1808," Bexar Papers Collection, 1776–1836, DBCAH.

81. R. R. de la Vega (1851.0801), "El jefe politico de Colima participa haber desarrollado en aquel territorio la epidemia de viruelas," GD 127, Gobernación, Caja 391, Expediente 1, Mexico City.

82. Miguel Barrera, "In Spite of Having My Residence on American Soil, the Doctor Refused to Hear My Arguments and Vaccinated Me," Filed in Rio Grande City, September 18, 1916, RG 59, Department of State Decimal Files, 1910–1920, 158.1208/13 Enclosure VI, NACP.

83. If Barrera was as old as he claimed and he was vaccinated at the age this was normally done in Mexico, this would date the original vaccination to 1853, before the liberal reforms of 1857 and the civil war that enveloped the Juarez presidency. The Barrera family would have probably been a family resident in a fairly urban area and committed to a version of modernity. I chose 1853 based on the average age of vaccination mentioned in Angela Thompson's survey of vaccination in Guanajuato; see Thompson, *Las otras guerras de México* (Guanajuato: Universidad Autónoma de Guanajuato, 1997), 6–10.

84. Books, articles, and monographs that examine Porfirian investments in modernity are too numerous to detail here. This discussion of modernity, northern

Mexico, and the Porfiriato builds on a recent survey by Robert Buffington and William French, "The Culture of Modernity," in *The Oxford History of Mexico*, ed. William Beezley (New York: Oxford University Press, 2000), 397–431.

85. William E. French, "Prostitutes and Guardian Angels: Women, Work, and Family in Porfirian Mexico," *Hispanic American Historical Review* 72, no. 3 (1992): 529–53.

86. Miguel E. Bustamante, "Vigesimoquinto aniversario de la eradicación de la viruela en Mexico," *Gaceta Medica de Mexico* 113, no. 12 (December 1977): 556.

87. Hamilton, "Report of Investigation on Trip along Lower Mexican Border," 1–7. See also Brown, "Trabajadores nativos y extranjeros en el México Porfiriano."

88. C. L. Baker, American Smelting and Refining Corporation, "Health and Starvation Conditions. Encloses Letter from C.L. Baker," RG 59, State Department, Decimal Subject Files, 158.12/19, Treasury, NACP.

89. Angela Thompson mentioned that among some rural residents in Guanajuato, the mark of smallpox was proof of a peasant's strength and therefore distinction. See Angela T. Thompson, "To Save the Children: Smallpox Inoculation, Vaccination, and Public Health in Guanajuato, Mexico, 1797–1840," *Americas (Academy of Franciscan History)* 49, no. 4 (1993): 431–55, esp. 438–42. See also Thompson, *Las otras guerras de México*. In the survey of epidemics in twentieth-century Peru, Marcos Cueto mentioned that many Quechua women used the presence of smallpox scars on men as proof of their resilience and physical strength. See Cueto, "Indigenismo and Rural Medicine in Peru: The Indian Sanitary Brigade and Manuel Nuñez Buitron," *Bulletin of the History of Medicine* 65, no. 1 (1991): 22–41.

90. Ibid.

91. The "Good Government" plank meant a middle-class slate of candidates with no Mexicans, no African Americans, and hopefully no machine politicians. This reform rhetoric supported the establishment of the white man's primary in Texas. Darlene Clark Hine, *Black Victory: The Rise and Fall of the White Primary in Texas*, new ed. (Columbia: University of Missouri, 2003). For the disenfranchisement of Mexican electors in South Texas, see Montejano, *Anglos and Mexicans*, 136. "Good" meant exclusively white and middle class.

92. See Evan Anders, *Boss Rule in South Texas: The Progressive Era* (Austin: University of Texas Press, 1982), 220–35.

93. Jorge Olivares, Rio Grande City resident, "Complaint Regarding Treatment at Rio Grande Station of Mexicans by Inspectors and Doctors Filed in Rio Grande City," May 9, 1917 (trans. J. H. Decker, the consular clerk for Leoncio Revelas), RG 59, State Department Decimal Files, 158.1208/13, Enclosure, NACP.

94. Elliott Young, "Deconstructing *La Raza*: Identifying the *Gente Decente* of Laredo, 1904–1911," *Southwestern Historical Quarterly* 98, no. 2 (1994): 227–59.

95. Ibid.

96. Jorge Olivares, Rio Grande City resident, "Complaint Regarding Treatment at

Rio Grande Station of Mexicans by Inspectors and Doctors Filed in Rio Grande City," May 9, 1917, RG 59, State Department Decimal Files, 158.1208/13, Enclosure, NACP.

97. Ibid. The rhetoric is similar to that in the *Plan de San Diego*. For a facsimile of the manifesto, see Montejano, *Anglos and Mexicans*, 126.

98. Enclosure, Deposition of Efraím Domínguez, Ygnacio Bonillas, "Complaint No. 2," May 22, 1917, RG 59, State Department Decimal Files, 1910–1920, 158.1208/7, NACP.

99. Ibid. The original sentence clause follows: "Teniendo que tolerar que medio lo desnudasen para revisarle sus ropas interiores no obstante el perfecto estado de limpieza visible aun desde lejos."

100. Ibid., 3.

101. Ibid.

102. "Ephraím Dominguez, Ygnacio Bonillas, "Complaint No. 2," May 22, 1917, RG 59, State Department Records, Decimal Files, 1910–1920, 158.1208/7, NACP.

103. Ibid.

104. Ibid.

105. "Ciudadanos Mexicanos" is an odd choice of words. Miguel Barrera and Jorge Olivares implied through their use of a consul for the de facto regime in Mexico an attachment to the mechanisms of the emerging post-Revolutionary state. The long-term benefits of this attachment to these two citizens may have been suspect, given that they were residents of the United States.

106. Ygnacio Bonillas, "Complaint No. 2," May 22, 1917, RG 59, State Department Decimal Files, 1910–1920, 158.1208/7, NACP. The key passage in Spanish follows: "Un informe en el que expone los malos tratamientos de que son objetos los ciudadanos Mexicanos por parte de las autoridades sanitarias del lado Americano."

107. Ignacio Bonillas, Embajada de Mexico en los Estados Unidos, "The Mexican Consul Reports a Concrete Case of Lack of Consideration on the Part of Sanitation Authorities toward Mexican Citizens and Dwells on the Fact That Such Are Frequent," May 7, 1917, RG 59, State Department Files, Mexico, Decimal Files, 1910–1920, 158.1208/3, NACP.

108. Ibid.

109. Ibid.

110. Edward Flannery, Inspector, Rio Grande City Station, "Letter Regarding Charge That I Treat Immigrants with Discourtesy," June 11, 1917, RG 59, State Department Decimal Files, 1910–1920, Enclosure X, 158.1208/11, NACP.

111. Ibid.

112. Ibid.

113. Leoncio Revelas, Mexican Consul, Rio Grande City, "Response to Investigation in Rio Grande City by W. M. Spivey, State Quarantine Officer," June 11, 1917, RG 59, State Department Decimal Files, 1910–1920, 158.1208/11, Enclosure IV, NACP; Reynolds, "Deposition Taken from Leoncio P. Revelas."

114. See Anders, *Boss Rule in South Texas*, 200–240.

115. See Allwyn Barr, *From Reconstruction to Reform: Politics in Texas, 1876–1906* (Austin: University of Texas Press, 1971), 95–170.

116. Montejano, *Anglos and Mexicans*, 128–39.

117. Ibid.

118. Ibid.

119. Ibid.

120. Ibid.

121. Ibid.

122. E. P. Reynolds, "Deposition on Complaints by Mexican Consul Leoncio Revelas, taken by E. P. Reynolds, Inspector in Charge," June 6, 1917, RG 59, State Department Decimal Files, 1910–1920, Enclosure IX, 158.1208/11, NACP.

123. Ibid.

124. For a discussion of consent and compulsory vaccination, see chapter 7.

125. J. P. Reynolds, "Letter to Spivey, in Reference to Certain Charges Brought against Me by Mexican Consul, by Dr. John H. Hunter," RG 59, State Department Decimal Files, 1910–1920, Enclosure VII, 158.1208/11, NACP.

126. The evidence gathered by Inspector J. P. Reynolds in his investigation of Rio Grande City complicates this assertion. Judging by the complaints filed by Consul Revelas and the deposition filed by Juana Garza, the assistant surgeon, John Hunter, did indeed communicate to incoming Mexican arrivals that they had to submit to vaccination if they wanted to enter the United States. Juana Garza, in her deposition, was shocked that she and her children were deported back to Mexico after all three members of her family were vaccinated against smallpox. Consul Revelas registered this shock and, based on other information, charged Dr. Hunter with deceit because a number of deportees were vaccinated and then deported. Reynolds, "Deposition Taken from Leoncio P. Revelas."

127. J. P. Reynolds, "Letter to Spivey, in Reference to Certain Charges Brought against Me by Mexican Consul, by Dr. John H. Hunter," RG 59, State Department Decimal Files, 1910–1920, Enclosure VII, 158.1208/11, NACP.

128. J. P. Reynolds, Chief Inspector, Brownsville Station, "Final Report Regarding Complaints at Rio Grande City—J. P. Reynolds," May 26, 1917, RG 59, State Department, Decimal Files, 1910–1920, Enclosure XII, 158.1208/13, Enclosure II, NACP.

129. Ibid.

130. Ibid.

131. Reynolds, "Deposition Taken from Leoncio P. Revelas."

132. Ibid.

133. The full quote follows: "In Camargo and its neighborhood, there are some people who are not satisfied with the way they have been treated when applying for admission in this country." See Leoncio Revelas, "Response to Investigation in Rio Grande City by W. M. Spivey, State Quarantine Officer," June 11, 1917, RG 59, State Department Decimal Files, 1910–1920, Enclosure IV, 158.1208/11, NACP.

134. Ibid.

135. "Reports Complaint by Mexican Consul in Eagle Pass Regarding Vaccination Inspection by Medical Inspector at Quarantine Station," RG 59, State Department Decimal Subject Files, 1910–1920, Treasury Department, 158.125/89, NACP.

136. Ibid.

137. Acting Secretary of Labor John Abercrombie, "Inspector Charles Parker, Enclosure II Deposition, Inspector Chris Parker," June 9, 1918, in "Investigation Subsequent to Complaint by Mexican Consul Regarding Vaccination of Two Sisters, Eagle Pass," June 8, 1918, RG 59, State Department Decimal Files, 158.125/90, NACP.

138. Ibid.

139. Miguel E. Bustamante, "Aniversario de la eradicación de la viruela," *Gaceta Médica de México* 113, no. 12 (December 1977): 556.

140. United States Shipping Board, "Protests Regarding Certificate of Smallpox Vaccination in Tampico," February 24, 1921, RG 59, State Department Decimal Subject Files, "Sanitary Conditions in Mexico," 158.1201/24, NACP.

141. Summerlin, "Revaccinating Whenever Deemed Expedient," April 9, 1921, RG 59, State Department Decimal Subject Files, "Sanitary Conditions in Mexico," 158.1201/25, NACP.

142. For an inspiring look at eugenics and immigration exclusions in Mexico and Latin America, see Nancy Leys Stepan, *In the Hour of Eugenics: Race, Gender, and Nation in Latin America* (Ithaca: Cornell University Press, 1991). For a more focused account that develops the intellectual eugenic networks that linked social policy in Mexico and the United States, see Alexandra Minna Stern, "Buildings, Boundaries, and Blood: Medicalization and Nation-Building on the U.S.-Mexico Border, 1910–1930," *Hispanic American Historical Review* 79, no. 1 (1999): 41–81.

Seven. Between Border Quarantine and the Texas-Mexico Border

1. Don Gaspar, "Los Mexicanos en la carrera de Maratón," *Excelsior*, August 7, 1932, 4.

2. Lamberto Alvarez Gayou, "La influencia de la decimal olimpiada en la nueva educacion fisica de Mexico," Seccion subsecretaria de educacion publica, Caja 1, Expediente 21, Subserie Alvarez Gayou, Lamberto, 1931–1932, Folio 22–27, SEP Archive, Mexico City.

3. "Frijoles para los indigenas," *Excelsior*, July 22, 1932, 4.

4. Seymour Lowman, "the extension of free entry privilege to foreign participants in Olympic Games," has been received through the office of the Deputy Commissioner, Divisions of Customs Agents, Treasury Department, Washington, D.C., Seymour Lowman, "The extension of free entry privileges to foreign participants in Olympic Games, August 3, 1931," edited by Los Angeles Olympic Committee, *The Games of the Xth Olympiade, Los Angeles, 1932: Official Report* (Los Angeles: The Xth Olympiade Committee of the Games of Los Angeles), 225.

5. Complaints Regarding Inoculation of Mexican Olympic Team in El Paso, 1932, RG 59, State Department Decimal Subject Files, 158.1208, Mexican Embassy, NACP.

6. Ibid.

7. Robert N. McLean, "Goodbye Vicente," *Survey* 66 (May 1, 1931): 182–83 (italics in the original). For the response in Laredo, see Richard Boyce, "Immigration: Repatriation of Mexicans through Laredo, Texas," January 12, 1931, RG 90, State Department Decimal Files, 311.1215/19, NACP.

8. "Los Mexicanos en la carrera de Maratón."

9. Lamberto Alvarez Gayou, "Influencia de la decima olimpiada," Sección subsecretaria de educacion publica, Caja 1, Expediente 21, Subserie Alvarez Gayou, Lamberto, 1931–1932, Folio 22–27, SEP Archive, Mexico City.

10. Translation, *El Universal Grafico*, August 8, 1932, RG 59, State Department Decimal Files, 811.4063-olympic games/367, NACP.

11. "Editoriales breves: El desastre de las Olimpiadas," *Excelsior*, August 13, 1932, 5.

12. The full text in Spanish follows: "Que saben nuestros pobres indigenas de marathones, ni como han de vencer a deportistas preparados desde su niñez, sujetos a una alimentación especial, a un genero de vida adecuada, discipulos de famosos maestros y aleccionados en todos los secretos del 'arte' a que se dedican." In "Editoriales breves: El desastre de las Olimpiadas," 5.

13. Lamberto Alvarez Gayou, "La influencia de la decima olimpiada," Seccion subsecretaria de educacion publica, Caja 1, Expediente 21, Subserie Alvarez Gayou, Lamberto, 1931–1932, Folio 22–27, SEP Archive, Mexico City.

14. Gayou, "Influencia," 2

15. Editorial, "extreme health measures," *El Universal Grafico*, August 8, 1932, in Reuben Clark, "Alleged Inoculations of the Mexican Olympic Team, August 18, 1932," RG 59, State Department, Decimal Files, 811.4063-olympic games/367, NACP.

16. Ibid.

17. Dr. Allen claimed he administered smallpox vaccinations in the inspection stations at the bridge. Complaints regarding inoculation of Mexican Olympic team in El Paso, 1932, RG 59, State Department Decimal Subject Files, 158.1208, Mexican Embassy, NACP.

18. Editorial, *El Universal Grafico*, August 8, 1932.

19. Complaints regarding inoculation of Mexican Olympic team in El Paso, 1932.

20. Richard Allen, "Report of Inspection of Border Stations along the Rio Grande," September 1938, RG 90, USPHS General Classified Records, 1936–1944, Subject File 1850–95: El Paso Quarantine 1935–1939, NACP. In El Paso, Irving McNeil was born in 1867. In Presidio, the surgeon Francis Gibbons was born in 1871. In Del Rio, H. B. Ross was born in 1868. In Eagle Pass, Lea Hume was born in 1875. In Laredo, O. T. Arnold was born in 1865. In Zapata, W. A. Harper was born in 1866. In Roma, R. C. Hannah was born in 1869. In Rio Grande City, Dr. C. J. Martin was born in 1883. In Hidalgo, J. M. Hardy was born in 1873. In Thayer, Dr. Charles Buck was born

in 1869. In San Antonio, the immigration inspector Dr. Beal was born in 1867. For Irving McNeil, see Heritagequestonline.com, Series T624, Roll 1549, p. 136. http:// www.heritagequestonline.com/hqoweb/library/do/index (accessed March 12, 2012).

21. For an overview of vd efforts in the New Deal, see Brandt, *No Magic Bullet*, 122–61. For efforts to address infant mortality, see Richard A. Meckel, *"Save the Babies": American Public Health Reform and the Prevention of Infant Mortality, 1850–1920* (Baltimore: Johns Hopkins University Press, 1990), 178–220. For the usphs untreated syphilis treatment survey in Macon County, see Susan Reverby, *Examining Tuskegee: The Infamous Syphilis Study and Its Legacy* (Chapel Hill: University of North Carolina Press, 2010), 29–73. For tb and urban African American communities, see Samuel Roberts, *Infectious Fear: Politics, Disease, and the Health Effects of Segregation* (Chapel Hill: University of North Carolina Press, 2008), 169–201.

22. Charles Armstrong, "Typhus Fever on the San Juan Indian Reservation, 1920 and 1921," *Public Health Reports* 37, no. 12 (1922): 685–93.

23. Wilbur Sawyer, "Public Health Implications of Tropical and Imported Diseases," *American Journal of Public Health* 34, no. 1 (1944): 10–15.

24. Margaret Humphreys, "A Stranger to Our Camps: Typhus in American History," *Bulletin of the History of Medicine* 80, no. 2 (2006): 269–90.

25. Sawyer, "Public Health Implications"; C. R. Eskey, "Relation of Reported Cases of Typhus Fever to Location, Temperature, and Precipitation," *Public Health Reports* 63, no. 29 (July 16, 1948): 941–48.

26. Nathan King, "Compensation and Duties of Attendants," December 31, 1920, rg 90, usphs, Laredo Quarantine, 1923–1939, nc 34-E10, Box 259, nacp.

27. Ibid.

28. Ibid.

29. Joe I. Sanders, "Annual Report Del Rio Quarantine," June 30, 1940, rg 90, usphs General Classified Records, 1936–1944, Subject File 1850–15: Del Rio Station, nacp.

30. L. Lumsden, "Recent Inspections of El Paso, Eagle Pass, and Laredo, TX," November 7, 1934, rg 90, usphs Decimal Files, 1930–1935, Subject File 1850–95: Quarantine Stations, Decimal File, 711.129, nacp.

31. F. A. Carmelia, "Note to Medical Inspector in Charge of Laredo Station," September 12, 1935, rg 90, usphs Decimal Files, 1850–15, Laredo Quarantine, 1923–1939,nacp.

32. Lumsden, "Recent Inspections."

33. P. J. Gorman, "Narrative Report Covering Transaction by US Quarantine Station, Laredo, Texas, July 7, 1938." rg 90 usphs, Decimal Files 1935–1939, Subject File 1850–15: Laredo Quarantine Station, nacp.

34. Richard Allen, "Of Quarantine Operations at El Paso, Texas during Fiscal Year June 30, 1936," rg 59, usphs Decimal Files, Subject File 1850–95: El Paso Quarantine,

NACP Richard Allen, "Of Quarantine Operations at El Paso, Texas during Fiscal Year June 30, 1938," RG 59, USPHS Decimal Files, Subject File 1850–95: El Paso Quarantine, NACP.

35. Irving McNeil,, "Response to April 22 Letter," April 26, 1936, RG 59, USPHS Decimal Files, Subject File 1850–95: El Paso Quarantine, NACP.

36. Richard Allen, "Of Quarantine Operations at El Paso, Texas during Fiscal Year June 30, 1936."

37. Richard Allen, AA Surgeon in Charge, "To C. L. Williams Regarding Fumigation Baths," November 4, 1938, RG 59, USPHS General Classified Records, 1936–1944, Subject File 1850–95: El Paso Quarantine, NACP.

38. Richard Allen, "Of Quarantine Operations at El Paso, Texas during Fiscal Year June 30, 1936," RG 59, USPHS Decimal Files, 1850–95: El Paso Quarantine, NACP.

39. Ibid.

40. P. J. Gorman, Surgeon in Charge in Laredo, "Responding to Letter of May 31, 1935 Activities in Eagle Pass Quarantine Station," RG 90, USPHS General Classified Records, 1936–1944, Subject File 1850–15: Laredo Quarantine Files, NACP.

41. Ibid.

42. Ibid.

43. Lea Hume, "Annual Report Eagle Pass Quarantine Station," July 7, 1936, RG 90, USPHS, General Classified Records, 1936–1944, Subject File 1850–1915: Eagle Pass Quarantine, NACP.

44. Lumsden, "Recent Inspections."

45. Richard Allen, "Inspection Trip of Border Ports East of El Paso," February 22, 1943, RG 90, USPHS, General Classified Records, 1936–1944, Subject File 1850–95: El Paso Quarantine, NACP.

46. Richard Allen, "Report of Inspection Trip to Ports East of El Paso," November 1941, RG 90, USPHS, General Classified Records, 1936–1944, Subject File 1850: El Paso Quarantine, NACP.

47. Breckinridge Long, "Guarding against Typhus Fever," p. 1, RG 59 State Department Decimal Files, 1940–1945, 158.09-typhus/1, NACP.

48. Breckinridge Long, *America and the Holocaust*, www.pbs.org/wgbh/amex/holocaust/peopleevents/pandeAMEX90.html (accessed March 23, 2011).

49. Sawyer, "Public Health Implications," 12.

50. Ibid.

51. Don Aubertine, USPHS Inspector, "Letter to Colonel Walter Harrison, USPHS District 5 Supervisor, USPHS San Francisco Office," May 18, 1944, RG 90 USPHS General Classified Records, 1936–1944, Subject File 1850: Mexico–Mexico, NACP.

52. Thomas Parran, "Letter to Colonel Walter Harrison USPHS District 5 Supervisor, USPHS San Francisco Office," May 9, 1944, RG 90 USPHS, General Classified Records, 1936–1944, Decimal Files, Subject File 1850: Mexico, NACP.

53. Carlos Ortiz-Mariotte and Felipe Malo-Juvera, "Control of Typhus Fever in Mexican Villages and Rural Populations through the Use of DDT," *American Journal of Public Health* 35, no. 11 (1945): 1191–95.

54. Mireya Loza, "Pedro del Real Pérez," in Bracero History Archive, Item No. 152, braceroarchive.org/items/show/152 (accessed March 23, 2011).

55. Myrna Parra-Mantilla, "Elías Espino," in Bracero History Archive, Item No. 7, braceroarchive.org/items/show/7 (accessed March 23, 2011).

56. Fernanda Carrillo, "Faye Terrazas," in Bracero History Archive, Item No. 50, braceroarchive.org/items/show/50 (accessed March 24, 2011).

57. Anaís Acosta, "Alberto Magallón Jiménez," in Bracero History Archive, Item No. 153, braceroarchive.org/items/show/153 (accessed March 24, 2011).

58. Meckel, *"Save the Babies,"* 198–221.

59. Colgrove, *States of Immunity*, 1–76.

60. Summerlin, "Revaccinating Whenever Deemed Expedient," April 9, 1921, RG 59, State Department Decimal Subject Files, 158.1201/25, NACP.

61. For Nogales, Douglas, and Naco, see H. S. Cummings, "Re: Smallpox in Arizona," July 28, 1923, RG 90, USPHS Central Files, 1897–1923, File No. 2796, Smallpox, Box 254, NACP. For Ajo and San Fernando, see John M. Hardy, AA Surgeon, San Fernando, "Not Been a Known Case of Smallpox in This Section of Mexico," June 25, 1923, RG 90, USPHS Central Files, 1897–1923, File No. 2796, Smallpox, Box 254, NACP.

62. Dr. W. E. Quinn, La Botica Internacional, Monclova, Coahuila, "Smallpox and Texas-Mexicans in Monclova," August 15, 1918, RG 90, USPHS Central Files, 1897–1923, File No. 2796, NACP.

63. "Compulsory Vaccination Approved by Council," *El Paso Herald*, August 30, 1923, 1.

64. Ibid.

65. Ibid.

66. Linda Gordon, *Heroes of Their Own Lives: The Politics and History of Family Violence, Boston, 1880–1960* (New York: Viking, 1988).

67. *El Paso Herald*, August 20, 1923, 13.

68. Although this clause of the constitution was never mentioned directly in the debate, references were made to the clauses of the Fourteenth Amendment: "Providing that no state shall make or enforce any law abridging the privileges or immunities of citizenship, nor deprive any person of life, liberty or property without due process of law." *Henning Jacobson v. Commonwealth of Massachusetts*, 197 U.S. 11, 25 S. Ct. 358.

69. Brandt, *No Magic Bullet*, 52–94.

70. Robyn Muncy, *Creating a Female Dominion in American Reform* (New York: Oxford University Press, 2006), 93–122.

71. For more on the history of vaccination in Texas, see Texas State Historical Association, "Vaccination," in The Handbook of Texas Online, www.tsha.utexas.edu/handbook/online/articles/view/LL/jc11.html (accessed March 29, 2001). For Richard

Dudley's public anti-Klan campaign and defeat of P. E. Gardener for the mayoralty of El Paso, see Lay, *War, Revolution, and the Ku Klux Klan*, 130–48, 141–44.

72. See H. S. Cumming, "Smallpox in Dallas," November 1922, RG 90, USPHS Central Files, 1897–1923, File No. 2796, Box 254, Civilian Records, NACP.

73. Hammonds, *Childhood's Deadly Scourge*, 10.

74. For 1918, see J. C. Perry, "Response to W. B. Pratt, Secretary, State Board of Health, Tucson," April 18, 1918, RG 90, USPHS Central Files, 1897–1923, Subject File 3655–Vaccination, April 1918–May 1918, Box 363, NACP. For 1922, see H. S. Cumming, "Re: Parran's Arrival on Scene Stems Tide of Opposition," December 2, 1922, RG 90, USPHS Central Files, 1897–1923, File No. 2796, Smallpox, 1922–1923, Box 254, NACP.

75. Dr. Spears finished his advertisement with the following quote by Blackstone: "No laws are binding on the human subject which assault the body or violate the conscience." See "Leo Spears, Still Not Vaccinated," n.d., Enclosure, Dr. Tracy Love, "Assistance by Thomas Parran," November 28, 1922, RG 90, USPHS Central Files, 1897–1923, File No. 2796, Smallpox, 1922–1923, Box 254, NACP. Regarding the advertisement, Dr. Love mentioned that he would "take up with [Dr. Parran] the question of any possible means whereby such advertisement may be suppressed."

76. "Chiropractor Is Forcibly Vaccinated for Fighting Order," *El Paso Times*, August 6, 1923, 1.

77. For Oregon, see Robert Davis Johnston, "The Myth of the Harmonious City: Will Daly, Lora Little, and the Hidden Face of Progressive Era Portland," *Oregon Historical Quarterly* 99, no. 3 (Fall 1994): 269–87.

78. "Ciudad Juarez. Fighting Mosquito Pest in Ciudad Juarez," February 9, 1923, RG 59, State Department Decimal Subject Files, "Malaria in Mexico," 158.124/3, NACP.

79. Texas State Medical Association, "El Paso Solves the Vaccination Question," *Texas State Journal of Medicine* 19, no. 2 (1923): 318.

80. The extent to which El Paso's Good Government League was able to disenfranchise the Mexican vote can be seen in records for 1922. In 1922, approximately 15,000 voters had Anglo surnames, leaving approximately 4,000 voters with Spanish surnames, for a total of 19,040 residents who paid their poll taxes. The census estimated in 1920 that approximately 48,000 of the city residents were born in Mexico or of Mexican parents. Lay's study of the demographics of El Paso's registered voters is shocking. See Lay, *War, Revolution, and the Ku Klux Klan*, 81.

81. Walker, "Union Labor–Carpenters Discuss Compulsory Vaccination," *El Paso Herald*, August 28, 1923, 8.

82. Dr. Hugh Crouse, the medical association writer, claimed that this was the rallying cry of the Christian Scientists and the chiropractors. See Texas State Medical Association, "El Paso Solves the Vaccination Question," 318. The extent of the Carpenters' Union's statement can be seen in the "Union Labor" column in the *El Paso Herald*. H. J. Walker, "UNION LABOR—Carpenters Discuss Compulsory Vaccination," *El Paso Herald*, August 23, 1923, 8.

83. Stephen Gottschalk, *The Emergence of Christian Science in American Religious Life* (Berkeley: University of California Press, 1973), 248.

84. Ibid.

85. R. W. Still quoted in "Vaccination Battle Wages Bitter Arguments before City Council," *El Paso Herald*, August 23, 1923, 1.

86. For a good legal account of this dance between the AFL and the judiciary branch, read Christopher L. Tomlins, *The State and the Unions: Labor Relations, Law, and the Organized Labor Movement in America, 1880–1960* (New York: Cambridge University Press, 1985). For a history of activist responses to this embrace of legality, see David Montgomery, *The Fall of the House of Labor: The Workplace, the State, and American Labor Activism, 1865–1925* (New York: Cambridge University Press, 1987).

87. Joan Zimmerman, "The Jurisprudence of Equality: The Women's Minimum Wage, the First Equal Rights Amendment and Adkins v. Children's Hospital of New York," *Journal of American History* 78, no. 1 (June 1991): 190. The citation was brought to my attention in Eric Foner, *The Story of American Freedom* (New York: W. W. Norton, 1998), 180, 368.

88. Ibid., 97.

89. Walker, "UNION LABOR—Carpenters Discuss Compulsory Vaccination," 8. The Union Labor column was located on page 8 of the *El Paso Herald* every Wednesday.

90. Ibid.

91. Gompers cited in Mario T. García, *Desert Immigrants: The Mexicans of El Paso* (New Haven: Yale University Press, 1982), 100.

92. Ibid., 95.

93. Dr. Hugh Crouse was one of the early local eugenic advocates and health writers in El Paso. On March 15, 1916, Crouse addressed the Equal Suffrage Society on the topic of "keys to a new home." In this address, he argued "men and women should no longer regard the subject of eugenics as something not to be touched, and not until they face the problem unflinchingly will the future generations be benefited." See "Cleanliness Will Save Babies," *El Paso Morning Times*, March 16, 1916, 7.

94. For an account of the Frontier Klan 100 and evangelical Christian role in the movement to close the bridge between El Paso and Ciudad Juárez earlier, see Lay, *War, Revolution, and the Ku Klux Klan*, 5–8, 25–45. For an account of the reaction by businessmen in Ciudad Juárez to prohibition and the attempt to close the bridge, see Oscar Martinez, *Border Boomtown: Ciudad Juarez since 1848* (Austin: University of Texas Press, 1978).

95. Texas State Medical Association, "El Paso Solves the Vaccination Question," 318. For evidence of Major Tarbett's presence in El Paso, see "Ciudad Juarez. Fighting Mosquito Pest in Ciudad Juarez," February 9, 1923, RG 59, State Department Decimal Subject Files, Malaria in Mexico, 158.124/3, NACP.

96. "Health Experts Answer Brown Questionnaire: Vaccination Endorsed," *El Paso Herald*, August 20, 1923, 12.

97. Ibid. Victor Vaughan supported a syphilis test for food handlers in El Paso. The vaccination ordinance attracted more enthusiastic support from the respondents to Brown's questionnaire.

98. The code was proposed to the city council under Mayor Charles Davis in March 1923. Given the open council conflict over Klan influence in El Paso politics between 1922 and 1923, there was little legislative movement in the city council. Once Richard Dudley won election in the summer of 1923, he began his push for public works and building renovation. For the place of the Klan for middle-class white insurgent politics within the El Paso Democratic party, see Lay, "Imperial Outpost on the Border: El Paso's Frontier Klan 100," in *The Invisible Empire in the American West*, ed. Shawn Lay (Urbana: University of Illinois Press, 2004), 88–94.

99. His mayoral campaign was the final defeat of Klan-backed candidates in El Paso. Dudley and his aldermanic slate ran on an anti-Klan and pro–religious tolerance, probusiness platform and took all the seats on the city council. Prior to holding elected office, Dudley directed the construction of the Chihuahua and Pacific Railway and the Mexico & Northwestern Railway, eventually settling down in El Paso as the organizer of the Texas Bank and Trust. Between 1912 and 1918, Dudley served two terms as state senator. Arthur H. Leibson, "Dudley, Richard M.," Handbook of Texas Online, http://www.tshaonline.org/handbook/online/articles/fdu55 (accessed March 12, 2012). Published by the Texas State Historical Association.

100. "Forces Ready for Last Fight on Compulsory Vaccination: Will Decide Issue Thursday," *El Paso Herald*, August 21, 1923, 1.

101. "World War Furnishes Striking Proof of Value of Vaccination, Says Head of Texas Medicine," *El Paso Herald*, August 20, 1923, 12.

102. Besides militarizing the debate, the change of venue may have also protected the city council from informal political pressure by local citizens as audiences and witnesses to the hearing. Texas State Medical Association, "El Paso Solves the Vaccination Question," 318.

103. According to Shawn Lay, during the rise of evangelical Protestantism that accompanied southern white Protestant migration to El Paso, the city council took to staging public debates. See Lay, *War, Revolution, and the Ku Klux Klan*, 89–90. Lay completed spectacular work using the depositions and records available in the El Paso newspapers, highlighting the common membership of the Ku Klux Klan and the Good Government League in El Paso. Through the same records, he shows that El Paso Mayor Tom Lea was a member of the Klan since 1915, halfway through his first tenure as mayor of El Paso. Lay, *War, Revolution, and the Ku Klux Klan*, 25, 81, 141, 144.

104. Texas State Medical Association, "El Paso Solves the Vaccination Question," 318–20.

105. Ibid.

106. There was open skepticism over the extent of scientific certainty around con-

troversial and widely shared processes like death. This skepticism openly challenged the social power claimed by medical expertise. There were crossovers in language and organizing networks between antivivisectionists, the Society to Prevent Premature Burial, and abolitionists. See Martin S. Pernick, "Back from the Grave: Recurring Controversies over Defining and Diagnosing Death in History," in *Death: Beyond Whole-Brain Criteria*, ed. Richard M. Zaner (Amsterdam: Kluwer Academic, 1988), 37, 47–52.

107. Hammonds, *Childhood's Deadly Scourge*, 10.

108. Texas State Medical Association, "El Paso Solves the Vaccination Question."

109. Ibid., 320.

110. Ibid.

111. For a discussion of the opposite situation in England, see R. M. MacLeod, "Law, Medicine, and Public Opinion: The Resistance to Compulsory Health Legislation, 1870–1907," *Public Law* 167 (summer 1967): 107–28. Nadja Durbach, "'They Might as Well Brand Us': Working Class Resistance to Compulsory Vaccination in Victorian England," *Social History of Medicine* 13, no. 1 (2000): 45–62.

112. George J. Sánchez, "Race, Nation, and Culture in Recent Immigration Studies," *Journal of American Ethnic History* 18, no. 4 (1999): 69, 73, 82. The classic statement of this predicament can be found in Gutiérrez, *Walls and Mirrors*, 5–7.

113. *Buck v. Bell*, 274 U.S. 200 (1927).

114. *Henning Jacobson v. State of Massachusetts*, December 1904, 197 U.S. 11, 25 S. CT. 358.

115. "Protests regarding certificate of smallpox vaccination in Tampico," February 24, 1921, RG 59, State Department Decimal File, 158.1201/24, "Sanitary Conditions in Mexico," United States Shipping Board, NACP.

116. Summerlin, "Revaccinating Whenever Deemed Expedient," April 9, 1921, RG 59, State Department Decimal File, 158.1201/25, "Sanitary Conditions in Mexico," NACP.

117. Akers Folkman Company, "Seeks Information on Vaccination Requirements and Smallpox Epidemic in Mexico," January 24, 1931, RG 59, State Department Decimal File, 158.125/119, NACP.

118. United States Consul Ciudad Juárez, "Mexican Authorities Require Vaccination Certificates from Persons Entering Mexico through Ciudad Juarez on Account of Epidemic of Smallpox in El Paso," March 30, 1932, RG 59, State Department Decimal File, 158.125/121, Farnsworth, NACP.

119. "Burris Jackson Requests That Vaccination Requirement Be Waived for Lions International Convention," June 7, 1935, RG 59, State Department Decimal File, 158.125/155, NACP.

120. Gordon S. Reid, "Vaccination of Tourists Before Entering Mexico," April 8, 1939, RG 59, State Department Decimal File, 158.125/164.02, NACP.

121. For New York, see Judith Walzer Leavitt, "Be Safe, Be Sure: New York City's

Experience with Epidemic Smallpox," in Leavitt and Numbers, *Sickness and Health in America*, 555–74.

122. "Laredo y Nuevo Laredo: Se esta vacunando a los turistas," *La Prensa*, January 19, 1949, 1 (my translation).

123. J. V. Irons et al., "Outbreak of Smallpox in the Lower Rio Grande Valley of Texas in 1949," *American Journal of Public Health* 43, no. 1 (1953): 25–29.

124. Emilio Forto, "Actual Situation on the River Rio Grande: Information Rendered to Colonel H. J. Slocum of the American Forces at Brownsville," *Pan American Labor Press*, September 11, 1918, cited in Montejano, *Anglos and Mexicans*, 225.

125. Taylor, *American-Mexican Frontier, Nueces County* (New York: Russell and Russell, 1971), 310.

126. P. S. Taylor, Taylor Collection, No. 66-656, cited in Montejano, *Anglos and Mexicans*, 227.

127. E. E. Davis, *A Report on Illiteracy in Texas* (Austin: University of Texas Publications, 1923), cited in Montejano, *Anglos and Mexicans*, 228.

128. Rosa Linda Fregoso, "Dr. Hector Garcia and the American G.I. Forum," Onda Latina: Digitizing the Mexican American Experience, www.laits.utexas.edu/onda_latina/program?sernum=MAE_82_01_mp3&term=hector%20garcia (accessed March 26, 2011).

129. United States Public Health Service, "Principal Causes of Death in United States Registration Area: Census Bureau Summarizes Mortality Statistics," *Public Health Reports* 34, no. 27 (1919): 1474–75.

130. Ibid. The death rate for diarrhea was 79 per 100,000; the death rate for heart disease was 153.2 per 100,000; the death rate for pneumonia was 149.9 per 100,000; and the death rate for tuberculosis was 148 per 100,000. This did not include Texas. Ibid., 1474.

131. Ibid., 1475.

132. "No clasificaran a Mexicanos entre raza de color," *El Continental*, October 7, 1936, 1.

133. For the geographic diversity of racial segregation in Texas, see Montejano, *Anglos and Mexicans*. For an examination of these three racial categories at work in one industry in Texas, see Foley, *White Scourge*.

134. "Alarming Mortality in Mexican Colony in This City," *La Prensa*, June 26, 1926, 1.

135. Ibid.

136. Foley, *White Scourge*, 1–19; Montejano, *Anglos and Mexicans*, 229.

137. Clara Rodriguez, *Changing Race: Latinos, the Census, and the History of Ethnicity in the United States* (New York: New York University Press, 2000).

138. "7 mil Mexicanos contra 2 mil Americanos," *La Prensa (San Antonio)*, January 12, 1930, 4.

139. "Mexicana centenaria presa en El Paso por ejercer de partera sin licencia," *La Prensa*, August 31, 1935.

140. Ibid.

141. Mario García, "Mexican Americans and the Politics of Citizenship: The Case of El Paso, 1936," *New Mexico Historical Review* 59, no. 2 (1984): 188–89.

142. Editorial, "A que precio este grocero insulto a 60,000 Pasenos," *El Continental*, October 7, 1936, 1.

143. Ibid.

144. Hine, *Black Victory*, 114–25.

145. García, "Mexican Americans and the Politics of Citizenship," 191.

146. *El Continental (El Paso)*, October 6, 1936, cited in ibid.

147. "Las protestas se llevaran hasta Washington," *El Continental*, October 8, 1936, 1–2.

148. Ibid.

149. Pablo Delgado, "Letter to the editor," *El Paso Herald-Post*, October 8, 1936, cited in García, "Mexican Americans and the Politics of Citizenship," 191.

150. La Union Latina, "Memorial al Presidente Roosevelt," *La Prensa (Los Angeles)*, October 31, 1936, 2.

151. "Las clasificaciones raciales," *La Prensa (San Antonio)*, October 15, 1936, 3.

152. "Digna actitud de Mexicanos," *La Prensa (San Antonio)*, October 10, 1936.

153. Urias, "A que precio este terrible insulto," 1," *El Continental*, October 107, 1936, 1.

154. Ibid.

155. "La mortalidad infantil ha aumentado en El Paso," *El Continental*, June 5, 1935, 4.

156. "Se mueren los niños," *El Continental*, June 5, 1936, 4.

157. "Son Mexicanos," *El Continental*, June 10, 1935.

158. "Mortalidad," *El Continental*, June 20, 1935.

159. "Han muerto muchos niños en El Paso, dicen autoridades," *El Continental*, July 20, 1935, 4.

160. "Se necesita clinica en el sur de El Paso," *El Continental*, October 13, 1937.

161. Herbert Biberman, "Sanitation, not discrimination," Film Still, Silver City, 1954. Cover photograph, ed. Deborah Silverton Rosenfelt, Michael Wilson, *Salt of the Earth* (New York: Feminist Press of the City University of New York, 1978). This phrase is visible on a banner being waved by women re-creating the 1951 Empire Zinc Strike at Silver City, N.M.

162. George Cox, *The Latin American Health Problem in Texas*, Texas State Department of Health, Division of Maternal and Child Health, Austin, 1940, p. 4, in Rare Books Collection, Nettie Lee Benson Rare Books and Manuscripts Library, Austin. Roberts, *Infectious Fear*, 28.

163. Cox, *Latin American Health Problem*, 10.

164. Ibid.

165. Ibid.

166. Ibid., 8.

167. Victor Ehlers, "The Creation of a Sanitary District Dedicated to the American-Mexican Boundary, October 27, 1938," RG 59, State Department Decimal Files, 711.129 Sanitary/1, NACP.

168. J. W. H Beck, Will M. Martin, T. J. Holbrook, W. K. Hopkins, Margie Neal, A. Paov, Albert Stone, and K. M. Regan, "Request for International Health Commission," November 10, 1934, RG 59, State Department Decimal Files, 1930–1939, 711.129/2, NACP.

169. See Morris Sheppard, "Re: A Survey to Create an International Health Commission," RG 59, State Department Decimal Files, 1930–1939, 711.129/1, NACP. Thomas Connolly, "Proposal for Establishment of an International Public Health Commission—Letter October 27, 1934 from Texas Senate Chamber Stating Reasons for—[?] Transmitted for Comment and Return," RG 59, State Department Decimal Files, 1930–1939, 711.129/1 Sanitary/1, 711.129 Sanitary/1, NACP.

170. J. W. Beck et al., "Request for International Health Commission," November 10, 1934, RG 59, State Department Decimal Files, 711.129/2, NACP.

171. Cordell Hull, "Re: Plan to Safeguard Health along the American-Mexican Border, December 8, 1934," RG 59, State Department Decimal Files, 711.129/1, NACP.

172. Dr. Richard Allen, "Report on Inspection Stations West of the El Paso Border," February 3, 1942 (declassified April 17, 2008), RG 90, USPHS General Classified Records, 1936–1944, Subject File: El Paso Quarantine Station, 1850–95, NACP.

173. Julie Collins-Dogrul, "Managing U.S. Mexico 'Border Health': An Organizational Field Approach," *Social Science and Medicine* 63 (2006): 3202–3.

174. Richard Allen, "Report of Inspection Trip to Ports East of El Paso, November 1941," RG 90, USPHS, Subject File 1850–95: El Paso Quarantine, NACP.

175. Rosalinda Fregoso, "Dr. Hector Garcia: The American G.I. Forum," November 27, 1981, from Onda Latina: Digitizing the Mexican American Experience, www .laits.utexas.edu/onda_latina/program?sernum=MAE_82_01_mp3&term=hector% 20garcia (accessed August 25, 2011).

Epilogue

1. New Spain did have a royal medical licensing program under the Royal Protomedicato. The Protomedicato did not survive Mexican independence, and it disappeared in 1831. See Jose Ortiz Monasterio, "Agonia y muerte del protomedicato de Nueva España, 1831. La categoría socioprofesional de los médicos," *Historias* 57 (January 2004): 34–50.

2. Samuel Ryan Curtis, *Mexico under Fire*, ed. Joseph Chance (Fort Worth: Texas Christian University Press, 1994), 9, 1.

3. Ibid., 24.

4. Humphreys, *Intensely Human*, 119–40.

5. The concerted efforts of volunteer and army physicians and the National Sanitary Commission reduced the level of deaths by disease to 10 percent of Union soldiers. Antiseptic measures and sanitary measures like privies reduced the toll of infections that started in camps. This was a drastic improvement on the 13 percent casualty rate in the U.S.-Mexico War.

6. William Cronon, *Nature's Metropolis: Chicago and the Great West* (New York: W. W. Norton, 1992), 55–74.

7. John Hunter Pope, "The Condition of the Mexican Population of Western Texas in Its Relation to Public Health," in *Public Health Papers and Reports*, vol. 6, ed. American Public Health Association (Boston: Franklin Press, Rand and Avery, 1881), 163.

8. For an examination of community-based movements separate from the federal dimensions of public health policies, see Zamora, *The World of the Mexican Worker*, 86–109.

9. This quarantine guard predated the establishment of the Border Patrol by forty-two years. For a discussion of the medical dimensions of the Border Patrol, see Alexandra Minna Stern, "Nationalism on the Line: Masculinity, Race, and the Creation of the Border Patrol, 1910–1924," in Truett and Young, *Continental Crossroads*, 299–323.

10. "Transnational" refers to those processes that are anchored in and transcend two or more states. This use of the term comes from Gina Perez, *Near Northwest Side Story: Migration, Displacement and Puerto Rican Families* (Berkeley: University of California Press, 2004), 13. The original definition comes from Michael Kearney, "The Local and the Global: The Anthropology of Transnationalism and Globalization," *Annual Review of Anthropology* 24: 548.

11. See Milton Rosenau, "Smallpox—Some Peculiarities of Camp Jenner Epidemic," in *Annual Report of the Surgeon General of the United States Marine Hospital Service for the Fiscal Year 1896* (Washington, D.C.: Government Printing Office, 1896), 234–44; J. J. Kinyoun, "The Serum Therapy of Variola and Vaccinia," in *Annual Report of the Supervising Surgeon General of the United States Marine Hospital Service for the Fiscal Year 1896* (Washington, D.C.: Government Printing Office, 1899), 766. For the military dimensions of Eagle Pass, see Leiker, *Racial Borders*, 113–20.

12. Jerrold Michael and Thomas R. Bender, "Fighting Smallpox on the Texas Border: An Episode from PHS's Proud Past," *Public Health Reports* 99, no. 6 (1984): 579–82. For Tuskegee, see James Jones, *Bad Blood: The Tuskegee Syphilis Experiment* (New York: Free Press, 1993), and Susan Reverby, *Examining Tuskegee: The Infamous Syphilis Study and Its Legacy* (Chapel Hill: University of North Carolina Press, 2010).

13. See James Cassedy, "The Registration Area and American Vital Statistics," *Bulletin of the History of Medicine* 39 (1965): 223

14. "Alarming Mortality in Mexican Colony in This City," *La Prensa* (San Antonio), June 26, 1926, 1.

15. Pauline Kibbe, ed. Carlos Cortes, *Latin Americans in Texas* (New York: Arno Press, 1974), 155–56.

16. Emma Tenayuca, *Emma Tenayuca: La Pasionaria, La Profeta* (San Antonio: Esperanza Peace and Justice Center, 1997), 8.

17. George I. Sanchez, "Migrant Labor Camp," George Isidore Sanchez Papers, Nettie Lee Benson Library, www.lib.utexas.edu/photodraw/sanchez/raw/sanmig21.html (accessed July 10, 2011).

18. Salvador Franco Urias, "A que precio este terrible insult a 60,000 paseños,"*El Continental (El Paso)*, October 7, 1936, 1.

19. Wald, *Contagious*, 4–11.

20. The term "nativism" comes from Higham, *Strangers in the Land*, xi. Medicalized nativism comes from Kraut, *Silent Travelers*, 3.

21. Michael Savage, "Deadly Swine Flu Epidemic and Illegal Mexican Immigrants and Epidemics," YouTube, www.youtube.com/watch?v=YwHCO_trqhM& feature=watch_response_rev (accessed July 14, 2011); Rush Limbaugh, "Why Swine Flu Is Worse in Mexico," *The Rush Limbaugh Show*, http://www.rushlimbaugh.com/ daily/2009/04/28/why_swine_flu_is_worse_in_mexico (accessed March 13, 2012).

22. James McKinley, "Mexican Child Visiting U.S. 1st to Die Here of Swine Flu," *New York Times*, April 29, 2009, www.nytimes.com/2009/04/30/health/30toddler. html?sq=swine flu (accessed July 14, 2011).

23. Julio Frenk, "Mexico's Fast Diagnosis," *New York Times*, April 30, 2009, www .nytimes.com/2009/05/01/opinion/01frenk.html (accessed March 13, 2012).

24. For the sudden shift in the relative status of ethnic minorities in the political order, see the election of Barack Obama to the presidency of the United States.

25. Sheryll Gay Stolberg, "Obama, Armed with Details, Says Health Plan Is Necessary," *New York Times*, September 10, 2009, www.nytimes.com/2009/09/10/us /politics/10obama.html?ref=politics (accessed July 14, 2011). "Joe Wilson Says Outburst Spontaneous," CNN Politics, articles.cnn.com/2009-09-10/politics/obama .heckled.speech_1_illegal-immigrants-illegal-aliens-rep-joe-wilson?_s=PM:POLITICS (accessed July 14, 2011).

26. Rosenberg, *Cholera Years*, 137–38, 148.

BIBLIOGRAPHY

Archives Consulted

Alabama Department of Archives and History, Montgomery

Alabama Governors Papers, 1894–1896
Place Names, Vertical File Tuscaloosa

National Archives and Records Administration, College Park, Maryland (NACP)

RECORD GROUP 59, U.S. DEPARTMENT OF STATE
Sanitary Files, 711.129, 1910–1920
Sanitary Files, 711.129, 1920–1929
Sanitary Files, 711.129, 1930–1934
Sanitary Files, 711.129, 1935–1939
Sanitary Files, 711.129, 1940–1945
Decimal Files, 1910–1920, Enclosure XII.158.1208
Decimal Files, Mexico, 158.008/12
Decimal Records of the State Department, 1910–1920, 158.129, Sanitary Files, Mexico Decimal Files, 1910–1920, Complaints against Quarantine, 158.1208/7
Classified Decimal Subject Files, 1935–1939
Decimal Subject Files, entry 158.1208/18, "General Complaints by Mexico against administration of quarantine laws and regulations, 1920–1930"
Sanitary Files, 1930–1934, Decimal File 711.129
Decimal Files, 1930–1934, 811.4063-olympic games/367
Decimal Subject Files, 1920–1929, entry 158.1208
Decimal Subject Files, entry 158.125/27, Ciudad Porfirio Diaz
Decimal Subject Files, entry 158.125/90, Department of Labor
Decimal Subject Files, 1935–1940, entry 158.125/155
Classified Decimal Files, 711.129/1, Sanitation, 1940–1945

RECORD GROUP 90, UNITED STATES PUBLIC HEALTH SERVICE

Subject Files No. 2796—Smallpox. United States Public Health Service Central Files, 1897–1923

Subject Files No. 2126—Typhus. United States Public Health Service Central Files, 1897–1923

Subject File No. 3655—Vaccination, El Paso Quarantine, United States Public Health Service Central Files, 1923–1939

Laredo Quarantine, United States Public Health Service Files, 1923–1939

Subject File 1850–15: Del Rio Quarantine Station, General Classified Records, 1936–1944

Subject File 1850–1915: Eagle Pass Quarantine Station, General Classified Records, 1936–1944

Subject File 1850–95: El Paso Quarantine Station, General Classified Records, 1936–1944

Subject File 1850–15: Laredo Quarantine Station, General Classified Records, 1936–1944

Subject File 1850–95: Quarantine Stations, General Classified Records, 1936–1944

Quarantine Stations, Decimal File 711.129, 1924–1929

Quarantine Stations, Decimal File 711.129, 1930–1935

National Archives and Record Administration, Washington, D.C. (NAB)

Mexico City

ARCHIVO SECRETARÍA DE EDUCACIÓN PÚBLICA

Colección Lamberto Alvarez Gayou, Sección Subsecretaría de Educación Publica

ARCHIVO DE LA UNIVERSIDAD IBERO-AMERICANA,
UNIVERSIDAD IBERO-AMERICANA

Colección Porfirio Díaz

ARCHIVO GENERAL DE LA NACIÓN (AGN)

Grupo Documental 127 Gobernación, Caja 391, Expediente 1

Grupo Documental 127 Gobernación, Caja 405, Expediente 6, AGN 2

Grupo Documental 127 Gobernación, Caja 405, Expediente 12, 1

Grupo Documental 3000 Relaciones Exteriores, Siglo XIX, Nueva Orleans

Texas

TEXAS STATE ARCHIVES AND LIBRARY (TSAL), AUSTIN

Laredo Smallpox Epidemic, Governor Joseph D. Sayers Collection 301-175, 1

Papers of Governor Oran Milo Roberts

Governor Joseph Sayers Collection

TEXAS STATE DEPARTMENT OF HEALTH, DIVISION OF MATERNAL AND CHILD
HEALTH, NETTIE LEE BENSON RARE BOOKS AND MANUSCRIPTS LIBRARY, AUSTIN

DOLPH BRISCOE CENTER FOR AMERICAN HISTORY (DBCAH), AUSTIN
Bexar Archives, 1770–1836, Dolph Briscoe Center for American History
Texana Collection, Dolph Briscoe Center for American History

BORDER HERITAGE CENTER OF THE EL PASO PUBLIC LIBRARY, EL PASO

C. L. SONNICHSEN SPECIAL COLLECTION, UNIVERSITY OF TEXAS AT EL PASO
LIBRARY, EL PASO

Newspapers and Periodicals

American Flag
Annual Report of the Surgeon General of the United States Marine Hospital Service
Birmingham Age-Herald
Brownsville Journal
Chaparral
Christian Recorder
Cincinnati Enquirer
Columbia State
Correo de Laredo
Dallas Morning News
El Centinela de Brownsville
El Continental
El Diputado de Laredo
El Figaro de Laredo
El Mutualista de Laredo
El Paso City and County Labor Advocate
El Paso del Norte
El Paso Herald
El Paso Morning Times
El Paso Times
Everybody's Magazine
Evolución de Laredo
Fort Worth Star Telegram
Frank Leslie's Illustrated Weekly
Gaceta Medica de Mexico
Houston Post
La Bandera de Brownsville
La Colonia Mexicana
La Prensa

Laredo Daily Times
Laredo Times
Las Dos Americas
Los Angeles Times
Mexican Herald
Miami Daily News
New Orleans Picayune
New York Herald
New York Medical Recorder
Outlook
San Antonio Daily Express
San Antonio Express
Survey: Social, Charitable, Civic: A Journal of Constructive Philanthropy
Texas Medical Journal
Texas Sanitarian
Texian Advocate
Tuscaloosa Times
Washington Bee
Washington Post
Weekly Abstract of Sanitary Reports

Digital Archives

America's Historical Newspapers (www.readex.com/readex/?content=96)
African American Newspapers (www.readex.com/readex/product.cfm?product
    =308)
African American Newspapers: The 19th Century (www.accessible-archives.com
    /collections/african-american-newspapers/)
Hispanic American Newspapers (www.readex.com/readex/product.cfm?product
    =249)
Online Handbook of Texas (www.tshaonline.org/handbook/online)

Books and Articles

Aceves Pastrana, Maria. "Conflictos y negociaciones en las expediciones de bal-
    mis." *Estudios Novohispanos* 17 (1997): 171–200.
Agamben, Giorgio. *Homo Sacer: Sovereign Power and Bare Life*. Stanford: Stanford
    University Press, 1998.
Agostoni, Claudia. *Monuments of Progress: Modernization and Public Health in
    Mexico City, 1876–1910*. Boulder: University of Colorado Press, 2003.
Aguílar Camin, Hector, and Lorenzo Meyer. *In the Shadow of the Mexican Revo-
    lution: Contemporary Mexican History, 1910–1985*. Austin: University of Texas
    Press, 1993.

Aguirre-Molina, Marilyn, Noilyn Abesamis, and Michelle Castro. "The State of the Art: Latinas in the Health Literature." In *Latina Health in the United States: A Public Health Reader*, edited by Marilyn Aguirre-Molina and Carlos W. Molina, 3–22. San Francisco: Jossey Bass, 2003.

Alanis Enciso, Fernando Saúl. "La Labor Consular Mexicana en Estados Unidos: El caso de Eduardo Ruiz, 1921." *Secuencia: Revista de Historia y Ciencias Sociales* (2002): 41–61.

Alchon, Suzanne Austin. *Native Society and Disease in Colonial Ecuador*. New York: Cambridge University Press, 1991.

Alden, Dauril. "Out of Africa: The Slave Trade and the Transmission of Smallpox to Brazil, 1560–1831." *Journal of Interdisciplinary History* 18, no. 2 (1987): 195–224.

Alexander, Charles C. *The Ku Klux Klan in the Southwest*. Louisville: University of Kentucky Press, 1964.

Almaguer, Tomás. *Racial Fault Lines: The Historical Origins of White Supremacy in California*. Berkeley: University of California Press, 1994.

Alonso, Ana María. *Thread of Blood: Colonialism, Gender, and Revolution on Mexico's Northern Frontier*. Tucson: University of Arizona Press, 1995.

———. "U.S. Military Intervention, Revolutionary Mobilization, and Popular Ideology in the Chihuahuan Sierra, 1916–1917." In *Rural Revolt in Mexico: U.S. Intervention and the Domain of Subaltern Politics*, edited by Daniel Nugent, 207–36. Durham: Duke University Press, 1998.

Alonzo, Armando C. *Tejano Legacy: Rancheros and Settlers in South Texas, 1734–1900*. Albuquerque: University of New Mexico Press, 1998.

American Public Health Association. "The Typhus Rocky Mountain Spotted Fever Group of Infections in the Eastern and Southeastern States." *American Journal of Public Health* 21, no. 5 (May 1931): 540–42.

Anders, Evan. *Boss Rule in South Texas: The Progressive Era*. Austin: University of Texas Press, 1982.

Anderson, Benedict. *Imagined Communities: Reflections on the Origin and Spread of Nationalism*. New York: Verso, 1991.

Anderson, Warwick. "The Trespass Speaks: White Masculinity and Colonial Breakdown." *American Historical Review* 102 (December 1997): 1343–71.

Andreas, Peter. "Borderless Economy, Barricaded Border." *North American Chronicle of Latin America* 33, no. 3 (1999): 14–21.

Andrews, Bridie, and Andrew Cunningham, eds. *Western Medicine as Contested Knowledge*. New York: Manchester University Press, 1997.

Archer, Mattie Austin. "Municipal Government of San Fernando de Bexar." M.A. thesis, University of Texas at Austin, 1903.

Argüello, Ana Rosa Suárez, ed. *En el nombre del Destino Manifiesto: Guía de ministros y embajadores de Estados Unidos en México, 1825–1993*. Mexico: Instituto Mora, Secretaria de Relaciones Exteriores, 1998.

Arnold, David. *Colonizing the Body: State Medicine and Epidemic Disease in Nine-teenth-Century India*. Berkeley: University of California Press, 1993.

Arreola Valenzuela, Arturo. "Comunicaciones y cambios estructurales durante el porfiriato." In *Durango (1840–1915): Banca, transportes, tierra e industria*, edited by Mario Cerutti, 35–58. Monterrey, Nuevo León: Universidad Autonoma de Nuevo León, 1995.

Ayers, Edward. *The Promise of the New South: Life after Reconstruction*. New York: Oxford University Press, 1992.

Azize-Vargas, Yamila. "The Emergence of Feminism in Puerto Rico, 1870–1930." In *Unequal Sisters: A Multicultural Reader in U.S. Women's History*, edited by Vicki L. Ruiz and Ellen C. Du Bois, 268–76. New York: Routledge, 1994.

Balibar, Étienne. "The Nation Form: History and Ideology." In *Race, Nation, Class*, edited by Étienne Balibar and Immanuel Wallerstein, 86–105. New York: Routledge, Kegan and Paul, 1992.

Balogh, Brian. "Reorganizing the Organizational Synthesis: Federal-Professional Relations in Modern America." *Studies in American Political Development* 5, no. 1 (1991): 119–72.

Bannon, John Francis. *Bolton and the Spanish Borderlands*. Norman: University of Oklahoma Press, 1964.

Barbachano, Arturo Erosa. "El gobierno de Juarez y la salud publica de Mexico." *Salud Publica de Mexico* 19, no. 3 (1977): 375–81.

Barr, Alwynn. "Black State Conventions." In The Online Handbook of Texas, edited by Texas State Historical Collections, Austin, 2004. (www.tshaonline.org /handbook/online/articles/pkb01)

———. *From Reconstruction to Reform: Politics in Texas, 1876–1906*. Austin: University of Texas Press, 1971.

Bator, Paul Adolphus. "The Health Reformers versus the Common Canadian: The Controversy over Compulsory Vaccination against Smallpox in Toronto and Ontario, 1900–1920." *Ontario History* 75 (1988): 348–73.

Beardsley, Edward H. *A History of Neglect: Health Care for Blacks and Millworkers in the Twentieth-Century South*. Knoxville: University of Tennessee Press, 1987.

Beck, Ulrich. *World Risk Society*. Malden, Mass.: Polity Press, 1999.

Beezley, William. *Insurgent Governor: Abraham Gonzalez and the Mexican Revolution in Chihuahua*. Lincoln: University of Nebraska Press, 1973.

———. *Judas at the Jockey Club and Other Incidences in Porfirian Mexico*. Lincoln: University of Nebraska Press, 1987.

Benavides García, Raymundo. *Historia de la salud pública en Nuevo León, 1820–1950*. Monterrey: Universidad Autonoma de Nuevo León, 1998.

Bender, Thomas, ed. *The Antislavery Debate: Capitalism and Abolitionism as a Problem in Historical Interpretation*. Berkeley: University of California Press, 1992.

Benjamin, Thomas. *La Revolución: Mexico's Great Revolution as Memory, Myth, and History.* Austin: University of Texas Press, 2000.

Benjamin, Thomas, and William McNellie. *Other Mexicos: Essays on Regional Mexican History, 1876–1911.* Albuquerque: University of New Mexico Press, 1984.

Bersani, Leo. "Is the Rectum a Grave? Sexuality and the AIDS Epidemic." *October* 43 (1987): 197–222.

Birn, Anne-Emanuelle. "Local Health and Foreign Wealth: The Rockefeller Foundation's Public Health Programs in Mexico, 1924–1951." Ph.D. diss., Johns Hopkins University, 1993.

———. "A Revolution in Rural Health? The Struggle over Local Health Units in Mexico, 1928–1940." *Journal of the History of Medicine and Allied Sciences* 53, no. 1 (1998): 43–76.

———. "Six Seconds per Eyelid: The Medical Inspection of Immigrants at Ellis Island, 1892–1914." *Dynamis* 17, no. 281–316 (1997).

———. "Wa(i)ves of Influence: Rockefeller Public Health in Mexico, 1920–50." *Studies in History and Philosophy of Biological and Biomedical Sciences* 31, no. 3 (2000): 381–95.

Birn, Anne-Emmanuel, and A. Solorzano. "Public Health Policy Paradoxes: Science and Politics in the Rockefeller Foundation's Hookworm Campaign in Mexico in the 1920s." *Social Science and Medicine* 49, no. 9 (1999): 1197–1213.

Blackwelder, Julia Kirk. *Women of the Depression: Caste and Culture in San Antonio, 1929–1939.* College Station: Texas A&M University Press, 1984.

Bloom, Khalid. *Mississippi Valley's Great Yellow Fever Epidemic of 1878.* Baton Rouge: Louisiana State University Press, 1993.

Blum, Edward. "The Crucible of Disease: Trauma, Memory and National Reconciliation in the Yellow Fever Epidemic of 1878." *Journal of Southern History* 69, no. 4 (2003): 791–820.

Bolton, Herbert E. "The Epic of Greater America." *American Historical Review* 38 (April 1933): 448–74.

———. "The Mission as a Frontier Institution in the Spanish American Colonies." *American Historical Review* 23 (October 1917): 42–61.

Boyd, James. "Slave Narratives, a Folk History of Slavery in the United States from Interviews with Former Slaves. Texas Narratives, Volume XVI, Part 2—Ex-Slave Stories (Texas)." In *Born in Slavery: Slave Narratives from the Federal Writers' Project, 1936–1938*, 117–25. Washington, D.C.: Government Publication Office, 1937.

Brandt, Allan M. "AIDS in Historical Perspective: Four Lessons from the History of Sexually Transmitted Diseases." In *Sickness and Health in America: Readings in the History of Medicine and Public Health*, 3rd ed., rev., edited by Judith Walzer Leavitt and Ronald Numbers, 426–32. Madison: University of Wisconsin Press, 1997.

————. *No Magic Bullet: The Social History of Venereal Disease in the United States since 1880.* New York: Oxford University Press, 1987.

Breeden, James O. "Disease as a Factor in Southern Distinctiveness." In *Disease and Distinctiveness in the American South,* edited by Todd L. Savitt and James Harvey Young, 1–28. Knoxville: University of Tennessee Press, 1988.

Brieger, Gert H. "Sanitary Reform in New York City: Stephen Smith and the Passage of the Metropolitan Health Bill." In *Sickness and Health in America: Readings in the History of Medicine and Public Health,* 3rd ed., rev., edited by Judith Walzer Leavitt and Ronald Numbers, 437–51. Madison: University of Wisconsin Press, 1997.

Briggs, Charles, and Clara Mantini Briggs. *Stories in the Time of Cholera: Racial Profiling during a Medical Nightmare.* Berkeley: University of California Press, 2004.

Brooks, Francis. "Revising the Conquest of Mexico." *Journal of Interdisciplinary History* 24, no. 1 (1993): 1–29.

Brown, Jonathan C. "Trabajadores nativos y extranjeros en el Mexico Porfiriano." *Siglo XIX: Cuadernos de Historia* 3, no. 9 (1994): 7–49.

Bruton, Peter. "The National Board of Health, 1879–1884." Ph.D. diss., University of Maryland, 1975.

Buffington, Robert M., and William E. French. "The Culture of Modernity." In *The Oxford History of Mexico,* edited by Michael C. Meyer and William Beezley, 397–431. New York: Oxford University Press, 2000.

Bustamante, Miguel E. *La fiebre amarilla en México y su origen en América.* Monografía numero 2. Mexico City: Secretaria de Salubridad y Asistencia, Instituto de Salubridad y Enfermedades Tropicales, 1958.

————. "Vigesimoquinto aniversario de la eradicación de la viruela en Mexico." *Gaceta Médica de México* 113, no. 12 (1977): 556.

Bustos-Aguilar, Pedro. "Mister Don't Touch the Banana: Notes on the Popularity of the Ethnosexed Body South of the Border." *Critique of Anthropology* 15, no. 2 (1995): 149–70.

Butler, Judith. *Bodies That Matter: Notes on the Discursive Limits of "Sex."* New York: Routledge, 1993.

Cain, Louis P. "Raising and Watering a City: Ellis Sylvester Chesbrough and Chicago's First Sanitation System." In *Sickness and Health in America: Readings in the History of Medicine and Public Health,* 3rd ed., rev., edited by Judith Walzer Leavitt and Ronald Numbers, 531–41. Madison: University of Wisconsin Press, 1997.

Camarillo, Albert. *Chicanos in a Changing Society: From Mexican Pueblos to American Barrios in Santa Barbara and Southern California, 1848–1930.* Cambridge: Harvard University Press, 1979.

Camin, Héctor Aguilar, and Lorenzo Meyer. *In the Shadow of the Mexican Revolution: Contemporary Mexican History*. Austin: University of Texas Press, 1993.

Campbell, Randolph. *Grassroots Reconstruction in Texas, 1865–1880*. Baton Rouge: Louisiana State University Press, 1997.

Cantor, David. "Cortisone and the Politics of Drama, 1949–1955." In *Medical Innovations in Historical Perspective*, edited by John Pickstone, 165–84. New York: St. Martin's, 1992.

Capers, Gerald M. *Biography of a River Town*. Chapel Hill: University of North Carolina Press, 1938.

———. "Yellow Fever in Memphis in the 1870s." *Mississippi Valley Historical Review* 24, no. 4 (1938): 483–502.

Cardenas, Enrique. "A Macroeconomic Interpretation of Nineteenth-Century Mexico." In *How Latin America Fell Behind: Essays on the Economic Histories of Mexico and Brazil, 1800–1914*, edited by Stephen Haber, 65–93. Stanford: Stanford University Press, 1997.

Carrigan, Jo Ann. *The Saffron Scourge: A History of Yellow Fever in Louisiana*. Lafayette: Center for Louisiana Studies, University of Southwestern Louisiana, 1994.

———. "Yellow Fever: Scourge of the South." In *Disease and Distinctiveness in the American South*, edited by Todd L. Savitt and James Harvey Young, 55–78. Knoxville: University of Tennessee Press, 1988.

Casanueva, Fernando. "Una peste de viruelas en la región de la frontera de guerra hispanoamericana en el reino de Chile, 1791." *Revista de Historia* 26 (1992): 31–65.

Cassedy, James. "The Registration Area and American Vital Statistics: Development of a Health Resource, 1885–1915." *Bulletin of the History of Medicine* 39, no. 5 (1965): 221–31.

Castañeda, Antonia. "Sexual Violence in the Politics and Policies of Conquest: Amerindian Women and the Spanish Conquest of Alta California." In *Building with Our Hands: New Directions in Chicana Studies*, edited by Adela de la Torre and Beatriz M. Pesquera, 16–33. Berkeley: University of California Press, 1993.

Caulfield, Sueann. "Getting into Trouble: Dishonest Women, Modern Girls, and Women-Men in the Conceptual Language of Vida Policial, 1925–1927." *Signs: Journal of Women in Culture and Society* 19, no. 1 (1993): 146–75.

———. *In Defense of Honor: Sexual Morality, Modernity, and Nation in Early-Twentieth-Century Brazil*. Durham: Duke University Press, 2000.

Cell, John W. *The Highest Stage of White Supremacy: The Origins of Segregation in South Africa and the American South*. Cambridge: Cambridge University Press, 1982.

Cerutti, Mario. "Comercio, guerras y capitales en torno al Rio Bravo." In *El Norte de Mexico y Texas, 1848–1880*, edited by Mario Cerutti, 13–114. Mexico, Distrito Federal: Instituto de Investigaciones Jose Luis Mora, 1999.

———. "Durango (1840–1915): Banca, transportes, tierra e industria." In *Historia económica de Mexico Norte* edited by Mario Cerutti. Monterrey, Nuevo León: Universidad Autonoma de Nuevo Leon, 1995.

———. "El prestamo prebancario en el noreste de Mexico: La actividad de los grandes comerciantes de Monterrey (1850–1890)." In *Banca y poder en Mexico (1800–1925)*, edited by Leonor Ludlow and Carlos Marichal, 119–64. Mexico City: Enlace/Historia, 1985.

Chalhoub, Sidney. *Cidade febril: Corticos e epidemias na corte imperial*. São Paulo: Companhia das Letras, 1996.

———. "The Politics of Disease Control: Yellow Fever and Race in Nineteenth-Century Rio de Janeiro." *Journal of Latin American Studies* 25 (1993): 441–63.

Cheeseman, Bruce S. "Richard King: Pioneering Market Capitalism on the Frontier." In *Ranching in South Texas: A Symposium*, edited by Joe S. Graham. Kingsville: Texas A&M University Press, 1994.

Cheng, Lucie, and Edna Bonacich. *Labor Immigration under Capitalism: Asian Immigrant Workers in the United States before World War II*. Berkeley: University of California Press, 1984.

Chomsky, Aviva. *West Indian Workers and the United Fruit Company in Costa Rica, 1870–1940*. Baton Rouge: Louisiana State University Press, 1997.

Chong, Nilda. *The Latino Patient: A Cultural Guide for Health Care Providers*. Yarmouth, Me.: Intercultural Press, 2002.

Chowning, Margaret. "Reassessing the Prospects for Profit in Nineteenth-Century Mexican Agriculture from a Regional Perspective: Michoacan, 1810–1860." In *How Latin America Fell Behind: Essays on the Economic Histories of Mexico and Brazil, 1800–1914*, edited by Stephen Haber, 179–214. Stanford: Stanford University Press, 1997.

Churchill, Larry, and Keith Wailoo. "Genetic Research as Therapy: Implications of 'Gene Therapy' for Informed Consent." *Journal of Law, Medicine and Ethics* 26, no. 1 (1998): 38–47.

Cirillo, Vincent. "More Fatal than Powder and Shot: Dysentery in the United States Army during the Mexican War, 1846–1848." *Perspectives in Biology and Medicine* 52, no. 3 (2009): 400–405.

Clark, Margaret. *Health in the Mexican-American Culture: A Community Study*, 3rd ed. Berkeley: University of California Press, 1973.

Cliff, Andrew. *Deciphering Global Epidemics: Analytical Approaches to the Disease Records of World Cities, 1888–1912*. New York: Cambridge University Press, 1998.

Coatsworth, John. *Growth against Development: The Economic Impact of Railroads in Porfirian Mexico*. DeKalb: Northern Illinois University Press, 1981.

Cohen, Cathy. *The Boundaries of Blackness: AIDS and the Breakdown of Black Politics*. Chicago: University of Chicago Press, 1999.

Coleman, William. *Yellow Fever in the North: The Method of Epidemiology.* Madison: University of Wisconsin Press, 1987.

Colgrove, James. *States of Immunity: The Politics of Vaccination in Twentieth-Century America.* Berkeley: University of California Press, 2006.

Collingwood, R. G. *The Idea of History.* London: Oxford University Press, 1946.

Collins-Dogrul, Julie. "Managing U.S. Mexico 'Border Health': An Organizational Field Approach." *Social Science and Medicine* 63 (2006): 3199–3211.

Cooper, Frederick. *Beyond Slavery: Explorations of Race, Labor, and Citizenship in Postemancipation Societies.* Chapel Hill: University of North Carolina Press, 2000.

———. "Urban Space, Industrial Time, and Wage Labor in Africa." In *Struggles for the City: Migrant Labor, Capital, and the State in Urban Africa,* edited by Frederick Cooper and Sara Berry, 7–50. Beverly Hills, Calif.: Sage, 1983.

Cotter, John Vincent. "Mosquitoes and Disease in the Lower Rio Grande Valley, 1846–1986." Ph.D. diss., University of Texas at Austin, 1986.

Craib, Raymond. "A Nationalist Metaphysics: State Fixations, National Maps, and the Geo-Historical Imagination in Nineteenth-Century Mexico." *Hispanic American Historical Review* 82, no. 1 (2002): 33–68.

Crussi, Miguel Gonzalez. *There Is a Life Elsewhere.* New York: Riverhead Books, 1999.

Cruz Soto, Rosalba. "La prensa de Durango en el porfiriato." *Revista Mexicana de Ciencias Políticas y Sociales* 28, no. 109 (1982): 55–67.

Cueto, Marcos. *El regreso de las epidemias: Salud y sociedad en el Perú del siglo XX.* Lima: Instituto de Estudios Peruanos, 1997.

———, ed. *Missionaries of Science: The Rockefeller Foundation and Latin America.* Bloomington: Indiana University Press, 1994.

Cumming, James G., and Harold F. Sentner. "The Prevention of Endemic Typhus in California." *Journal of the American Medical Association* 69 (July–December 1917): 98–102.

Cunningham, Roger D. "'A Lot of Fine Sturdy Black Warriors': Texas African American 'Immunes' in the Spanish American War." *Southwestern Historical Quarterly* 108, no. 3 (2005): 344–67.

Curtin, Phillip D. *Death by Migration: Europe's Encounter with the Tropical World in the Nineteenth Century.* New York: Cambridge University Press, 1989.

Davis, David Brion. "Reflections on Abolitionism and Ideological Hegemony." In *The Antislavery Debate: Capitalism and Abolitionism as a Problem in Historical Interpretation,* edited by Thomas Bender, 161–80. Berkeley: University of California Press, 1992.

De Kruif, Paul. *Microbe Hunters,* 3rd ed. New York: Harcourt, Brace & World, 1966.

De León, Arnoldo. *They Called Them Greasers: Anglo Attitudes toward Mexicans in Texas, 1821–1900.* Austin: University of Texas Press, 1983.

De León, Arnoldo, and Kenneth Stewart. *Tejanos and the Numbers Game: A Socio-*

Historical Interpretation of the Federal Censuses, 1850–1900. Albuquerque: University of New Mexico Press, 1989.

Delaney, David. *Race, Place, and the Law.* Austin: University of Texas Press, 1998.

Derby, Lauren Hutchinson. "Gringo Chickens with Worms: Food and Nationalism in the Dominican Republic." In *Close Encounters of Empire: Writing the Cultural History of U.S.–Latin American Relations,* edited by Gilbert Joseph, 451–93. Durham: Duke University Press, 1998.

Deutsch, Sarah. *No Separate Refuge: Women and Men on the Anglo-Hispanic Frontier, 1880–1940.* Oxford: Oxford University Press, 1989.

Dittmer, John. *Local People: The Struggle for Civil Rights in Mississippi, Blacks in the New World.* Urbana: University of Illinois Press, 1994.

Douglas, Mary. *Purity and Danger.* London: Routledge, Kegan and Paul, 1969.

Dowell, Greensville. *Yellow Fever and Malaria, Embracing a History of Epidemic Yellow Fever in Texas.* Philadelphia: Medical Publication Associations, 1876.

Duffy, John. "The Social Impact of Disease in the Late Nineteenth Century." In *Sickness and Health in America: Readings in the History of Medicine and Public Health,* 3rd ed., rev., edited by Judith Walzer Leavitt and Ronald Numbers, 418–25. Madison: University of Wisconsin Press, 1997.

Duran, Toribio. "Dr. Zervan and the Inactivity and Inefficiency of His Care." In *A Century of Medicine in San Antonio,* edited by Pat Ireland Nixon, 18–19. San Antonio: Pat Ireland Nixon, 1936.

Durbach, Nadja. *Bodily Matters: The Anti-Vaccination Movement in England, 1853–1907.* Durham: Duke University Press, 2005.

———. "'They Might as Well Brand Us': Working Class Resistance to Compulsory Vaccination in Victorian England." *Social History of Medicine* 13, no. 1 (2000): 45–62.

Eisenhower, John S. *So Far from God: The U.S. War with Mexico.* New York: Random House, 1989.

Ellis, John. "Businessmen and Public Health in the Urban South during the Nineteenth Century: New Orleans, Memphis, and Atlanta." *Bulletin of the History of Medicine* 44, no. 3 (May/June 1970): 197–212.

———. "Businessmen and Public Health in the Urban South during the Nineteenth Century: New Orleans, Memphis, and Atlanta." *Bulletin of the History of Medicine* 44, no. 4 (July/August 1970): 346–71.

———. *Yellow Fever and Public Health in the New South.* Lexington: University Press of Kentucky, 1992.

Engelstein, Lorna. "Morality and the Wooden Spoon: Russian Doctors View Syphilis, Social Class, and Sexual Behavior, 1890–1905." In *The Making of the Modern Body: Sexuality and Society in the Nineteenth Century,* edited by Catherine Gallagher and Thomas Laqueur, 169–207. Berkeley: University of California Press, 1987.

Epstein, Steven. *Impure Science: AIDS, Activism, and the Politics of Knowledge.* Berkeley: University of California Press, 1996.

Espinosa, Mariola. *Epidemic Invasions: Yellow Fever and the Limits of Cuban Independence.* Chicago: University of Chicago Press, 2009.

Estrella, Eduardo. "Ciencia ilustrada y saber popular en el conocimiento de la quina en el Siglo XVIII." In *Saberes andinos: Ciencia y tecnología en Bolivia, Ecuador y Peru,* edited by Marcos Cueto, 37–58. Lima: Instituto de Estudios Peruanos, 1995.

Fabri Dos Anjos, Marcio. "Medical Ethics in the Developing World: A Liberation Theology Perspective." *Journal of Medicine and Philosophy* 21 (1995): 629–37.

Fairchild, Amy. *Science at the Borders: Immigrant Medical Inspection and the Shaping of the Modern Industrial Labor Force.* Baltimore: Johns Hopkins University Press, 2003.

Falcón, Romana. "Force and the Search for Consent: The Role of the *Jefaturas Politicas* of Coahuila in National State Formation." In *Everyday Forms of State Formation: Revolution and the Negotiation of Rule in Modern Mexico,* edited by Gilbert M. Joseph and Daniel Nugent, 125–31. Durham: Duke University Press, 1994.

Farley, John. *Bilharzia, a History of Imperial Tropical Medicine.* New York: Cambridge University Press, 1991.

Farmer, Paul. *AIDS and Accusation: Haiti and the Geography of Blame.* Berkeley: University of California Press, 1992.

———. *Infections and Inequalities: The Modern Plague:* Berkeley: University of California Press, 1999.

Fenn, Elizabeth. *Pox Americana: The Great Smallpox Epidemic of 1775–82.* New York: Hill and Wang, 2001.

Foley, Neil. "The New South in the Southwest: Anglos, Blacks and Mexicans in Central Texas, 1880–1930." Ph.D. diss., University of Michigan, 1990.

———. *The White Scourge: Mexicans, Blacks, and Poor Whites in Texas Cotton Culture, 1880–1940.* American Crossroads. Berkeley: University of California Press, 1996.

Foner, Eric. *A Short History of Reconstruction, 1863–1877.* New York: Harper & Row, 1990.

———. *The Story of American Freedom.* New York: W. W. Norton, 1998.

Foucault, Michel. *Birth of the Clinic: An Archaeology of Medical Perception.* New York: Vintage, 1994.

———. *Discipline and Punish: The Birth of the Prison.* New York: Vintage Books, Publisher, 1977.

———. "The Subject and Power." *Critical Inquiry* 8, no. 4 (1982): 777–95.

Fraser, Gertrude Jacinta. *Dialogues of Birth, Race, and Memory: African American Midwifery in Green County, Virginia.* Cambridge: Harvard University Press, 1998.

Fraser, Nancy. "Struggle over Needs: Outline of a Socialist-Feminist Critical Theory of Late Capitalist Political Culture." In *Unruly Practices: Power, Discourse, and Gender in Contemporary Social Theory*, edited by Nancy Fraser, 171–83. Minneapolis: University of Minnesota Press, 1989.

———. *Unruly Practices: Power, Discourse, and Gender in Contemporary Social Theory*. Minneapolis: University of Minnesota Press, 1989.

French, William E. *A Peaceful and Working People: Manners, Morals, and Class Formation in Northern Mexico*. Albuquerque: University of New Mexico Press, 1996.

———. "Prostitutes and Guardian Angels: Women, Work, and Family in Porfirian Mexico." *Hispanic American Historical Review* 72, no. 3 (1992): 529–53.

Frost, Richard H. "The Pueblo Indian Smallpox Epidemic in New Mexico, 1898–1899." *Bulletin of the History of Medicine* 64 (1990): 417–45.

Fry, Gladys Marie. *Night Riders in Black Folk History*. Knoxville: University of Tennessee Press, 1975.

Gabbert, Ann R. "They Die Like Dogs: Disease Mortality among U.S. Forces in the Mexican War." *Military History of the West* 31, no. 1 (2001): 27–50.

Gallagher, Catherine, and Thomas Laqueur, eds. *The Making of the Modern Body: Sexuality and Society in the Nineteenth Century*. Berkeley: University of California Press, 1987.

Gamble, Vanessa Northington. *Making a Place for Ourselves: The Black Hospital Movement, 1920–1945*. New York: Oxford University Press, 1995.

———. "Roots of the Black Hospital Reform Movement." In *Sickness and Health in America: Readings in the History of Medicine and Public Health*, 3rd ed., rev., edited by Judith Walzer Leavitt and Ronald Numbers, 369–91. Madison: University of Wisconsin Press, 1997.

García, Gervasio Luis. "Strangers in Paradise?: Puerto Rico en la Correspondencia de los Consules Norteamericanos, 1869–1900." *Boletín del Centro de Investigaciones Históricas* 9 (1997): 27–55.

García, María Cristina. *Havana USA: Cuban Exiles and Cuban Americans in South Florida, 1959–1994*. Berkeley: University of California Press, 1996.

Garcia, Mario. "Mexican Americans and the Politics of Citizenship: The Case of El Paso, 1936." *New Mexico Historical Review* 59, no. 2 (1984): 187.

———. *Mexican Americans: Leadership, Ideology, and Identity, 1930–1960*. New Haven: Yale University Press, 1989.

Garcia, Richard. *The Rise of the Mexican American Middle Class: San Antonio, 1929–1941*. College Station: Texas A&M University Press, 1991.

García Canclini, Nestor. *Cultura y comunicación: Entre Lo global y lo local*. Buenos Aires: Ediciones de Periodismo y Comuniciación, 1997.

———. *Las culturas populares en el capitalismo*. Havana: Casa de las Americas, 1984.

García Muñiz, Humberto. "U.S. Consular Activism in the Caribbean, 1783–1903:

With Special Reference to St. Kitts-Nevis' Sugar Depression, Labor Turmoil, and Its Proposed Acquisition by the United States." *Revista Mexicana del Caribe* 3, no. 5 (1998): 32–79.

Garcilazo, Jeffrey Marcos. "Traqueros: Mexican Railroad Workers in the United States." Ph.D. diss., University of California–Santa Barbara, 1995.

Garrett, Laurie. *The Coming Plague: Newly Emerging Diseases in a World out of Balance*. New York: Farrar, Straus and Giroux, 1994.

Garrison, George. "Robert M. Swearingen." *Texas State Historical Association* 8, no. 3 (1923): 225–31.

Garza-Falcón, Leticia Magda. *Gente Decente: A Borderlands Response to the Rhetoric of Dominance*. Austin: University of Texas Press, 1998.

Gillens, Martin. "'Race Coding' and White Opposition to Welfare." *American Political Science Review* 90, no. 3 (1996): 593–604.

Gilly, Adolfo. "Chiapas and the Rebellion of the Enchanted World." In *Rural Revolt in Mexico: U.S. Intervention and the Domain of Subaltern Politics*, edited by Daniel Nugent, 261–333. Durham: Duke University Press, 1998.

Going, Allen J. "Critical Months in Alabama Politics, 1895–1896." *Alabama Review* 5, no. 2 (1952): 269–81.

Goldstein, Brandt. *Storming the Court: How a Band of Law Students Sued the President—and Won*. New York: Scribner, 2005.

Gomez, Jose. "Higiene: Un alimento en tela de juicio que puede ser peligroso." *Gaceta Medica de Mexico* 23, no. 6 (1888): 138–40.

González, Deena J. "La Tules of Image and Reality: Euro-American Attitudes and Legend Formation on a Spanish-Mexican Frontier." In *Building with Our Hands: New Directions in Chicana Studies*, edited by Adela de la Torre and Beatriz M. Pesquera, 75–90. Berkeley: University of California Press, 1993.

———. "Malinche as Lesbian: A Reconfiguration of 500 Years of Resistance." *California Sociologist* 14, nos. 1–2 (1991): 91–97.

Gonzalez, Gilbert. *Mexican Consuls and Labor Organizing: Imperial Politics in the American Southwest*. Austin: University of Texas Press, 1999.

Gonzalez, Jovita. *Dew on the Thorn*. Houston: Arte Publico, 1997.

Goodman, James E. *Stories of Scottsboro*. New York: Pantheon, 1994.

Gordon, Linda. *The Great Arizona Orphan Abduction*. Cambridge: Harvard University Press, 1999.

———. *Heroes of Their Own Lives: The Politics and History of Family Violence, Boston, 1880–1960*. New York: Viking, 1988.

Gorman, James. "The Altered Human Is Already Here." *New York Times*, April 6, 2004.

Gottschalk, Stephen. *The Emergence of Christian Science in American Religious Life*. Berkeley: University of California Press, 1973.

Gracia, Diego. "The Historical Setting of Latin American Bioethics." *Journal of Medicine and Philosophy* 21 (1996): 593–609.

Gregory, Steven, and Roger Sanjek, eds. *Race*. New Brunswick: Rutgers University Press, 1994.

Griswold del Castillo, Richard. *The Los Angeles Barrio, 1850–1890*. Berkeley: University of California Press, 1979.

———. *The Treaty of Guadalupe Hidalgo: A Legacy of Conflict*. Norman: University of Oklahoma Press, 1990.

Guarnizo, Luis Eduardo, and Alejandro Portes. "Assimilation and Transnationalism: Determinants of Transnational Political Action among Contemporary Migrants." *American Journal of Sociology* 108, no. 6 (2003): 1211–48.

Guerin-Gonzales, Camille. *Mexican Workers and American Dreams: Immigration, Repatriation, and California Farm Labor, 1900–1939*. New Brunswick: Rutgers University Press, 1994.

Gutiérrez, David. *Walls and Mirrors: Mexican Americans, Mexican Immigrants, and the Politics of Ethnicity*. Berkeley: University of California Press, 1995.

Gutiérrez, Elena Rebeca. "The Racial Politics of Reproduction: The Social Construction of Mexican-Origin Women's Fertility." Ph.D. diss., University of Michigan, 2000.

Gutiérrez, Ramón. "The Erotic Zone: Sexual Trangression on the U.S.–Mexican Border." In *Mapping Multiculturalism*, edited by Avery F. Gordon and Christopher Newfield, 253–62. Minneapolis: University of Minnesota Press, 1996.

———. *When Jesus Came, the Corn Mothers Went Away: Marriage, Sexuality, and Power in Colonial New Mexico, 1500–1848*. Stanford: Stanford University Press, 1991.

Gutiérrez-Jones, Carl. *Rethinking the Borderlands: Between Chicano Culture and Legal Discourse*. Berkeley: University of California Press, 1995.

Haas, Lisbeth. *Conquests and Historical Identities in California, 1769–1936*. Berkeley: University of California Press, 1996.

Haas, Peter. "Do Regimes Matter: Epistemic Communities and Mediterranean Pollution Control." *International Organization* 43, no. 1 (1989): 377–403.

———. "Introduction: Epistemic Communities and International Policy Coordination." *International Organization* 46, no. 1 (1992): 1–36.

Haber, Stephen. *How Latin America Fell Behind: Essays on the Economic Histories of Mexico and Brazil, 1800–1914*. Stanford: Stanford University Press, 1997.

Haber, Stephen, and Laura Pulido. "La industrializacion de Mexico: Historiografia y analisis." *Historias* 42, no. 3 (1993): 649–88.

Hacking, Ian. *The Taming of Chance*. New York: Cambridge University Press, 1990.

Hall, Linda B., and Donald M. Coerver. *Revolution on the Border: The United States and Mexico, 1910–1920*. Albuquerque: University of New Mexico Press, 1988.

Haller, John S. "The Physician versus the Negro: Medical and Anthropological Concepts of Race in the Late Nineteenth Century." *Bulletin of the History of Medicine and Allied Sciences* 44, no. 2 (1970): 154–67.

Halperin, David. *Saint Foucault*. New York: Oxford University Press, 1995.

Hammonds, Evelynn. *Childhood's Deadly Scourge: The Campaign to Control Diphtheria in New York City, 1880–1930*. Baltimore: Johns Hopkins University Press, 1998.

Haney-Lopez, Ian. *Racism on Trial: The Chicano Fight for Justice*. Cambridge: Belknap Press of Harvard University Press, 2003.

———. *White by Law: The Legal Construction of Race*. Critical America. New York: New York University Press, 1996.

Hansen, Bert. "American Physicians' 'Discovery' of Homosexuals, 1880–1900: A New Diagnosis in a Changing Society." In *Sickness and Health in America: Readings in the History of Medicine and Public Health*, 3rd ed., rev., edited by Judith Walzer Leavitt and Ronald Numbers, 13–31. Madison: University of Wisconsin Press, 1997.

———. "New Images of a Medicine: Visual Evidence for the Widespread Popularity of Therapeutic Discoveries in America after 1885." *Bulletin of the History of Medicine* 73, no. 4 (1999): 629–78.

Haraway, Donna J. "Universal Donors in a Vampire Culture: It's All in the Family: Biological Kinship Categories in the Twentieth-Century United States." In *Uncommon Ground: Rethinking the Human Place in Nature*, edited by William Cronon, 323–66. New York: W. W. Norton, 1997.

Harrison, Mark. *Public Health in British India: Anglo-Indian Preventive Medicine, 1859–1914*. New York: Cambridge University Press, 1994.

Hart, John Mason. *Empire and Revolution: Americans in Mexico since the Civil War*. Berkeley: University of California Press, 2006.

Harvey, David. *Justice, Nature, and the Geography of Difference*. New York: Blackwell, 1996.

Haskell, Thomas I. "Capitalism and the Origins of the Humanitarian Sensibility, Part 1." In *The Antislavery Debate: Capitalism and Abolitionism as a Problem in Historical Interpretation*, edited by Thomas Bender, 107–35. Berkeley: University of California Press, 1992.

———. "Capitalism and the Origins of the Humanitarian Sensibility, Part 2." In *The Antislavery Debate: Capitalism and Abolitionism as a Problem in Historical Interpretation*, edited by Thomas Bender, 136–60. Berkeley: University of California Press, 1992.

Hasson, Gail Snowden. "The Medical Activities of the Freedmen's Bureau in Reconstruction Alabama, 1865–1868." Ph.D. diss., University of Alabama, 1982.

Headrick, Daniel R. *The Tools of Empire: Technology and European Imperialism in the Nineteenth Century*. New York: Oxford University Press, 1981.

Herbert, C. "Rat Worship and Taboo in Mayhew's London." *Representations* 23 (1988): 1–24.

Hewitt, Nancy A. "'The Voice of Virile Labor': Labor Militancy, Community Solidarity and Gender Identity among Tampa's Latin Workers, 1880–1921." In *Work Engendered: Toward a New History of American Labor,* edited by Ava Baron, 144–67. Ithaca: Cornell University Press, 1991.

Higham, John. *Strangers in the Land: Patterns of American Nativism, 1860–1925.* New Brunswick: Rutgers University Press, 1988.

Hill, Elmer, et al. "Evaluation of County Wide DDT Dusting Operations in Murine Typhus Control, 1946–1949." *American Journal of Public Health* 41, no. 4 (1951): 398–401.

Hine, Darlene Clark. *Black Women in White: Racial Conflict and Cooperation in the Nursing Profession.* Bloomington: Indiana University Press, 1989.

Holt, Thomas. "The Essence of the Contract: The Articulation of Race, Gender, and Political Economy in British Emancipation Policy." In *Beyond Slavery: Explorations of Race, Labor, and Citizenship in Postemancipation Societies,* edited by Frederick Cooper, Thomas Holt, and Rebecca Scott, 33–59. Chapel Hill: University of North Carolina Press, 2000.

Hondagneu-Sotelo, Pierrette. *Domestica: Immigrant Workers Cleaning and Caring in the Shadow of Affluence.* Berkeley: University of California Press, 2001.

———. "Regulating the Unregulated? Domestic Workers' Social Networks." *Social Problems* 41 (1994): 50–64.

Hopkins, Donald. *Princes and Peasants: A History of Smallpox.* Chicago: University of Chicago Press, 1983.

Huerkamp, Claudia. "The History of Smallpox Vaccination in Germany: A First Step in the Medicalization of the General Public." *Journal of Contemporary History* 20, no. 4 (1985): 617–85.

Humphreys, Margaret. *Intensely Human: The Health of the Black Soldier in the American Civil War.* Baltimore: Johns Hopkins University Press, 2008.

———. "A Stranger to Our Camps: Typhus in American History." *Bulletin of the History of Medicine* 80, no. 2 (2006): 269–90.

———. *Yellow Fever and the South.* Baltimore: Johns Hopkins University Press, 1992.

Hunter, Tera. *To 'Joy My Freedom: Black Southern Women's Lives and Labor in the South after the Civil War.* Cambridge: Harvard University Press, 1996.

Ileto, Reynaldo. "Cholera and the Origins of the American Sanitary Order." In *Imperial Medicine and Indigenous Societies,* edited by David Arnold, 125–48. Manchester: Manchester University Press, 1987.

Irey, Robert. "Soldiering, Suffering, and Dying in the Mexican War." *Journal of the West* 11, no. 2 (1972): 285–98.

Irons, J. V., et al. "Outbreak of Smallpox in the Lower Rio Grande Valley of Texas in 1949." *American Journal of Public Health* 43, no. 1 (1953): 25–29.

Jacobson, Mathew Frye. *Special Sorrows: The Diasporic Imagination of Irish, Polish, and Jewish Immigrants in the United States.* Cambridge: Harvard University Press, 1995.

———. *Whiteness of a Different Color: European Immigrants and the Alchemy of Race.* Cambridge: Harvard University Press, 1998.

Jacoby, Karl. "Between North and South: The Alternative Borderlands of William Ellis and the African American Colony of 1895." In *Continental Crossroads: Remapping U.S.-Mexico Borderlands History,* edited by Elliott Young, 209–39. Durham: Duke University Press, 2005.

———. "From Plantation to Hacienda: The Mexican Colonization Movement in Alabama." *Alabama Heritage,* no. 35 (1995): 34–43.

James, Winston. *Holding Aloft the Banner of Ethiopia: Caribbean Radicalism in Early Twentieth-Century America.* New York: Verso, 1998.

Johnson, Susan Lee. *Roaring Camp: The Social World of the California Gold Rush.* New York: Random House, 2000.

Jones, Margaret. "The Ceylon Malaria Epidemic of 1934–35: A Case Study of Colonial Medicine." *Social History of Medicine* 13, no. 1 (2000): 87–109.

Jordan, Thomas. "'An Awful Visitation of Providence': The Irish Famine of 1845–49." *Journal of the Royal Society of Health* 117, no. 4 (1997): 216–22.

Joseph, Gilbert M. "The United States, Feuding Elites, and Rural Revolt in Yucatan, 1836–1915." In *Rural Revolt in Mexico: U.S. Intervention and the Domain of Subaltern Politics,* edited by Daniel Nugent, 173–205. Durham: Duke University Press, 1998.

Kaplan, Amy, and Donald E. Pease, ed. *Cultures of United States Imperialism.* Durham: Duke University Press, 1993.

Katz, Friedrich. "From Alliance to Dependency: The Formation and Deformation of an Alliance between Francisco Villa and the United States." In *Rural Revolt in Mexico: U.S. Intervention and the Domain of Subaltern Politics,* edited by Daniel Nugent, 239–59. Durham: Duke University Press, 1998.

———. *The Life and Times of Pancho Villa.* Stanford: Stanford University Press, 1998.

———. *The Secret War in Mexico: Europe, the United States, and the Mexican Revolution.* Chicago: University of Chicago Press, 1981.

Katz, Jay. *Experimentation with Human Beings.* New York: Russell Sage Foundation, 1972.

Kaufmann, Martin. "The American Anti-Vaccinationists and Their Arguments." *Bulletin of the History of Medicine* 41, no. 5 (1967): 463–77.

Kearney, Milo, and Anthony Knopp. *Boom and Bust: The Historical Cycles of Matamoros and Brownsville.* Austin: Eakin Press, 1991.

Keller, Morton. *Regulating a New Society: Public Policy and Social Change in America, 1900–1933.* Cambridge: Harvard University Press, 1994.

Kelton, Paul. "Not All Disappeared: Disease and Southeastern Indian Survival, 1500–1800." Ph.D.diss., University of Oklahoma, 1998.

Kim, Richard "Korean Immigrant (Trans)nationalism: Diaspora, Ethnicity, and State-making, 1903–1945." Ph.D. diss., University of Michigan, 2002.

Kiple, Kenneth F., and Virginia Himmelsteib King. *Another Dimension to the Black Diaspora: Diet, Disease, and Racism.* New York: Cambridge University Press, 1981.

Knee, Stuart. *Christian Science in the Age of Mary Baker Eddy.* Westport, Conn.: Greenwood, 1994.

Knight, Alan. *The Mexican Revolution.* Vol. 1, *Porfirians, Liberals, Peasants.* Cambridge: Cambridge University Press, 1986.

Kolchin, Peter. "Whiteness Studies: The New History of Race in America." *Journal of American History* 89, no. 1 (2002): 154–73.

Koreck, Maria Teresa. "Space and Revolution in Northeastern Chihuahua." In *Rural Revolt in Mexico: U.S. Intervention and the Domain of Subaltern Politics,* edited by Daniel Nugent, 147–71. Durham: Duke University Press, 1998.

Kouri, Emilio. "Interpreting the Expropriation of Indian Pueblo Lands in Porfirian Mexico: The Unexamined Legacies of Andres Molina Enriquez." *Hispanic American Historical Review* 82, no. 1 (2002): 69–117.

Krasner, Stephen D. "Regimes and the Limits of Realism: Regimes as Autonomous Variables." In *International Regimes,* edited by Stephen Krasner, 358–68. Ithaca: Cornell University Press, 1983.

———. "Structural Causes and Regime Consequences: Regimes as Intervening Variables." In *International Regimes,* edited by Stephen D. Krasner, 1–21. Ithaca: Cornell University Press, 1983.

Kraut, Alan. *Silent Travelers: Germs, Genes, and the Immigrant Menace.* New York: Basic Books, 1995.

Krieger, Nancy. "The Making of Public Health Data: Paradigms, Politics, and Policy." *Journal of Public Health Policy* 13 (1992): 412–27.

Kuhlenbeck, Hartwig. "Dangers Associated with the Use of Living 'Attenuated' Typhus Vaccine." *American Journal of Public Health* 36, no. 9 (1946): 1027–29.

Kunitz, Stephen. *Disease and Social Diversity: The European Impact on the Health of Non-Europeans.* New York: Oxford University Press, 1994.

———. *Disease Change and the Role of Medicine: The Navajo Experience.* Berkeley: University of California Press, 1983.

———. "Premises, Premises: Comments on the Comparability of Classifications." *Journal of the History of Medicine and Allied Sciences* 54, no. 2 (1999): 241–60.

Lacour, Claudia Brodsky. "The 'Interest' of the Simpson Trial: Spectacle, National History, and the Notion of Disinterested Judgment." In *Birth of a Nation'hood: Gaze, Script, and Spectacle in the O. J. Simpson Case,* edited by Toni Morrison. New York: Pantheon, 1997.

Lain Entralgo, Pedro. "From Galen to Magnetic Resonance: History of Medicine in Latin America." *Journal of Medicine and Philosophy* 21 (1996): 571–91.

Larrazolo, Margarita. *Coahuila 1893: Una respuesta a la centralización política.* México: Instituto Nacional de Estudios Históricos de la Revolución Mexicana, 1997.

Lay, Shawn. *War, Revolution, and the Ku Klux Klan: A Study of Intolerance in a Border City.* El Paso: Texas Western Press, 1985.

Leavitt, Judith Walzer. "Be Safe, Be Sure: New York City's Experience with Epidemic Smallpox." In *Sickness and Health in America: Readings in the History of Medicine and Public Health,* 3rd ed., rev., edited by Judith Walzer Leavitt and Ronald Numbers, 555–74. Madison: University of Wisconsin Press, 1997.

———. *The Healthiest City: Milwaukee and the Politics of Health Reform.* Princeton: Princeton University Press, 1982.

———. *Typhoid Mary: Captive to the Public's Health.* Boston: Beacon, 1996.

———. "Typhoid Mary Strikes Back: Bacteriological Theory and Practice in Early Twentieth-Century Public Health." In *Sickness and Health in America: Readings in the History of Medicine and Public Health,* 3rd ed., rev., edited by Judith Walzer Leavitt and Ronald Numbers, 543–54. Madison: University of Wisconsin Press, 1997.

Leavitt, Judith Walzer, and Ronald L. Numbers, eds. *Sickness and Health in America: Readings in the History of Medicine and Public Health,* 3rd ed., rev. Madison: University of Wisconsin Press, 1997.

Lederer, Susan. *Subjected to Science: Human Experimentation in America before the Second World War.* Baltimore: Johns Hopkins University Press, 1995.

Lee, Erika. "Enforcing the Borders: Chinese Exclusion along the U.S. Borders with Canada and Mexico, 1882–1924." *Journal of American History* 89, no. 1 (2002): 54–87.

———. "Immigrants and Immigration Law: A State of the Field Assessment." *Journal of American Ethnic History* 18, no. 4 (1999): 85–114.

Lee, Sharon M. "Racial Classifications in the United States Census: 1890–1990." *Ethnic and Racial Studies* 16, no. 1 (1993): 75–94.

Leiker, James N. *Racial Borders: Black Soldiers along the Rio Grande.* College Station: Texas A&M University Press, 2002.

Lerner Sigal, Victoria. "Espionaje y Revolución Mexicana." *Historia Mexicana* 44, no. 4 (1995): 617–43.

Lewis, Earl. "To Turn as on a Pivot: Writing African Americans into a History of Overlapping Diasporas." *American Historical Review* 100, no. 3 (June 1995): 765–87.

Leyva, Yolanda Chavez. "'¿Que son los niños?': Mexican Children along the U.S.-Mexico Border, 1880–1930." Ph.D. diss., University of Arizona, 1999.

Limerick, Patricia. *The Legacy of Conquest: The Unbroken Past of the American West.* New York: W. W. Norton, 1987.

Limón, Jose E. *Dancing with the Devil: Society and Cultural Poetics in Mexican-American South Texas.* Madison: University of Wisconsin Press, 1994.

Lipsitz, George. "The Possessive Investment in Whiteness: Racialized Social Democracy and the 'White' Problem in American Studies." *American Quarterly* 47,
no. 3 (1995): 369–87.

———. "Response: Toxic Racism." *American Quarterly* 47, no. 3 (1995): 416–27.

Lloyd, Jane-Dale. "Rancheros and Rebellion: The Case of Northwestern Chihua-
hua, 1905–1909." In *Rural Revolt in Mexico: U.S. Intervention and the Domain of
Subaltern Politics*, edited by Daniel Nugent, 107–32. Durham: Duke University
Press, 1998.

Lowe, Lisa. "Heterogeneity, Hybridity, Multiplicity: Asian American Differences."
In *Immigrant Acts: On Asian American Cultural Politics*, edited by Lisa Lowe,
60–83. Durham: Duke University Press, 1997.

Luckingham, Bradford. *Epidemic in the Southwest, 1918–1919.* El Paso: Texas Western Press, 1984.

Macfadden, David Fancher. "International Cooperation and Pandemic Disease: Regimes and the Role of Epistemic Communities in Combatting Cholera, Smallpox
and Aids." Ph.D. diss., Claremont Graduate School, 1995.

MacLeod, Robert. "Law, Medicine, and Public Opinion: The Resistance to Compulsory Health Legislation, 1870–1907." *Public Law* 167 (summer 1967): 107–28.

Marichal, Carlos. "Obstacles to the Development of Capital Markets in Nineteenth-
Century Mexico." In *How Latin America Fell Behind: Essays on the Economic
Histories of Mexico and Brazil, 1800–1914*, edited by Stephen Haber, 118–45. Stan-
ford: Stanford University Press, 1997.

Markel, Howard. "Caring for the Foreign Born: The Health of Immigrant Children
in the United States, 1890–1925." *Archives of Pediatric and Adolescent Medicine*
152, no. 10 (1998): 1020–27.

———. "'The Eyes Have It': Trachoma, the Perception of Disease, the United States
Public Health Service, and the American Jewish Immigration Experience, 1897–
1924." *Bulletin of the History of Medicine* 74, no. 3 (2000): 525–60.

———. "For the Welfare of Children: The Origins of the Relationship between U.S.
Public Health Workers and Pediatricians." *American Journal of Public Health* 90,
no. 6 (2000): 893–99.

———. *Quarantine! East European Jewish Immigrants and the New York City Epidemics of 1892.* Baltimore: Johns Hopkins University Press, 1999.

———. "Symposium: Workshop on the BRCA1 Breast Cancer Gene in the Jewish
Population: Di Goldine Medina (the Golden Land): Historical Perspectives of
Eugenics and the East European (Ashkenazi) Jewish-American Community,
1880–1925." *Health Matrix: Journal of Law-Medicine* 7 (winter 1997): 49–62.

Marks, Cheryl. *Farewell—We're Good and Gone: The Great Black Migration. Blacks
in the Diaspora.* Bloomington: Indiana University Press, 1989.

Martin, Biddy. "Lesbian Identity and Autobiographical Difference." In *The Lesbian
and Gay Studies Reader*, edited by Henry Abelove et al., 274–93. New York: Routledge, 1993.

Martin, Emily. *Flexible Bodies: Tracking Immunity in American Culture from the Days of Polio to the Age of Aids.* Boston: Beacon, 1994.

Martinez, Oscar Jaquez. *Border Boom Town: Ciudad Juarez since 1848.* Austin: University of Texas Press, 1978.

Massey, Sara. *Black Cowboys of Texas.* College Station: Texas A&M University Press, 2000.

Masur, Kate. "A Rare Phenomenon of Philological Vegetation: The Word 'Contraband' and the Meanings of Emancipation in the United States." *Journal of American History* 93, no. 4 (2007): 1050–84.

McBride, David. *From TB to AIDS: Epidemics among Urban Blacks since 1900.* Albany: State University of New York Press, 1991.

———. *Integrating the City of Medicine: Blacks in Philadelphia Health Care, 1910–1965.* Philadelphia: Temple University Press, 1989.

McCaa, Robert. "Spanish and Nahuatl Views on Smallpox and Demographic Catastrophe in Mexico." *Journal of Interdisciplinary History* 25, no. 3 (1995): 397–431.

McCaffrey, James M. "Santa Anna's Greatest Weapon: The Effect of Disease on the American Soldier in the Mexican War." *Military History of the West* 24, no. 2 (1994): 111–21.

McCallister-Linn, Brian. *Guardians of Empire: The U.S. Army and the Pacific, 1902–1940.* Chapel Hill: University of North Carolina Press, 1997.

McCamant, T. J. "Typhus Fever." *Texas State Journal of Medicine* 19 (1923): 42.

McClain, Charles. *In Search of Equality: The Chinese Struggle against Discrimination in Nineteenth-Century America.* Berkeley: University of California Press, 1994.

McClenahan, Heather. "A Diarist's Tale: Roby Mcfarland's Tampa, 1887–1888." *Tampa Bay History* 15, no. 1 (1993): 5–29.

McLean, Charles. *In Search of Equality: The Chinese Struggle against Discrimination in Nineteenth-Century America.* Berkeley: University of California Press, 1994.

Meade, Teresa. "Civilizing Rio de Janeiro: The Public Health Campaign and the Riot of 1904." *Journal of Social History* 20 (1986): 301–22.

Meckel, Richard A. *"Save the Babies": American Public Health Reform and the Prevention of Infant Mortality, 1850–1920.* Baltimore: Johns Hopkins University Press, 1990.

Meyer, Melissa L. "'We cannot get a living as we used to': Dispossession and the White Earth Anishinaabeg, 1889–1920." *American Historical Review* 96, no. 2 (1991): 368–95.

Meyers, William K. *Forge of Progress: Popular Politics in the Comarca Lagunera, 1880–1920.* Albuquerque: University of New Mexico Press, 1991.

———. "La Comarca Lagunera: Work, Protest, and Popular Mobilization in North Central Mexico." In *Other Mexicos: Essays on Regional Mexican History, 1876–*

1911, edited by Thomas Benjamin and William McNeelie, 243–74. Albuquerque: University of New Mexico Press, 1984.

———. "Politics, Vested Rights, and Economic Growth in Porfirian Mexico: The Company Tlahualilo in the Comarca Lagunera." *Hispanic American Historical Review* 57, no. 3 (1977): 435.

Michael, Jerrold, and Thomas R. Bender. "Fighting Smallpox on the Texas Border: An Episode from the PHS's Proud Past," *Public Health Reports* 99, no. 6 (1984): 579–82

Miguel, Guadalupe San. *Let All of Them Take Heed: The Mexican American Pursuit of Educational Equality, 1848–1980.* Austin: University of Texas Press, 1991.

Mihesuah, Devon A. "American Indians, Anthropologists, Pothunters, and Repatriation: Ethical, Religious, and Political Differences." *American Indian Quarterly* 20, no. 2 (1996): 229–38.

———. "Commonality of Difference: American Indian Women and History." *American Indian Quarterly* 20, no. 1 (1996): 15–28.

———. "A Few Cautions at the Millennium on the Merging of Feminist Studies with American Indian Women's Studies." *Signs* 25, no. 4 (2000): 124–27.

———. "Indigenous Scholars versus the Status Quo: Criticism and Interpretation." *American Indian Quarterly* 26 (2002): 145–50.

———. "Suggested Guidelines for Institutions with Scholars Who Conduct Research on American Indians." *American Indian Culture and Research Journal* 17, no. 3 (1993): 1131–40.

———. "The Texas Cherokees: A People between Two Fires, 1819–1840." *Journal of the West* 32, no. 1 (1993): 83.

———. "Voices, Interpretations, and the 'New Indian History': Comment on the American Indian Quarterly's Special Issue on Writing about American Indians." *American Indian Quarterly* 20, no. 1 (1996): 91–109.

Miranda, Francisco. "The Public Health Department in Mexico City." *American Journal of Public Health* (1930): 1125–30.

Molina, Carlos, and Marilyn Aguirre-Molina, eds. *Latina Health in the United States: A Public Health Reader.* San Francisco: Jossey-Bass, 2003.

Montejano, David. *Anglos and Mexicans in the Making of Texas, 1836–1986.* Austin: University of Texas Press, 1986.

Montgomery, David. *The Fall of the House of Labor: The Workplace, the State, and American Labor Activism, 1865–1925.* New York: Cambridge University Press, 1987.

Moon, Graham, and Kelvyn Jones. *Health, Disease and Medical Society: A Critical Medical Geography.* New York: Routledge, Kegan and Paul, 1987.

Morantz Sanchez, Regina Markell. *Conduct Unbecoming a Woman: Medicine on Trial in Turn-of-the-Century Brooklyn.* New York: Oxford University Press, 1999.

———. "Review: Drawing Blood: Technology and Disease Identity in Twentieth-Century America." *Journal of Interdisciplinary History* 29, no. 1 (1998): 150–53.

———. *Sympathy and Science: Women Physicians in American Medicine.* New York: Oxford University Press, 1985.

Mora-Torres, Juan. *The Making of the Mexican Border: The State, Capitalism, and Society in Nuevo León, 1848–1910.* Austin: University of Texas Press, 2001.

Morrison, Toni. "On the Backs of Blacks." *Time* 142 (1993): 57.

Mort, Frank. *Dangerous Sexualities: Medico-Moral Politics in England since 1830.* New York: Routledge, Kegan and Paul, 1987.

Mullan, Fitzhugh. *Plagues and Politics: The Story of the United States Public Health Service.* New York: Basic Books, 1989.

Murray, Edward S., et al. "Brill's Disease IV: Study of 26 Cases in Yugoslavia." *American Journal of Public Health* 41, no. 11 (1951): 1359–69.

Needell, Jeffrey D. "The Revolta Contra Vacina of 1904: The Revolt against 'Modernization' in Belle-Epoque Rio de Janeiro." *Hispanic American Historical Review* 67 (1987): 233–69.

Negrón-Montaner, Frances. "Jennifer's Butt." *Aztlan* 22 (1997): 181–94.

Ngai, Mae M. "The Architecture of Race in American Immigration Law: A Reexamination of the Immigration Act of 1924." *Journal of American History* 86, no. 1 (1999): 67–92.

———. "Legacies of Exclusion: Illegal Chinese Immigration During the Cold War Years." *Journal of American Ethnic History* 18, no. 1 (1998): 3–35.

———. "Review: Laws Harsh as Tigers: Chinese Immigrants and the Shaping of American Immigration Law." *Political Science Quarterly* 111, no. 4 (1996): 734–35.

Nixon, Pat Ireland. *A Century of Medicine in San Antonio.* San Antonio: Pat Ireland Nixon, 1936.

Norwood, Stephen Harlan. *Labor's Flaming Youth: Telephone Operators and Worker Militancy, 1878–1923.* Urbana: University of Illinois Press, 1990.

Novak, William J. *The People's Welfare: Law and Regulation in Nineteenth-Century America.* Chapel Hill: University of North Carolina Press, 1996.

Nugent, Daniel, ed. *Rural Revolt in Mexico: U.S. Intervention and the Domain of Subaltern Politics.* American Encounters/Global Interactions. Durham: Duke University Press, 1998.

Numbers, Ronald. *Almost Persuaded: American Physicians and Compulsory Health Insurance, 1912–1920.* Baltimore: Johns Hopkins University Press, 1978.

Ogawa, Mariko. "Uneasy Bedfellows: Science and Politics in the Refutation of Koch's Bacterial Theory of Cholera." *Bulletin of the History of Medicine* 74 (2000): 671–707.

Omi, Michael, and Howard Winant. *Racial Formation in the United States: From the 1960s to the 1990s.* 2nd ed. New York: Routledge, Kegan and Paul, 1994.

Omran, A. R. "The Epidemiologic Transition: A Theory of the Epidemiology of Population Change." *Millbank Memorial Quarterly* 49 (1971): 509–38.

Ong, Aihwa. "Making the Biopolitical Subject: Cambodian Immigrants, Refugee Medicine, and Cultural Citizenship in California." *Social Science and Medicine* 50, no. 9 (1995): 1243–57.

O'Phelan Godoy, Scarlett. "Vivir y morir en el mineral de Hualgayoc a fines de la colonia." *Jahrbuch für Geschichte von Staat, Wirtschaft und Gesellschaft Lateinamerikas* 30 (1993): 75–127.

Ortiz-Mariotte, Carlos, and Felipe Malo-Juvera. "Control of Typhus Fever in Mexican Villages and Rural Populations through the Use of DDT." *American Journal of Public Health* 35, no. 11 (1945): 1191–95.

Osagie, Iyonolu Folayan. *The Amistad Revolt: Memory, Slavery, and the Politics of Identity in the United States and Sierra Leone.* Athens: University of Georgia Press, 2000.

Osorio, Ruben. "Villismo: Nationalism and Popular Mobilization in Northern Mexico." In *Rural Revolt in Mexico: U.S. Intervention and the Domain of Subaltern Politics,* edited by Daniel Nugent, 89–106. Durham: Duke University Press, 1998.

Packard, Randall M. *White Plague, Black Labor: Tuberculosis and the Political Economy of Health and Disease in South Africa.* Berkeley: University of California Press, 1989.

Painter, Nell Irvin. *Exodusters: Black Migration to Kansas after Reconstruction.* New York: W. W. Norton, 1992.

Pani, Erika. "Dreaming of a Mexican Empire: The Political Projects of the 'Imperialistas.'" *Hispanic American Historical Review* 82, no. 1 (2002): 1–32.

Paredes, Américo. "On Ethnographic Work among Minority Groups: A Folklorist's Perspective." *New Scholar: New Directions in Chicano Scholarship* 6 (1977): 1–31.

Parran, Thomas. "Public Health Implications of Tropical and Imported Diseases: Strategy against the Global Spread of Disease." *American Journal of Public Health* 34, no. 1 (1944): 1–13.

Pastrana, Patricia Aceves, and Alba Morales Cosme. "Conflictos y negociaciones en las expediciones de balmis." *Estudios Novohispanos* 17 (2007): 171–200.

Pearcy, Thomas L. "The Smallpox Outbreak of 1779–1782: A Brief Comparative Look at Twelve Borderland Communities." *Journal of the West* 36, no. 1 (1997): 26–37.

Peavy, James E. *History of Public Health in Texas.* Austin: Texas State Department of Health, 1974.

Pegler Gordon, Anna. *In Sight of America: Photography and the Development of U.S. Immigration Policy.* American Crossroads. Berkeley: University of California Press, 2010.

Pérez, Emma. "Speaking from the Margin: Uninvited Discourse on Sexuality and Power." In *Building with Our Hands: New Directions in Chicana Studies*, edited by Adela de la Torre and Beatriz Pesquera, 57–71. Berkeley: University of California Press, 1994.

Pernick, Martin S. "Back from the Grave: Recurring Controversies over Defining and Diagnosing Death in History." In *Death: Beyond Whole-Brain Criteria*, edited by Richard M. Zaner, 17–74. Amsterdam: Kluwer Academic, 1988.

———. *The Black Stork: Eugenics and the Death of "Defective" Babies in American Medicine and Motion Pictures since 1915*. New York: Oxford University Press, 1999.

———. *A Calculus of Suffering: Pain, Professionalism, and Anesthesia in Nineteenth-Century America*. New York: Columbia University Press, 1985.

———. "Eugenics and Public Health in American History." *American Journal of Public Health* 87, no. 11 (1997): 1767–72.

———. "The Patient's Role in Medical Decisionmaking: A Social History of Informed Consent in Medical Therapy." In *Making Health Care Decisions: The Ethical and Legal Obligations of Informed Consent in the Patient-Practitioner Relationship*. Vol. 3: *Appendices Studies on the Foundation of Informed Consent*, edited by Morris A. Abram, 1–37. Washington, D.C.: Superintendents of Documents, Government Printing Office, 1982.

———. "Race, Labor, and Fevers in the Pre-Canal USA: Brief Remarks on Some Unexamined Issues." Paper presented at the conference Beyond Walter Reed: Yellow Fever, Public Health, Race, and Free Labor in Post-Emancipation Societies, February 18, 2000, William L. Clements Library, University of Michigan, Ann Arbor.

Pickstone, John. Introduction to *Medical Innovations in Historical Perspective*, 1–16. New York: St. Martin's, 1992.

———, ed. *Medical Innovations in Historical Perspective*. New York: St. Martin's, 1992.

Plotz, Harry. "Endemic Typhus Fever in Jamaica, B.W.I." *American Journal of Public Health* 33 (1943): 812–14.

Pohl, Lynn Marie. "Long Waits, Small Spaces, and Compassionate Care: Memories of Race and Medicine in a Mid-Twentieth-Century Southern Community." *Bulletin of the History of Medicine and Allied Sciences* 74, no. 1 (2000): 107–37.

Poovey, Mary. *Making a Social Body: British Cultural Formation, 1830–1864*. Chicago: University of Chicago Press, 1995.

Porter, Dorothy. "Enemies of the Race: Biology, Environmentalism, and Public Health in Edwardian England." *Victorian Studies*, 34, no. 2 (winter 1991): 159–78.

Portes, Alejandro. "Conclusion: Theoretical Convergences and Empirical Evidence in the Study of Immigrant Transnationalism." *International Migration Review* 37, no. 3 (2003): 874–93.

———. "Global Villagers: The Rise of Transnational Communities." *American Prospect* 25 (1996): 74–78.

———. "Immigration Theory for a New Century: Some Problems and Opportunities." *International Migration Review* 31, no. 4 (winter 1997): 799–825.

———. "Immigration's Aftermath." *American Prospect* 13 (2002): 35–38.

———. "Latin American Class Structures: Their Composition and Change during the Neoliberal Era." *Latin American Research Review* 38 (2003): 41–84.

———. "Mental Illness and Help-Seeking Behavior among Mariel Cuban and Haitian Refugees in South Florida." *Journal of Health and Social Behavior* 33, no. 4 (1992): 283–99.

———. "Morning in Miami: A New Era for Cuban-American Politics." *American Prospect* 38 (1998): 28–33.

———. "Neoliberalism and the Sociology of Development: Emerging Trends and Unanticipated Facts." *Population and Development Review* 23, no. 2 (1997): 229–60.

———. "The Party or the Grass Roots: A Comparative Analysis of Urban Political Participation in the Caribbean Basin." *International Journal of Urban and Regional Research* 18, no. 3 (1994): 491–510.

———. "Should Immigrants Assimilate?" *Public Interest* 116 (1994): 18–34.

———. "Social Capital: Its Origins and Applications in Modern Sociology." *Annual Review of Sociology* 24, no. 1 (1998): 1–25.

———. "What Shall I Call Myself? Hispanic Identity Formation in the Second Generation." *Ethnic and Racial Studies* 19, no. 3 (1996): 523–78.

Poyo, Gerald E. *With All, and for the Good of All: The Emergence of Popular Nationalism in the Cuban Communities of the United States, 1848–1898.* Durham: Duke University Press, 1989.

Quinby, Griffith E. "Epidemiologic and Serologic Appraisal of Murine Typhus in the United States, 1948–1951." *American Journal of Public Health* 43, no. 2 (1953): 160–64.

Raat, Dirk. *Revoltosos: Mexico's Rebels in the United States.* College Station: Texas A&M University Press, 1981.

Rabinowitz, Howard. *Race Relations in the Urban South, 1865–1900.* Urbana-Champaign: University of Illinois Press, 1980.

Ramirez, Susana. *La salud del imperio: Real expedición filantrópica de la vacuna.* Madrid: Fundación Jorge Juan, 2002.

Ramos, Julio. "A Citizen Body: Cholera in Havana, 1833." *Dispositio/n* 46 (1996): 179–96.

Rappaport, Joanne. *The Politics of Memory: Native Historical Interpretation in the Colombian Andes.* Durham: Duke University Press, 1990.

Redkey, Edwin. *Black Exodus: Black Nationalist and Back-to-Africa Movements, 1890–1910.* New Haven: Yale University Press, 1970.

Reilly, Philip. *The Surgical Solution: Involuntary Sterilization in the United States*. Baltimore: Johns Hopkins University Press, 1991.

Reverby, Susan. "More Than a Metaphor: An Overview of the Scholarship of the Study." In *Tuskegee's Truths: Rethinking the Tuskegee Study*, edited by Susan Reverby, 1–11. Chapel Hill: University of North Carolina Press, 2000.

Reynolds, Alfred W. "The Alabama Negro Colony in Mexico, 1894–1896." *Alabama Review* 5, no. 4 (October 1952): 243–68.

———. "The Alabama Negro Colony in Mexico, 1894–1896," *Alabama Review* 6, no. 1 (January 1953): 31–58

Rickard, E. R., and E. G. Riley. "A State-Wide Survey of Typhus Fever in Florida." *American Journal of Public Health* 38, no. 4 (1948): 541–44.

Rigau Perez, José G. "The Introduction of Smallpox Vaccine in 1803 and the Adoption of Immunization as a Government Function in Puerto Rico." *Hispanic American Historical Review* 69, no. 3 (1989): 393–423.

———. "Surgery at the Service of Theology: Postmortem Cesarean Sections in Puerto Rico and the Royal Cedula of 1804." *Hispanic American Historical Review* 75, no. 3 (1995): 377–91.

———. "Smallpox Epidemics in Puerto Rico during the Pre-Vaccine Era (1518–1803)." *Journal of the History of Medicine* 37, no. 4 (1982): 423–38.

Rigau Perez, Jose G., and Luis A. Perera Díaz. "¡Hay Bilharzia! By Klock, Ildefonso, and Mateo Serrano: Medical Images of Poverty and Development in Puerto Rico and the 1950s." *Puerto Rican Health Sciences Journal* 15, no. 1 (1996): 33–44.

Riley, Denise. *Am I That Name?: Feminism and the Category of "Women" in History*. Minneapolis: University of Minnesota Press, 1988.

Roberts, Dorothy. *Killing the Black Body: Race, Reproduction and the Meaning of Liberty*. New York: Random House, 1999.

Rodriguez, Clara E. *Changing Race: Latinos, the Census, and the History of Ethnicity in the United States*. New York: New York University Press, 2000.

Rodriguez, Maria Guadalupe. "La Banca Porfiriana en Durango." In *Durango (1840–1915): Banca, transportes, tierra e industria*, edited by Mario Cerutti, 7–34. Monterrey, Nuevo León: Universidad Autonoma de Nuevo León, 1995.

Roediger, David. *The Wages of Whiteness: Race and the Making of the American Working Class*. New York: Verso, 1991.

Rogers, Naomi. "Dirt, Flies and Immigrants: Explaining the Epidemiology of Poliomyelitis, 1910–1916." In *Sickness and Health in America: Readings in the History of Medicine and Public Health*, 3rd ed., rev., edited by Judith Walzer Leavitt and Ronald Numbers, 309–22. Madison: University of Wisconsin Press, 1997.

Rogin, Michael. "How the Working Class Saved Capitalism: The New Labor History and the Devil and Miss Jones." *Journal of American History* 89, no. 1 (2002): 87–114.

Rolph-Trouillot, Michel. *Haiti, State against Nation: The Origins and Legacy of Duvalierism.* New York: Monthly Review Press, 1990.

———. *Silencing the Past: Power and the Production of History.* Boston: Beacon, 1997.

Romero, Mary. *Maid in the USA.* New York: Routledge, 1992.

Romo, David Dorado. *Ringside Seat to a Revolution: An Underground Cultural History of El Paso and Ciudad Juarez.* El Paso: Cinco Puntos, 2005.

Romo, Ricardo. *East Los Angeles: History of a Barrio.* Austin: University of Texas Press, 1983.

Rosales, Francisco Arturo. *Pobre Raza!: Violence, Justice, and Mobilization among México Lindo Immigrants, 1900–1936.* Austin: University of Texas Press, 1999.

Rosen, George. "Problems in the Application of Statistical Analysis to Questions of Health: 1700–1880." *Bulletin of the History of Medicine* 29, no. 1 (1955): 27–45.

Rosenbaum, Robert J. *Mexicano Resistance in the Southwest: "The Sacred Right of Self-Preservation."* Austin: University of Texas Press, 1981.

Rosenberg, Charles E. *The Care of Strangers: The Rise of America's Hospital System.* New York: Basic Books, 1987.

———. *The Cholera Years: The United States in 1832, 1849, and 1866,* 2nd ed. Chicago: University of Chicago Press, 1987.

———. "Florence Nightingale on Contagion: The Moral Universe of the Hospital." In *Explaining Epidemics: Essays in the History of Medicine.* New York: Cambridge University Press, 1992.

———. "Social Class and Medical Care in Nineteenth-Century America: The Rise and Fall of the Dispensary." In *Sickness and Health in America: Readings in the History of Medicine and Public Health,* 3rd ed., rev., edited by Judith Walzer and Ronald Numbers Leavitt, 309–22. Madison: University of Wisconsin Press, 1997.

Rosenberg, Charles E., and Janet Golden, eds. *Framing Disease: Studies in Cultural History.* New Brunswick: Rutgers University Press, 1992.

Rosenberg, Charles E., and Morris J. Vogel, eds. *The Therapeutic Revolution: Essays in the Social History of American Medicine.* Philadelphia: University of Pennsylvania Press, 1979.

Rosenzweig, Gabriel. *Trabajando por México fuera de México: Testimonios de miembros del Servicio Exterior Mexicano.* Mexico: Secretaria de Relaciones Exteriores, 1995.

Rosner, David, and Gerald Markowitz. "The Early Movement for Occupational Safety and Health, 1900–1917." In *Sickness and Health in America: Readings in the History of Medicine and Public Health,* 3rd ed., rev., edited by Judith Walzer Leavitt and Ronald Numbers, 467–81. Madison: University of Wisconsin Press, 1997.

———, ed. *Dying for Work: Worker's Safety and Health in Twentieth-Century America.* Bloomington: Indiana University Press, 1987.

Ross, Paul. "Mexico's Superior Health Council and the American Public Health Association: The Transnational Archive of Porfirian Public Health, 1887–1910." *Hispanic American Historical Review* 89, no. 4 (2009): 573–603.

Rousey, Dennis C. "Aliens in the Wasp Nest: Ethnocultural Diversity in the Antebellum Urban South." *Journal of American History* 79, no. 1 (1992): 152–64.

———. "Black Policemen in Memphis: A Post-Reconstruction Anomaly." *Journal of Southern History* 51, no. 3 (1985): 374.

Ruiz, Vicki L. "The Flapper and the Chaperone: Historical Memory among Mexican-American Women." In *Seeking Common Ground: Multidisciplinary Studies of Immigrant Women in the United States*, edited by Donna Gabaccia, 143–57. Westport, Conn.: Greenwood, 1992.

Rumbaut, Ruben. "The Americans: Latin American and Caribbean Peoples in the United States." In *The Americas: New Interpretive Essays*, edited by Alfred Stepan, 310–27. New York: Oxford University Press, 1992.

Said, Edward. *Orientalism*. New York: Vintage Books, 1979.

Sale, Maggie Montesinos. *The Slumbering Volcano: American Slave Ship Revolts and the Production of a Rebellious Masculinity*. New Americanists. Durham: Duke University Press, 1997.

Salyer, Lucy. *Laws Harsh as Tigers: Chinese Immigrants and the Shaping of Modern Immigration Law*. Studies in Legal History. Chapel Hill: University of North Carolina Press, 1995.

Sánchez, George J. *Becoming Mexican American: Ethnicity, Culture, and Identity in Chicano Los Angeles, 1900–1945*. New York: Oxford University Press, 1994.

———. "Face the Nation: Race, Immigration, and the Rise of Nativism in Late Twentieth Century America." *International Migration Review* 31, no. 4 (1997): 1009–21.

———. "'Go After the Women': Americanization and the Mexican Immigrant Woman, 1915–1929." In *Unequal Sisters: A Multicultural History of United States Women's History*, edited by Vicki L. Ruiz and Ellen C. DuBois, 284–97. New York: Routledge, 1994.

———. "Race, Nation, and Culture in Recent Immigration Studies." *Journal of American Ethnic History* 18, no. 4 (1999): 66–76.

———. "Reading Reginald Denny: The Politics of Whiteness in the Late Twentieth Century." *American Quarterly* 47, no. 3 (1995): 388–93.

———. "Y tu, que? (Y2K): Latino History in the New Millennium." In *Latinos Remaking America*, edited by Marcelo Suarez Orozco and Mariela M. Paez, 45–59. Berkeley: University of California Press, 2002.

Sánchez, Rosaura. *Telling Identities: The Californio Testimonios*. Minneapolis: University of Minnesota Press, 1995.

Sandoval, Chela. "U.S. Third World Feminism: The Theory and Method of Oppositional Consciousness in the Postmodern World." *Genders* 10 (spring 1991): 1–24.

Saragoza, Alex. *The Monterrey Elite and the Mexican State, 1910–1940*. Austin: University of Texas Press, 1990.

Sassen, Saskia. "Miami: A New Global City? (Consequences of Internationalization of Miami)." *Contemporary Sociology* 22, no. 4 (1993): 471–78.

———. *The Mobility of Labor and Capital: A Study of International Investment and Labor Flow*. Cambridge: Cambridge University Press, 1986.

Satter, Beryl. *Each Mind a Kingdom: American Women, Sexual Purity, and the New Thought Movement*. Berkeley: University of California Press, 1999.

Sauer, Norman J. "Forensic Anthropology and the Concept of Race: If Races Don't Exist, Why Are Forensic Anthropologists So Good at Identifying Them?" *Social Science and Medicine* 34, no. 2 (1992): 107–11.

Savitt, Todd L. "Black Health on the Plantation: Masters, Slaves, and Physicians." In *Sickness and Health in America: Readings in the History of Medicine and Public Health*, 3rd ed., rev., edited by Judith Walzer Leavitt and Ronald Numbers, 351–68. Madison: University of Wisconsin Press, 1997.

———. *Medicine and Slavery: The Diseases and Health Care of Blacks in Antebellum Virginia*. Urbana: University of Illinois Press, 1978.

———. "The Use of Blacks for Medical Experimentation and Demonstration in the Old South." *Journal of Southern History* 48 (1982): 331–48.

Sawyer, Wilbur. "Public Health Implications of Tropical and Imported Diseases." *American Journal of Public Health* 34, no. 1 (1944): 7–15.

Saxton, Alexander. *The Indispensable Enemy: Labor and the Anti-Chinese Movement in California*. Berkeley: University of California Press, 1971.

———. *The Rise and Fall of the White Republic: Class Politics and Mass Culture in Nineteenth-Century America*. New York: Verso, 1990.

Schell, William. *Integral Outsiders: The American Colony in Mexico City, 1876–1911*. Wilmington, Del.: SR Books, 2001.

Schlich, Thomas. "Medicalisation and Secularization: The Jewish Ritual Bath as a Problem of Hygiene." *Social History of Medicine* 8 (1995): 423–42.

Schweininger, Loren. *Black Property Owners in the South, 1790–1915*. Urbana: University of Illinois Press, 1990.

Scott, Joan W. "The Evidence of Experience." In *The Lesbian and Gay Studies Reader*, edited by Henry Abelove et al., 397–415. New York: Routledge, 1993.

———. *Gender and the Politics of History*. New York: Columbia University Press, 1988.

Scott, Rebecca. "Fault Lines, Color Lines, and Party Lines: Race, Labor, and Collective Action in Louisiana and Cuba, 1862–1912." In *Beyond Slavery: Explorations of Race, Labor, and Citizenship in Postemancipation Societies*, edited by Frederick Cooper, Thomas Holt, and Rebecca Scott, 61–105. Chapel Hill: University of North Carolina Press, 2000.

Shah, Nayan. *Contagious Divides: Epidemics and Race in San Francisco's Chinatown*. Berkeley: University of California Press, 2001.

———. "San Francisco's Chinatown: Race and the Cultural Politics of Public Health." Ph.D. diss., University of Chicago, 1995.

Silber, Nina. *Romance of Reunion: Northerners and the South, 1865–1900*. Chapel Hill: University of North Carolina Press, 1993.

Silva, Renan. *Las epidemias de viruela de 1782 y 1802 en le Nueva Granada: Contribucion a un analisis historico de los procesos de apropiacion de modelos culturales*. Calif: Universidad del Valle, 1992.

Skowronek, Stephen. *Building a New American State: The Expansion of National Administrative Capacities, 1877–1920*. New York: Cambridge University Press, 1982.

Slater, Jack. "Involuntary Sterilization: New Threat to the Poor." *Ebony*, 28, no. 12 (October 1973): 150–56.

Slusser, Cathy Bayless. "The Birth of an Infant Society: The Hillsborough County Medical Society Association." *Tampa Bay History* 10, no. 1 (1988): 4–18.

Smith, Dale C. "Gerhard's Distinction between Typhoid and Typhus and Its Reception in America, 1833–1860." *Bulletin of the History of Medicine* 34, no. 3 (1980): 368–84.

———. "Laveran's Germ: The Reception and Use of a Medical Discovery." *American Journal of Tropical Medicine and Hygiene* 34, no. 1 (1985): 2–20.

———. "The Rise and Fall of Typhomalarial Fever. I: Origins." *Journal of the History of Medicine* 37, no. 3 (1982): 183–220.

———. "The Rise and Fall of Typhomalarial Fever. II: Decline and Fall." *Journal of the History of Medicine and Allied Sciences* 37, no. 3 (July 1982): 287–320.

Smith, Mickey. "Soldiers on the Production Line." *Pharmacy in History* 37, no. 4 (1995): 183–88.

Smith, Susan L. *Sick and Tired of Being Sick and Tired: Black Women and the National Negro Health Movement, 1915–1950*. Philadelphia: University of Pennsylvania Press, 1995.

Smyth, Sydnia Keene. "The Antebellum Architecture of Tuscaloosa." Ph.D. diss., University of Alabama, 1929.

Solorzano, Armando Ramos, and Anne Emmanuel Birn. "Public Health Policy Paradoxes: Science and Politics in the Rockefeller Foundation's Hookworm Campaign in Mexico in the 1920s." *Social Science and Medicine* 49, no. 9 (1999): 1197–213.

Solorzano Ramos, Armando. *¿Fiebre dorada or fiebre amarilla? La Fundación Rockefeller en México (1911–1924)*. Guadalajara: Universidad de Guadalajara, 1997.

———. "The Rockefeller Foundation in Mexico: Nationalism, Public Health, and Yellow Fever (1911–1924)." University of Wisconsin–Madison, 1991.

Soriano, Miguel. "Estadistica del Hospital Juarez correspondiente a los meses de Julio, Agosto y Septiembre de 1888." *Gaceta Medica de Mexico* 23, no. 21 (1888): 433–52.

Sotiroff-Junker, Jacqueline. *A Bibliography on the Behavioural, Social, and Eco-*

nomic Aspects of Malaria and Its Control (Une bibliographie sur les aspects com-portementaux, sociaux, et économiques du paludisme et de la lutte antipaludique; Una bibliografia sobre los aspectos sociales,economicos, y de la conducta relativos al paludismo y la lucha antipaludica). Geneva, Switzerland: World Health Organization, 1978.

Stanley, Amy Dru. *From Bondage to Contract: Wage Labor, Marriage, and the Market in the Age of Slave Emancipation*. New York: Cambridge University Press, 1998.

Stepan, Nancy. *The Idea of Race in Science: Great Britain, 1800–1960*. London: Macmillan, in association with St. Anthony's College, Oxford, 1982.

———. "The Interplay between Socio-Economic Factors and Medical Science: Yellow Fever Research, Cuba, and the United States." *Social Studies of Science* 8, no. 4 (1978): 397–423.

Stepan, Nancy Leys. *In the Hour of Eugenics: Race, Gender, and Nation in Latin America*. Ithaca: Cornell University Press, 1991.

Stern, Alexandra Minna. *Eugenic Nation: Faults and Frontiers of Better Breeding in Modern America*. Berkeley: University of California Press, 2005.

———. "Buildings, Boundaries, and Blood: Medicalization and Nation-Building on the U.S.-Mexico Border, 1910–1930." *Hispanic American Historical Review* 79, no. 1 (1999): 41–81.

———. "Eugenics beyond Borders: Science and Medicalization in Mexico and the United States West, 1900–1950." Ph.D. diss., University of Chicago, 1999.

Stern, Alexandra Minna, and Howard Markel. "All Quiet on the Third Coast: Medical Inspections of Immigrants in Michigan." *Public Health Reports* 114, no. 2 (1999): 178–82.

———. "Which Face? Whose Nation? Immigration, Public Health, and the Construction of Disease at America's Ports and Borders, 1891–1928." *American Behavioral Scientist* 42, no. 9 (1999): 1314–31.

Stevenson, Lloyd G. "Science Down the Drain: On the Hostility of Certain Sanitarians to Animal Experimentation, Bacteriology, and Immunology." *Bulletin of the History of Medicine* 29, no. 1 (1955): 1–26.

Szczygiel, Bonj, and Robert Hewitt. "Nineteenth-Century Medical Landscapes: John Rauch, Frederick Law Olmsted, and the Search for Salubrity." *Bulletin of the History of Medicine* 74 (2000): 708–34.

Takaki, Ronald T. *Iron Cages: Race and Culture in Nineteenth-Century America*. New York: Oxford University Press, 1990.

Taylor, Henry Louis. "The Hidden Face of Racism." *American Quarterly* 47, no. 3 (1995): 396–408.

Taylor, Rex, and Annelie Rieger. "Medicine as Social Science: Rudolf Virchow on the Typhus Epidemic in Upper Silesia." *International Journal of Health Services* 4, no. 4 (1985): 547–59.

Taylor, William. *Magistrates of the Sacred: Priests and Parishioners in Eighteenth-Century Mexico*. Stanford: Stanford University Press, 1996.

Tenorio-Trillo, Mauricio. *Mexico at the World's Fair: Crafting a Modern Nation, 1876–1911*. New Historicism: Studies in Cultural Poetics. Berkeley: University of California Press, 1996.

Tesh, Sylvia Noble. *Hidden Arguments: Political Ideology and Disease Prevention Policy*. New Brunswick: Rutgers University Press, 1988.

Texas State Historical Association. "Dudley, Richard M." In The Online Handbook of Texas, www.tshaonline.org/handbook/online/articles/fdu55 (accessed February 22, 2012).

———. "Laredo Smallpox Riot." In The Online Handbook of Texas, www.tshaonline.org/handbook/online/articles/jcl01 (accessed February 22, 2012).

———. "Ochiltree, Thomas Peck." In The Online Handbook of Texas, www.tshaonline.org/handbook/online/articles/foco1 (accessed February 22, 2012).

———. "Riots." In The Online Handbook of Texas, www.tshaonline.org/handbook/online/articles/jcro2 (accessed February 22, 2012).

Texas State Medical Association. "El Paso Solves the Vaccination Question." *Texas State Journal of Medicine* 19, no. 2 (1923): 318–20.

———. "Texas Joins the National Registration Area." *Texas State Journal of Medicine* (1934): 410.

Thompson, Angela. *Las otras guerras de Mexico*. Guanajuato, Mexico: Universidad Autonoma de Guanajuato, 1997.

———. "To Save the Children: Smallpox Inoculation, Vaccination, and Public Health in Guanajuato, Mexico, 1797–1840." *The Americas: A Quarterly Review of Inter-American Cultural History* 49, no. 4 (1993): 431–55.

Thornton, Russell. *American Indian Holocaust and Survival: A Population History since 1492*. Norman: University of Oklahoma Press, 1987.

Tijerina, Andrés. *Tejano Empire: Life on the South Texas Ranchos*. College Station: Texas A&M University Press, 1998.

———. *Tejanos and Texas under the Mexican Flag*. College Station: Texas A&M University Press, 1994.

Tomes, Nancy. *The Gospel of Germs: Men, Women, and the Microbe in American Life*. Cambridge: Harvard University Press, 1998.

———. "The Private Side of Public Health: Sanitary Science, Domestic Hygiene, and the Germ Theory, 1870–1900." *Bulletin of the History of Medicine* 64, no. 4 (1990): 509–38.

Tomlins, Christopher L. *The State and the Unions: Labor Relations, Law, and the Organized Labor Movement in America, 1880–1960*. New York: Cambridge University Press, 1985.

Trouillot, Michel Rolph. *Silencing the Past: Power and the Production of History*. Baltimore: Johns Hopkins University Press, 1993.

Truett, Samuel Jefferson. "Neighbors by Nature: The Transformation of Land and Life in the U.S.-Mexico Borderlands, 1854–1910." Ph.D. diss., Yale University, 1997.

Truett, Samuel, and Elliott Young, eds. *Continental Crossroads: Remapping U.S.-Mexico Borderlands History*. Durham: Duke University Press, 2004.

U.S. Census Bureau. *Twelfth Census of the United States Taken in the Year 1900*. Vol. 2. Edited by Charles Merriam. New York: Norman Ross, 1997.

———. *Fourteenth Census of the United States, 1920*. Vol. 2, *1920 Population: General Report and Analytical Tables*. Edited by William Hunt. New York: Norman Ross, 2000.

———. *Sixteenth Census of the United States, 1940*. Vol. 2, *Population: Characteristics of the People*. Edited by Leon Truesdell. Washington, D.C.: Government Printing Office, 1943.

Urcioli, Bonnie. "The Political Topography of Spanish and English: The View from a New York City Puerto Rican Neighborhood." *American Ethnologist* 18, no. 2 (May 1991): 295–310.

Valencius, Conevery Bolton. *The Health of the Country: How American Settlers Understood Themselves and Their Land*. Cambridge: Harvard University Press, 2002.

Vargas, Zaragosa. *Labor Rights Are Civil Rights*. Princeton: Princeton University Press, 2007.

Vaughann, Meghan. "Slavery, Smallpox, and Revolution: 1792 in Ile de France." *Social History of Medicine* 13, no. 3 (2000): 411–28.

Vega, Bernardo. *Memoirs of Bernardo Vega*. New York: Monthly Review Press, 1984.

Vidaurreta, Alicia. "La Muerte en Buenos Aires, 1871." *Revista de Indias* 49, no. 186 (1989): 437–60.

Vila, Pablo. *Crossing Borders, Reinforcing Borders: Social Categories, Metaphors, and Narrative Identities on the U.S.-Mexico Frontier*. Austin: University of Texas Press, 2000.

Viner, Russell. "Abraham Jacobi and German Medical Radicalism in Antebellum New York." *Bulletin of the History of Medicine* 72 (1998): 434–63.

Vogel, Bernard. *American Indian Medicine*. Norman: University of Oklahoma Press, 1970.

Wailoo, Keith. *Drawing Blood: Technology and Disease Identity in Twentieth-Century America*. Baltimore: Johns Hopkins University Press, 1997.

———. *Dying in the City of Blues: Sickle Cell Anemia and the Politics of Race and Health*. Chapel Hill: University of North Carolina Press, 2001.

Wald, Priscilla. *Contagious: Cultures, Carriers, and the Outbreak Narrative*. John Hope Franklin Center Books. Durham: Duke University Press, 2008.

———. "Future Perfect: Grammar, Genes, and Geography." *New Literary History* 31, no. 4 (2000): 681–709.

———. "Our America: Nativism, Modernism, and Pluralism (Review of Walter Benn Michaels, *Our America*." *Modern Language Quarterly* 59, no. 1 (1998): 124–30.

———. "Review: Networking: Communicating with Bodies and Machines in the Nineteenth Century." *Perspectives in Biology and Medicine* 46, no. 3 (2003): 452–55.

———. "Terms of Assimilation: Legislating Subjectivity in the Emerging Nation." *Boundary 2* 19, no. 3 (1992): 777–805.

Walker, Richard. "California's Collision of Race and Class." In *Race and Representation: Affirmative Action*, edited by Robert Post and Michael Rogin, 281–306. New York: Zone Books, 1998.

Walkowitz, Judith. *Prostitution and Victorian Society: Women, Class, and the State*. New York: Cambridge University Press, 1980.

Warner, John Harley. *Against the Spirit of System: The French Impulse in Nineteenth-Century American Medicine*. Princeton: Princeton University Press, 1998.

———. "From Specificity to Universalism in Medical Therapeutics: Transformation in the Nineteenth-Century United States." In *Sickness and Health in America: Readings in the History of Medicine and Public Health*, 3rd ed., edited by Judith Walzer Leavitt and Ronald Numbers, 87–101. Madison: University of Wisconsin Press, 1997.

———. *The Therapeutic Perspective: Medical Practice, Knowledge, and Identity in America, 1820–1885*. Princeton: Princeton University Press, 1997.

Waters, Hazel. "The Great Famine and the Rise of Anti-Irish Racism." *Race and Class* 37, no. 1 (1995): 95–108.

Watkins, Susan. *After Ellis Island: Newcomers and Natives in the 1910 Census*. New York: Russell Sage Foundation, 1994.

Weber, David J. "John Francis Bannon and the Historiography of the Spanish Borderlands: Retrospect and Prospect." *Journal of the Southwest* 29 (winter 1987): 331–63.

———. "Turner, the Boltonians and the Borderlands." *American Historical Review* 91 (February 1986): 66–81.

Weindling, Paul. *Epidemics and Genocide in Eastern Europe, 1890–1945*. New York: Oxford University Press, 2000.

———. "From Medical Research to Clinical Practice: Serum Therapy for Diphtheria." In *Medical Innovations in Historical Perspective*, edited by John Pickstone, 72–82. New York: St. Martin's, 1992.

———. "Medicine and the Holocaust: The Case of Typhus." In *L'innovation en médicine: Études historiques et sociologiques/Medicine and Change: Historical and Sociological Studies of Medical Innovation*, edited by Ilana Lowy, 447–64. Montrouge, France: Editions John Libbey Eurotext, 1993.

Wheeler, Lieutenant Coronel Charles. "Control of Typhus in Italy 1943–1944 by Use of DDT." *American Journal of Public Health* 36, no. 2 (1944): 119–29.

White, Hayden. *Tropics of Discourse: Essays in Cultural Criticism.* Baltimore: Johns Hopkins University Press, 1978.

White, Richard. "Race Relations in the American West." *American Quarterly* 38 (1986): 396–416.

Widmer Sennauser, Rolf. "Politica sanitaria y lucha social en tiempos de viruelas: Corona, comercio y comunidades indigenas en Tehuantepec, 1795–1796." *Relaciones* 44 (Fall 1990): 33–74.

Wiebe, Robert H. *The Search for Order, 1877–1920.* New York: Hill and Wang, 1967.

Williams, Brackette. "Babies and Banks: The 'Reproductive Underclass' and the Raced, Gendered Masking of Debt." In *Race,* edited by Steven Gregory and Roger Sanjek, 348–64. New Brunswick: Rutgers University Press, 1999.

Williams, Walter. "Tragic Vision of Racial Problems." *American Quarterly* 47, no. 3 (1995): 409–15.

Wilson, Christopher. "Plotting the Border: John Reed, Pancho Villa and Insurgent Mexico." In *Cultures of United States Imperialism,* edited by Amy Kaplan and Donald Pease, 340–65. Durham: Duke University Press, 1993.

Wood, Joe. "Escape from Blackness: Notes on Creole America." *Village Voice* 39, no. 39 (December 1994): 25–34.

Wood, Peter H. *Black Majority: Negroes in Colonial South Carolina from 1670 through the Stono Rebellion.* New York: Knopf, 1974.

Worboys, Michael. "Vaccine Therapy and Laboratory Medicine in Edwardian England." In *Medical Innovations in Historical Perspective,* edited by John Pickstone, 84–102. New York: St. Martin's, 1992.

Young, Elliott. *Catarino Garza's Revolution on the Texas-Mexico Border.* American Encounters, Global Interaction. Durham: Duke University Press, 2004.

———. "Deconstructing *La Raza*: Identifying the *Gente Decente* of Laredo, 1904–1911." *Southwestern Historical Quarterly* 98, no. 2 (1994): 227–59.

———. "Imagining Alternative Modernities: Ignacio Martinez' Travel Narratives." In *Continental Crossroads: Remapping U.S.-Mexico Borderlands History,* edited by Samuel Truett and Elliott Young, 151–81. Durham: Duke University Press, 2004.

———. "Red Men, Princess Pocahontas, and George Washington: Harmonizing Race Relations in Laredo at the Turn of the Century." *Western Historical Quarterly* 29, no. 1 (1998): 48–85.

———. "Remembering Catarino Garza's 1891 Revolution: An Aborted Border Insurrection." *Mexican Studies/Estudios Mexicanos* 12, no. 2 (1996): 231–72.

Young, Oran R. *International Cooperation: Building Regimes for Natural Resources and the Environment.* Ithaca: Cornell University Press, 1989.

———. "Political Leadership and Regime Formation: On the Development of Institutions in International Society." *International Organizations* 45, no. 3 (1991): 281–308.

Young, T. Kue. *The Health of Native Americans: Toward a Biocultural Epidemiology.* New York: Oxford University Press, 1994.

Zamora, Emilio. *The World of the Mexican Worker in Texas, 1880–1930.* College Station: Texas A&M University Press, 1993.

INDEX

John Mckiernan-González is an assistant professor of history
at the University of Texas, Austin.

Library of Congress Cataloging-in-Publication Data
Mckiernan-González, John.
Fevered measures : public health and race at the
Texas-Mexico border, 1848–1942 / John Mckiernan-González.
   p. cm.
Includes bibliographical references and index.
ISBN 978-0-8223-5257-0 (cloth : alk. paper)
ISBN 978-0-8223-5276-1 (pbk. : alk. paper)
   1. Communicable diseases—Transmission—Mexican-
American Border Region—Prevention—History.
2. Public health—Mexican-American Border Region—
History. 3. Emigration and immigration—Health
aspects—Mexican-American Border Region—History.
4. Mexican-American Border Region—History. I. Title.
RA446.5.M49 M 35 2012
362.10972'1—dc23   2012011600

Made in the USA
Columbia, SC
14 October 2018